2012
YEAR BOOK OF
VASCULAR SURGERY®

The 2012 Year Book Series

Year Book of Anesthesiology and Pain Management™: Drs Chestnut, Abram, Black, Gravlee, Lien, Mathru, and Roizen

Year Book of Cardiology®: Drs Gersh, Cheitlin, Elliott, Gold, Graham, and Thourani

Year Book of Critical Care Medicine®: Drs Dries, Zanotti-Cavazzoni, Latenser, Martinez, Rincon, and Zwank

Year Book of Dermatology and Dermatologic Surgery™: Dr Del Rosso

Year Book of Diagnostic Radiology®: Drs Elster, Abbara, Oestreich, Offiah, Rosado de Christenson, Stephens, and Strickland

Year Book of Emergency Medicine®: Drs Hamilton, Bruno, Handly, Minczak, Mullin, Quintana, and Ramoska

Year Book of Endocrinology®: Drs Schott, Apovian, Clarke, Eugster, Meikle, Oetgen, Ovalle, Schteingart, and Toth

Year Book of Hand and Upper Limb Surgery®: Drs Yao, Adams, Isaacs, Lee, and Rizzo

Year Book of Medicine®: Drs Barker, Garrick, Gersh, Khardori, LeRoith, Panush, Talley, and Thigpen

Year Book of Neonatal and Perinatal Medicine®: Drs Fanaroff, Benitz, Donn, Neu, Papile, Polin, and Van Marter

Year Book of Neurology and Neurosurgery®: Drs Klimo, Minagar, Gandhi, House, Kevill, Liu, Mazia, Panagariya, Ragel, Riesenburger, Robottom, Schwendimann, Shafazand, Uhm, and Yang

Year Book of Obstetrics, Gynecology, and Women's Health®: Drs Dungan and Shulman

Year Book of Oncology®: Drs Arceci, Bauer, Chiorean, Gordon, Lawton, Murphy, Thigpen, and Tsao

Year Book of Ophthalmology®: Drs Rapuano, Cohen, Flanders, Hammersmith, Milman, Myers, Nagra, Nelson, Penne, Pyfer, Sergott, Shields, Talekar, and Vander

Year Book of Orthopedics®: Drs Morrey, Huddleston, Rose, Swiontkowski, and Trigg

Year Book of Otolaryngology-Head and Neck Surgery®: Drs Sindwani, Balough, Franco, Gapany, and Mitchell

Year Book of Pathology and Laboratory Medicine®: Drs Raab and Bissell

Year Book of Pediatrics®: Dr Stockman

Year Book of Plastic and Aesthetic Surgery™: Drs Miller, Gosman, Gurtner, Gutowski, Ruberg, Salisbury, and Smith

2012

The Year Book of VASCULAR SURGERY®

Editor-in-Chief
Gregory L. Moneta, MD
Professor and Chief of Vascular Surgery, Oregon Health and Science University; and Chief of Vascular Surgery, Oregon Health and Science University Hospital, Portland, Oregon

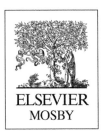

ELSEVIER
MOSBY

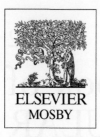

Vice President, Continuity: Kimberly Murphy
Editor: Teia Stone
Production Supervisor, Electronic Year Books: Donna M. Skelton
Electronic Article Manager: Emily Ogle
Illustrations and Permissions Coordinator: Dawn Vohsen

Composition by TNQ Books and Journals Pvt Ltd, India
Transferred to Digital Printing, 2012.

Editorial Office:
Elsevier
Suite 1800
1600 John F. Kennedy Blvd.
Philadelphia, PA 19103-2899

International Standard Serial Number: 0749-4041
International Standard Book Number: 978-0-323-08897-8

Printed and bound by CPI Group (UK) Ltd, Croydon, CR0 4YY

Transferred to digital print 2012

Associate Editors

David L. Gillespie, MD, RVT, FACS
Professor of Surgery, Chief Division of Vascular Surgery; University of Rochester School of Medicine and Dentistry, Rochester, New York

Benjamin W. Starnes, MD
Professor of Surgery and Chief, Division of Vascular Surgery; University of Washington, Seattle, Washington

Michael T. Watkins, MD
Associate Professor of Surgery, Harvard Medical School; and Director, Vascular Surgery Research Laboratory, Massachusetts General Hospital, Boston, Massachusetts

Contributors

Zachary M. Arthurs, MD
Assistant Professor, Department of Vascular Surgery, Uniformed Services University of Health Sciences, San Antonio Military Medical Center, San Antonio, Texas

Ankur Chandra, MD
Assistant Professor of Surgery, University of Rochester School of Medicine and Dentistry, Rochester, New York

Marc A. Passman, MD
Professor of Surgery, Section of Vascular Surgery and Endovascular Therapy, University of Alabama at Birmingham, Birmingham, Alabama

Joseph D. Raffetto, MD, FACS, FSVM
Assistant Professor of Surgery, Harvard Medical School, Brigham and Women's Hospital; Chief, Vascular Surgery Division, VA Boston Healthcare System, West Roxbury, Massachusetts

LTC Niten Singh, MD
Chief, Endovascular Surgery, Madigan Army Medical Center; and Associate Professor of Surgery, Uniformed Services University of Health Sciences, Tacoma, Washington

Table of Contents

Journals Represented

Journals represented in this YEAR BOOK are listed below.

AJNR American Journal of Neuroradiology
American Journal of Cardiology
American Journal of Epidemiology
American Journal of Kidney Diseases
American Journal of Medicine
American Journal of Surgery
Annals of Neurology
Annals of Surgery
Annals of Thoracic Surgery
Annals of Vascular Surgery
Archives of Surgery
British Journal of Surgery
Circulation
Dermatologic Surgery
Diabetes Care
European Heart Journal
European Journal of Vascular and Endovascular Surgery
Journal of Clinical Investigation
Journal of Neurological Sciences
Journal of Neurology, Neurosurgery, and Psychiatry
Journal of Pharmacology and Experimental Therapeutics
Journal of Stroke and Cerebrovascular Diseases
Journal of the American College of Cardiology
Journal of the American College of Radiology
Journal of the American College of Surgeons
Journal of Thoracic and Cardiovascular Surgery
Journal of Trauma
Journal of Ultrasound in Medicine
Journal of Vascular and Interventional Radiology
Journal of Vascular Surgery
Lancet
Neurology
Neurosurgery
Proceedings of the National Academy of Sciences of the United States of America
Scandinavian Cardiovascular Journal
Scandinavian Journal of Rheumatology
Southern Medical Journal
Stroke
Surgery
Thrombosis Research

STANDARD ABBREVIATIONS

The following terms are abbreviated in this edition: acquired immunodeficiency syndrome (AIDS), cardiopulmonary resuscitation (CPR), central nervous system (CNS), cerebrospinal fluid (CSF), computed tomography (CT), deoxyribonucleic acid (DNA), electrocardiography (ECG), health maintenance organization (HMO), human immunodeficiency virus (HIV), intensive care unit (ICU), intramuscular (IM), intravenous (IV), magnetic resonance (MR) imaging (MRI), ribonucleic acid (RNA), and ultrasound (US).

NOTE

The YEAR BOOK OF VASCULAR SURGERY® is a literature survey service providing abstracts of articles published in the professional literature. Every effort is made to assure the accuracy of the information presented in these pages. Neither the editors nor the publisher of the YEAR BOOK OF VASCULAR SURGERY® can be responsible for errors in the original materials. The editors' comments are their own opinions. Mention of specific products within this publication does not constitute endorsement.

To facilitate the use of the YEAR BOOK OF VASCULAR SURGERY® as a reference tool, all illustrations and tables included in this publication are now identified as they appear in the original article. This change is meant to help the reader recognize that any illustration or table appearing in the YEAR BOOK OF VASCULAR SURGERY® may be only one of many in the original article. For this reason, figure and table numbers will often appear to be out of sequence within the YEAR BOOK OF VASCULAR SURGERY®.

1 Basic Considerations

Safety and efficacy of dalcetrapib on atherosclerotic disease using novel non-invasive multimodality imaging (dal-PLAQUE): a randomised clinical trial

Fayad ZA, for the dal-PLAQUE Investigators (Translational and Molecular Imaging Inst, NY; et al)
Lancet 378:1547-1559, 2011

Background.—Dalcetrapib modulates cholesteryl ester transfer protein (CETP) activity to raise high-density lipoprotein cholesterol (HDL-C). After the failure of torcetrapib it was unknown if HDL produced by interaction with CETP had pro-atherogenic or pro-inflammatory properties. dal-PLAQUE is the first multicentre study using novel non-invasive multimodality imaging to assess structural and inflammatory indices of atherosclerosis as primary endpoints.

Methods.—In this phase 2b, double-blind, multicentre trial, patients (aged 18−75 years) with, or with high risk of, coronary heart disease were randomly assigned (1:1) to dalcetrapib 600 mg/day or placebo for 24 months. Randomisation was done with a computer-generated randomisation code and was stratified by centre. Patients and investigators were masked to treatment. Coprimary endpoints were MRI-assessed indices (total vessel area, wall area, wall thickness, and normalised wall index [average carotid]) after 24 months and ^{18}F-fluorodeoxyglucose (^{18}F-FDG) PET/CT assessment of arterial inflammation within an index vessel (right carotid, left carotid, or ascending thoracic aorta) after 6 months, with no-harm boundaries established before unblinding of the trial. Analysis was by intention to treat. This trial is registered at ClinicalTrials.gov, NCT00655473.

Findings.—189 patients were screened and 130 randomly assigned to placebo (66 patients) or dalcetrapib (64 patients). For the coprimary MRI and PET/CT endpoints, CIs were below the no-harm boundary or the adverse change was numerically lower in the dalcetrapib group than in the placebo group. MRI-derived change in total vessel area was reduced in patients given dalcetrapib compared with those given placebo after 24 months; absolute change from baseline relative to placebo was −4·01 mm^2 (90% CI −7·23 to −0·80; nominal p = 0·04). The PET/CT measure of index vessel most-diseased-segment target-to-background ratio (TBR) was not different between groups, but carotid artery analysis showed a 7% reduction in most-diseased-segment TBR in the dalcetrapib group compared with the placebo group (−7·3 [90% CI −13·5 to −0·8];

1

nominal p $= 0 \cdot 07$). Dalcetrapib did not increase office blood pressure and the frequency of adverse events was similar between groups.

Interpretation.—Dalcetrapib showed no evidence of a pathological effect related to the arterial wall over 24 months. Moreover, this trial suggests possible beneficial vascular effects of dalcetrapib, including the reduction in total vessel enlargement over 24 months, but long-term safety and clinical outcomes efficacy of dalcetrapib need to be analysed (Figs 2-4).

▶ Statins, through a combination of lipid-lowering and off-target effects, are the primary drugs for reducing cardiovascular risk in patients with elevated

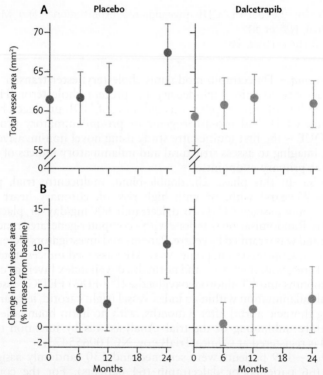

FIGURE 2.—Mean carotid total vessel area and percent increase in average carotid total vessel area (by MRI). (A) Raw mean data (90% CI) for total vessel area at baseline, 6, 12, and 24 months. Total vessel area increased after 24 months in the placebo group: model-derived, corrected average absolute change (24 months−baseline) was $5 \cdot 72$ mm^2 (90% CI $3 \cdot 30$−$8 \cdot 14$), p=$0 \cdot 0002$. However, in the dalcetrapib group, total vessel area did not change in the same period ($1 \cdot 71$ [$-0 \cdot 68$ to $4 \cdot 10$], p=$0 \cdot 24$). The average reduction in total vessel area on dalcetrapib (versus placebo), after correction of baseline, was $-4 \cdot 01$ ($-7 \cdot 23$ to $-0 \cdot 80$), p=$0 \cdot 04$. (B) Group mean data for percent change in total vessel area at 6, 12, and 24 months (relative to baseline). In patients assigned placebo, model-derived, corrected total vessel area increased in the initial 24 months: percent change total vessel area was $10 \cdot 8$ (90% CI $5 \cdot 8$−$15 \cdot 8$), p=$0 \cdot 001$. However, in patients assigned dalcetrapib, total vessel area did not increase in the same period ($4 \cdot 0$% [$0 \cdot 6$−$7 \cdot 3$], p=$0 \cdot 16$). The average percent change in total vessel area in the dalcetrapib group (versus placebo), after correction of baseline, was $-7 \cdot 1$% ($-12 \cdot 8$ to $-1 \cdot 3$), p=$0 \cdot 04$. (Reprinted from The Lancet, Fayad ZA, for the dal-PLAQUE Investigators. Safety and efficacy of dalcetrapib on atherosclerotic disease using novel non-invasive multimodality imaging (dal-PLAQUE): a randomised clinical trial. *Lancet*. 2011;378:1547-1559. Copyright 2011, with permission from Elsevier.)

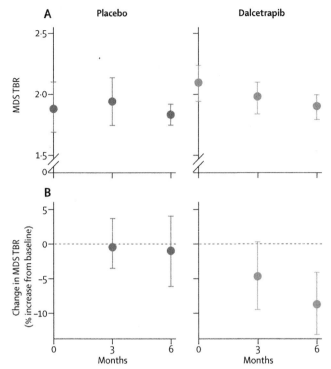

FIGURE 3.—Mean carotid MDS TBR and percent increase in average carotid most-diseased-segment TBR (by PET). MDS=most-diseased-segment. TBR=target-to-background ratio. (A) Raw mean data for average carotid MDS TBR at baseline, and at 3 and 6 months. In the placebo group, MDS TBR did not change after 6 months: model-derived, corrected average absolute change for MDS TBR (6 months–baseline) was $-0\cdot043$ (90% CI $-0\cdot14$ to $0\cdot06$), p=0·48. However, in the dalcetrapib group, MDS TBR decreased in the same period ($-0\cdot19$ [$-0\cdot29$ to $-0\cdot09$], p=0·001). The average reduction in MDS TBR on dalcetrapib (versus placebo), after correction for baseline, was $-0\cdot150$ ($-0\cdot29$ to $-0\cdot01$), p=0·08. (B) Group mean (90% CI) data for percent change in average carotid MDS TBR after 3 and 6 months (relative to baseline). In the placebo group, model-derived, corrected average MDS TBR did not change over the initial 6 months: percent change in MDS TBR was $3\cdot24$ (90% CI $-2\cdot18$ to $8\cdot66$), p=0·71. However, in the dalcetrapib group, MDS TBR decreased in the same period ($-7\cdot26\%$ [$-12\cdot50$ to $-2\cdot02$], p=0·003). The estimated average percent change in MDS TBR on dalcetrapib (versus placebo), after correction for baseline, was $-7\cdot35\%$ (90% CI $-13\cdot49$ to $-0\cdot76$), p=0·07. (Reprinted from The Lancet, Fayad ZA, for the dal-PLAQUE Investigators. Safety and efficacy of dalcetrapib on atherosclerotic disease using novel non-invasive multimodality imaging (dal-PLAQUE): a randomised clinical trial. *Lancet.* 2011;378:1547-1559. Copyright 2011, with permission from Elsevier.)

low-density lipoprotein cholesterol. Another potential approach is to reduce atherosclerotic plaque burden by raising high-density lipoprotein cholesterol (HDL-C). The importance of elevating HDL-C levels has been demonstrated in statin-treated patients where low HDL-C plasma concentrations continue to be an independent risk factor for cardiovascular events with high HDL-C levels associated with reduced plaque progression and reduced the frequency of cardiovascular events.[1,2] HDL-C can be increased using drugs that act on cholesterol ester transfer protein (CETP). The CETP inhibitor, torcetrapib, was found to effectively increase HDL-C but paradoxically was associated with increased mortality

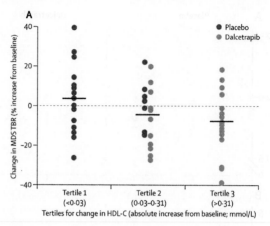

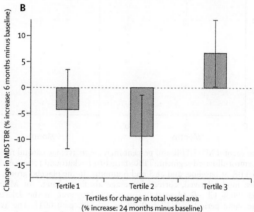

FIGURE 4.—Association between HDL-C and arterial inflammation as measured by MDS TBR on PET/CT and arterial inflammation and atherosclerotic burden HDL-C=high-density lipoprotein cholesterol. MDS=most-diseased-segment. TBR=target-to-background ratio. (A) Change in arterial inflammation (MDS TBR) over 6 months versus change in HDL-C over the same period grouped in tertiles (third tertile represents the greatest increase in HDL-C). (B) Early increases in arterial inflammation associated with subsequent increases in atherosclerotic burden. The change in carotid inflammation at 6 months was compared within subjects that were classified into tertiles according to the subsequent rate of change in total vessel area at 24 months. (Reprinted from The Lancet, Fayad ZA, for the dal-PLAQUE Investigators. Safety and efficacy of dalcetrapib on atherosclerotic disease using novel non-invasive multimodality imaging (dal-PLAQUE): a randomised clinical trial. *Lancet.* 2011;378:1547-1559. Copyright 2011, with permission from Elsevier.)

thought to be secondary to off-target effects, such as increased blood pressure and increased vascular inflammation.[3] Dalcetrapib is an inhibitor of CETP activity that also increases HDL-C. It has not been associated with clinically relevant increases in blood pressure, and pre-clinical experience in rodent models shows a decrease in atherosclerosis with dalcetrapib.[4] The authors sought to determine, using magnetic resonance imaging and positron emission tomography/computed tomography scanning, the effects of dalcetrapib on plaque morphology, progression and regression of atherosclerosis, and plaque inflammation. The primary goals of this study were to use this dual imaging approach to determine whether dalcetrapib results in an increase in atherosclerotic plaque progression or vascular inflammation compared with placebo. Coming on the heels of the failure of torcetrapib to be a clinically useful modulator of HDL cholesterol levels, the current study is encouraging for potential modulation of HDL cholesterol in the treatment of atherosclerosis. Dalcetrapib showed no evidence of pathologic effects related to the arterial wall over 24 months (Fig 4). There was a reduction in total vessel enlargement over 24 months (Figs 2 and 3), suggesting possible beneficial vascular effects at 24 months. Beneficial effects of dalcetrapib were associated with a 31% increase in HDL-C concentration and other potential favorable changes in the lipid profile. There are 2 large ongoing clinical trials of dalcetrapib. One is dal-PLAQUE 2. This assesses atherosclerotic disease progression using intravascular ultrasonography in the coronary arteries and measurements of intimal medial artery thickness in the carotid artery. The second is dal-OUTCOMES. It assesses cardiovascular morbidity and mortality and should eventually provide insights into the therapeutic effects of dalcetrapib and should also provide long-term information on the safety and ultimate clinical efficacy of dalcetrapib.[5,6]

G. L. Moneta, MD

References

1. Jafri H, Alsheikh-Ali AA, Karas RH. Meta-analysis: statin therapy does not alter the association between low levels of high-density lipoprotein cholesterol and increased cardiovascular risk. *Ann Intern Med.* 2010;153:800-808.
2. Wei L, Murphy MJ, MacDonald TM. Impact on cardiovascular events of increasing high density lipoprotein cholesterol with and without lipid lowering drugs. *Heart.* 2006;92:746-751.
3. Niesor EJ, Magg C, Ogawa N, et al. Modulating cholesteryl ester transfer protein activity maintains efficient pre-β-HDL formation and increases reverse cholesterol transport. *J Lipid Res.* 2010;51:3443-3454.
4. Okamoto H, Yonemori F, Wakitani K, Minowa T, Maeda K, Shinkai H. A cholesteryl ester transfer protein inhibitor attenuates atherosclerosis in rabbits. *Nature.* 2000;406:203-207.
5. Fayad ZA, Mani V, Woodward M, et al. Rationale and design of dal-PLAQUE: a study assessing efficacy and safety of dalcetrapib on progression or regression of atherosclerosis using magnetic resonance imaging and 18F-fluorodeoxyglucose positron emission tomography/computed tomography. *Am Heart J.* 2011;162:214-221.
6. Schwartz GG, Olsson AG, Ballantyne CM, et al; dal-OUTCOMES Committees and Investigators. Rationale and design of the dal-OUTCOMES trial: efficacy and safety of dalcetrapib in patients with recent acute coronary syndrome. *Am Heart J.* 2009;158:896-901.

HDL promotes rapid atherosclerosis regression in mice and alters inflammatory properties of plaque monocyte-derived cells
Feig JE, Rong JX, Shamir R, et al (New York Univ School of Medicine; et al)
Proc Natl Acad Sci U S A 108:7166-7171, 2011

HDL cholesterol (HDL-C) plasma levels are inversely related to cardiovascular disease risk. Previous studies have shown in animals and humans that HDL promotes regression of atherosclerosis. We hypothesized that this was related to an ability to promote the loss of monocyte-derived cells (CD68$^+$, primarily macrophages and macrophage foam cells) from plaques. To test this hypothesis, we used an established model of atherosclerosis regression in which plaquebearing aortic arches from apolipoprotein E-deficient (apoE$^{-/-}$) mice (low HDL-C, high non-HDL-C) were transplanted into recipient mice with differing levels of HDL-C and non-HDL-C: C57BL6 mice (normal HDL-C, low non-HDL-C), apoAI$^{-/-}$ mice (low HDL-C, low non-HDL-C), or apoE$^{-/-}$ mice transgenic for human apoAI (hAI/ apoE$^{-/-}$; normal HDL-C, high non-HDL-C). Remarkably, despite persistent elevated non-HDL-C in hAI/apoE$^{-/-}$ recipients, plaque CD68$^+$ cell content decreased by >50% by 1 wk after transplantation, whereas there was little change in apoAI$^{-/-}$ recipient mice despite hypolipidemia. The decreased content of plaque CD68$^+$ cells after HDL-C normalization was associated with their emigration and induction of their chemokine receptor CCR7. Furthermore, in CD68$^+$ cells laser-captured from the plaques, normalization of HDL-C led to decreased expression of inflammatory factors and enrichment of markers of the M2 (tissue repair) macrophage state. Again, none of these beneficial changes were observed in the apoAI$^{-/-}$ recipients, suggesting a major requirement for reverse cholesterol transport for the beneficial effects of HDL. Overall, these results establish HDL as a regulator in vivo of the migratory and inflammatory properties of monocyte-derived cells in mouse atherosclerotic plaques, and highlight the phenotypic plasticity of these cells.

▶ Epidemiology studies establish an inverse relationship between high-density lipoprotein cholesterol (HDL-C) and cardiovascular risk. In mouse models of atherosclerosis, HDL-C has been shown to be atheroprotective.[1] HDL-C may also have a role in regression of atherosclerosis. HDL-C has been infused into apolipoprotein E–deficient mice.[2] Infusion of HDL-C into human subjects has also been shown to reduce plaque size.[3] Based on these lines of evidence, the authors have postulated HDL-C may be an effective therapy to induce regression of established atherosclerosis. Their data indicate that HDL-C in vivo is a regulator of migratory and inflammatory properties of monocyte-derived cells found in mouse atherosclerotic plaques with a requirement for reverse cholesterol transport for the beneficial effects of HDL-C. These effects were independent of plasma non–HDL-C levels. Taken together, this indicates HDL-C may be an independent therapeutic target to promote atherosclerotic plaque regression through a mechanism of modifying the population of monocyte-derived cells in atherosclerotic plaques.

G. L. Moneta, MD

References

1. Rubin EM, Krauss RM, Spangler EA, Verstuyft JG, Clift SM. Inhibition of early atherogenesis in transgenic mice by human apolipoprotein AI. *Nature.* 1991; 353:265-267.
2. Shah PK, Yano J, Reyes O, et al. High-dose recombinant apolipoprotein A-I(milano) mobilizes tissue cholesterol and rapidly reduces plaque lipid and macrophage content in apolipoprotein e-deficient mice. Potential implications for acute plaque stabilization. *Circulation.* 2001;103:3047-3050.

3. Nissen SE, Tsunoda T, Tuzcu EM, et al. Effect of recombinant ApoA-I Milano on coronary atherosclerosis in patients with acute coronary syndromes: a randomized controlled trial. *JAMA*. 2003;290:2292-2300.

Antagonism of miR-33 in mice promotes reverse cholesterol transport and regression of atherosclerosis

Rayner KJ, Sheedy FJ, Esau CC, et al (New York Univ School of Medicine; Regulus Therapeutics, San Diego, CA; et al)
J Clin Invest 121:2921-2931, 2011

Plasma HDL levels have a protective role in atherosclerosis, yet clinical therapies to raise HDL levels have remained elusive. Recent advances in the understanding of lipid metabolism have revealed that miR-33, an intronic microRNA located within the *SREBF2* gene, suppresses expression of the cholesterol transporter ABC transporter A1 (ABCA1) and lowers HDL levels. Conversely, mechanisms that inhibit miR-33 increase ABCA1 and circulating HDL levels, suggesting that antagonism of miR-33 may be atheroprotective. As the regression of atherosclerosis is clinically desirable, we assessed the impact of miR-33 inhibition in mice deficient for the LDL receptor (*Ldlr*$^{-/-}$ mice), with established atherosclerotic plaques. Mice treated with anti-miR33 for 4 weeks showed an increase in circulating HDL levels and enhanced reverse cholesterol transport to the plasma, liver, and feces. Consistent with this, anti-miR33—treated mice showed reductions in plaque size and lipid content, increased markers of plaque stability, and decreased inflammatory gene expression. Notably, in addition to raising ABCA1 levels in the liver, anti-miR33 oligonucleotides directly targeted the plaque macrophages, in which they enhanced ABCA1 expression and cholesterol removal. These studies establish that raising HDL levels by anti-miR33 oligonucleotide treatment promotes reverse cholesterol transport and atherosclerosis regression and suggest that it may be a promising strategy to treat atherosclerotic vascular disease.

▶ Data from the Framingham Heart Study indicates that for every 1% increase in circulating high-density lipoprotein cholesterol (HDL-C) there is a 2% decrease in overall risk for development of coronary artery disease.[1] In mouse models of atherosclerosis, it has been found that overexpression of *apoA1*, which increases HDL levels, hinders plaque progression and promotes plaque regression.[2,3] These lines of evidence have stimulated an interest in therapies to raise HDL levels. However, despite the fact that HDL-raising strategies may be effective therapy for atherosclerosis, the underlying mechanisms that contribute to HDL regulation and its manipulation for therapy remain poorly understood. Studies of lipid metabolism such as this are becoming more directed toward enhancing HDL production and inducing regression of atherosclerosis. This study demonstrates that HDL generated by antagonism of miR-33 is functional and promotes removal of excess cholesterol from the atherosclerotic plaques into the reverse cholesterol transport pathway, thereby allowing for cholesterol excretion. Other effects of anti-miR33 included reduction in the lesion area, macrophage number, lipid content, and inflammatory gene expression. The study demonstrates for the first time that oligonucleotides can penetrate atherosclerotic plaque, reach lesion macrophages, and upgrade *ABCA1* expression. This enhances cholesterol removal and results in clinically relevant regression of atherosclerosis.

G. L. Moneta, MD

References

1. Wilson PW. High-density lipoprotein, low-density lipoprotein and coronary artery disease. *Am J Cardiol.* 1990;66:7A-10A.
2. Plump AS, Scott CJ, Breslow JL. Human apolipoprotein A-I gene expression increases high density lipoprotein and suppresses atherosclerosis in the apolipoprotein E-deficient mouse. *Proc Natl Acad Sci U S A.* 1994;91:9607-9611.
3. Rong JX, Li J, Reis ED, et al. Elevating high-density lipoprotein cholesterol in apolipoprotein E-deficient mice remodels advanced atherosclerotic lesions by decreasing macrophage and increasing smooth muscle cell content. *Circulation.* 2001;104:2447-2452.

Catalase and Superoxide Dismutase Conjugated with Platelet-Endothelial Cell Adhesion Molecule Antibody Distinctly Alleviate Abnormal Endothelial Permeability Caused by Exogenous Reactive Oxygen Species and Vascular Endothelial Growth Factor

Han J, Shuvaev VV, Muzykantov VR (Univ of Pennsylvania, Philadelphia)
J Pharmacol Exp Ther 338:82-91, 2011

Reactive oxygen species (ROS) superoxide anion (O_2^-) and hydrogen peroxide (H_2O_2) produced by activated leukocytes and endothelial cells in sites of inflammation or ischemia cause endothelial barrier dysfunction that may lead to tissue edema. Antioxidant enzymes (AOEs) catalase and superoxide dismutase (SOD) conjugated with antibodies to platelet-endothelial cell adhesion molecule-1 (PECAM-1) specifically bind to endothelium, quench the corresponding ROS, and alleviate vascular oxidative stress and inflammation. In the present work, we studied the effects of anti-PECAM/catalase and anti-PECAM/SOD conjugates on the abnormal permeability manifested by transendothelial electrical resistance decline, increased fluorescein isothiocyanate-dextran influx, and redistribution of vascular endothelial-cadherin in human umbilical vein endothelial cell (HUVEC) monolayers. Anti-PECAM/catalase protected HUVEC monolayers against H_2O_2-induced endothelial barrier dysfunction. Polyethylene glycol-conjugated catalase exerted orders of magnitude lower endothelial uptake and no protective effect, similarly to IgG/catalase. Anti-PECAM/catalase, but not anti-PECAM/SOD, alleviated endothelial hyperpermeability caused by exposure to hypoxanthine/xanthine oxidase, implicating primarily H_2O_2 in the disruption of the endothelial barrier in this model. Thrombin-induced endothelial permeability was not affected by treatment with anti-PECAM/AOEs or the NADPH oxidase inhibitor apocynin or overexpression of AOEs, indicating that the endogenous ROS play no key role in thrombin-mediated endothelial barrier dysfunction. In contrast, anti-PECAM/SOD, but not anti-PECAM/catalase, inhibited a vascular endothelial growth factor (VEGF)-induced increase in endothelial permeability, identifying a key role of endogenous O_2^- in the VEGF-mediated regulation of endothelial barrier function. Therefore, AOEs targeted to endothelial cells provide versatile molecular tools for testing the roles of specific ROS in vascular pathology and may be translated into remedies for these ROS-induced abnormalities.

▶ The literature is loaded with in vitro studies that suggest exogenous administration scavengers of reactive oxygen species might mediate endothelial dysfunction in vivo. A well-known problem with administration of the scavengers is their ability to localize near the cell membrane and penetrate the vascular cells. These investigators take a unique approach by conjugating well-known scavengers to reactive oxygen metabolites to a platelet endothelial cell adhesion molecule antibody. Theoretically this should direct the scavengers of reactive oxygen species in close location to the endothelium where they could be internalized or active at the surface of the cell membrane. It is important to note that superoxide dismutase has been conjugated to lipid moieties in the past that have shown little efficacy in managing tissue injury in vivo. The main difference between those studies and this one is that the platelet endothelial cell adhesion molecule antibody should specifically direct the scavengers to the endothelial cell membrane surface. These investigators document updates of their conjugated antibody into endothelial cells and show marked decrease in vascular permeability. The clinical correlation cannot be priced precisely to acute limb ischemia reperfusion because the authors administered the antibody before the exogenous stress (hydrogen peroxide) was administered. However, this experimental treatment strategy might be useful in in vivo models of organ transplantation or elective aneurysm repair.

M. T. Watkins, MD

Cilostazol suppression of arterial intimal hyperplasia is associated with decreased expression of sialyl Lewis X homing receptors on mononuclear cells and E-selectin in endothelial cells

Takigawa T, Tsurushima H, Suzuki K, et al (Univ of Tsukuba, Ibaraki, Japan; Dokkyo Med Univ, Koshigaya, Saitama, Japan)
J Vasc Surg 55:506-516, 2012

Background.—An inflammatory reaction in vascular tissue is a potential factor linking restenosis after angioplasty. Although cilostazol, a selective phosphodiesterase type 3 inhibitor that is a unique antiplatelet drug and vasodilator, has been reported to be anti-inflammatory, its effect on the inflammatory action of mononuclear cells homing to endothelial cells is not clearly understood. In this study, whether cilostazol inhibits neointimal formation and improves inflammatory actions by inhibiting sialyl

Lewis X (SLX) expression on mononuclear cells and E-selectin expression on endothelial cells was evaluated.

Methods.—The effect of cilostazol (1, 3, 10, 30 µM) on expression of E-selectin in human umbilical vein endothelial cells and SLX in rat mononuclear cells stimulated with lipopolysaccharide by immunofluorescence and real-time polymerase chain reaction (n = 3) was studied. Additionally, a double-balloon injury model was used on rat carotid arteries to evaluate vascular intimal hyperplasia. 0.1% cilostazol was administered 3 days before the first balloon injury, and the second balloon injury was performed 7 days after the first injury. Cilostazol administration was continued until rats were sacrificed 14 days after the second angioplasty. The expression of SLX on mononuclear cells and E-selectin on endothelial cells by immunofluorescence (n = 10) and real-time polymerase chain reaction (n = 5) were studied.

Results.—Cilostazol effectively inhibited the expression of SLX on mononuclear cells and E-selectin on endothelial cells. Cilostazol inhibited the migration of mononuclear cells in neointimal regions and neointimal hyperplasia after balloon injury. The numbers of macrophages and T-lymphocytes and the hyperplasia area in neointimal regions decreased from 71.06 ± 20.04, 1121 ± 244.4 cells per section, 206,400 ± 96,150 mm^2 to 29.65 ± 16.73, 374.2 ± 124.5 cells per section, and 101,900 ± 16,150 mm^2 due to the administration of cilostazol.

Conclusions.—These results demonstrate that the protective effect of cilostazol against neointimal hyperplasia may be mediated by its anti-inflammatory actions of mononuclear cells homing to endothelial cells by decreasing SLX and E-selectin expression.

▶ This study is brought to our readers' attention primarily because of the stunning effects reported on the way cilostazol modulated the intimal medial ratio and the measurements of the area of neointimal hyperplasia. Cilostazol is a selective type III phosphodiesterase inhibitor that has been used in humans to treat symptomatic peripheral vascular disease, specifically intermittent claudication. The expression of E-selectin, an important endothelial adhesion molecule, was found to be largely abrogated in rats after balloon angioplasty. On one hand, the data are very impressive because the authors present a combination of in vivo and in vitro analyses to support their conclusions. They also used a severe model of vascular injury, ie, a double balloon injury model, for the in vivo studies. In addition to the absence of intimal hyperplasia, there was a significant reduction of marker 5 and accumulation of T lymphocytes within the arterial wall. The majority of the data in this article supports the concept that cilostazol may have an effect on the vascular wall in the setting of significant injury. The authors did not, however, use an in vivo environment that reflects the kind of human condition often associated with vascular injury, ie, hypercholesterolemia, diabetes, or hypertension. If an evaluation of the effects of cilostazol on vascular injury in hypercholesterolemic or diabetic rats is as impressive as the data presented in normal mice, a clinical trial in humans may be in order.

M. T. Watkins, MD

Sterile inflammation of endothelial cell-derived apoptotic bodies is mediated by interleukin-1α

Berda-Haddad Y, Robert S, Salers P, et al (Aix-Marseille Univ, France; et al)

Proc Natl Acad Sci U S A 108:20684-20689, 2011

Sterile inflammation resulting from cell death is due to the release of cell contents normally inactive and sequestered within the cell; fragments of cell membranes from dying cells also contribute to sterile inflammation. Endothelial cells undergoing stress-induced apoptosis release membrane microparticles, which become vehicles for proinflammatory signals. Here, we show that stress-activated endothelial cells release two distinct populations of particles: One population consists of membrane microparticles (<1 μm, annexin V positive without DNA and no histones) and another larger (1−3 μm) apoptotic body-like particles containing nuclear fragments and histones, representing apoptotic bodies. Contrary to present concepts, endothelial microparticles do not contain IL-1α and do not induce neutrophilic chemokines in vitro. In contrast, the large apoptotic bodies contain the full-length IL-1α precursor and the processed mature form. In vitro, these apoptotic bodies induce monocyte chemotactic protein-1 and IL-8 chemokine secretion in an IL-1α-dependent but IL-1β−independent fashion. Injection of these apoptotic bodies into the peritoneal cavity of mice induces elevated serum neutrophil-inducing chemokines, which was prevented by cotreatment with the IL-1 receptor antagonist. Consistently, injection of these large apoptotic bodies into the peritoneal cavity induced a neutrophilic infiltration that was prevented by IL-1 blockade. Although apoptosis is ordinarily considered noninflammatory, these data demonstrate that nonphagocytosed endothelial apoptotic bodies are inflammatory, providing a vehicle for IL-1α and, therefore, constitute a unique mechanism for sterile inflammation.

▶ Although inflammation can be triggered by bacterial or viral infection, sterile inflammation is the most common cause of both acute and chronic diseases. During myocardial infarction stroke or acute renal failure, sterile inflammation occurs in response to cell necrosis. The study was designed to determine whether stressed human endothelial cells might be a source of interleukin 1 (IL-1). These investigators sought to determine whether stimuli thought to contribute to stroke, atherosclerosis, or vasculitis might be related to activation of IL-1 in endothelial cells. The investigators have determined that IL-1 is secreted by endothelial cells in microparticles that are only produced during cellular apoptosis. These studies provide convincing evidence that apoptotic cells can release substances that actually amplify the inflammatory response. It is important to note that these experiments were done in the absence of macrophages, thereby firmly implicating endothelial injury as the cause of the inflammatory stimulus. It is possible that atherosclerosis and autoimmune disorders such as lupus may be related to defective clearance of microparticles known to carry IL-1. These data support the concept that IL-1 family members may play a central role in inflammation induced by apoptotic/necrotic cell death and may be a potential therapeutic target.

M. T. Watkins, MD

Assessment of mouse hind limb endothelial function by measuring femoral artery blood flow responses

Wang C-H, Chen K-T, Mei H-F, et al (Chang Gung Univ College of Medicine, Taoyuan, Taiwan; Natl Yang-Ming Univ, Taipei, Taiwan)
J Vasc Surg 53:1350-1358, 2011

Objective.—Substantial progress has been made in cell therapy strategies and in gene- and cytokine-introduced angiogenesis using a variety of mouse models, such as hind limb ischemia models. Endothelial function is an important target in evaluating the effects and outcomes of these potential therapies. Although animal models have been established for estimating endothelium-dependent function by measuring the blood flow responses in carotid and renal arteries and the abdominal aorta, a model specific for an indicated hind limb by measuring femoral artery blood flow (FABF) has not yet been established.

Methods.—A 2-day protocol was designed, including exploration of the segmental femoral artery on the first day, and evaluation of endothelium-dependent vasodilatation function the next day. By placing a transonic flow probe around the left femoral artery, the FABF in response to endothelium-dependent and endothelium-independent vasodilatory stimulations was reproducibly measured. Hemodynamic measurements, including the left FABF and mean arterial pressure, were recorded.

Results.—In normal controls, the baseline left FABF averaged 0.12 ± 0.01 mL/min. Acetylcholine increased the FABF up to 0.41 ± 0.02 mL/min. Rose bengal-associated photochemical injury was titrated to cause endothelial dysfunction but without disturbing the integrity of the endothelial layer. The response to acetylcholine significantly decreased 10 minutes after photochemical injury and was further impaired after 1 and 24 hours. However, the response to nitroprusside was preserved. A femoral and iliac artery wire-injury model was also introduced to cause endothelial and smooth muscle cell injury. One day after the wire injury, the responses to acetylcholine and nitroprusside injections were both remarkably attenuated.

Conclusions.—This model can be widely used to analyze the in vivo endothelium-dependent vasodilatation function before and after a variety of therapeutic interventions on a mouse hind limb (Figs 1 and 4).

▶ Hind limb mouse models, such as those for inducing limb ischemia, are well established in the laboratory to study the effects of ischemia reperfusion on the limb and systemically. Evaluation of endothelial function is critical to understand the effects of the development of various cardiovascular diseases, the importance of atherosclerotic lesion formation, and the progression of atheromatous disease. However, current hind limb mouse models use remote arterial sites to study and

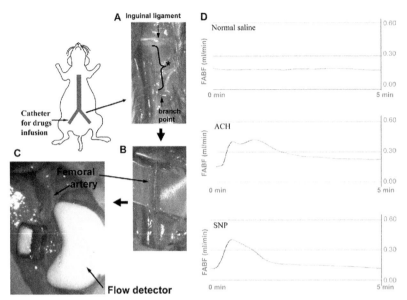

FIGURE 1.—A, A segment of the left femoral artery was chosen between the inguinal ligament and the first major branch. B, The femoral artery explored to a length of about 7 mm. C, The explored femoral artery was hooked up to a laser flow detector to measure the blood flow velocity. D, Injection of normal saline used as the control. Endothelium-dependent and endothelium-independent vasodilatation was assessed by injecting acetylcholine (*ACH*) and sodium nitroprusside (*SNP*), respectively, from a catheter inserted in the right femoral artery. *FABF*, Femoral artery blood flow. (Reprinted from the Journal of Vascular Surgery, Wang C-H, Chen K-T, Mei H-F, et al. Assessment of mouse hind limb endothelial function by measuring femoral artery blood flow responses. *J Vasc Surg*. 2011;53:1350-1358. Copyright 2011, with permission from The Society for Vascular Surgery.)

estimate endothelial-dependent and endothelial-independent mechanisms of blood flow responses and do not evaluate the endothelial function at the hind limb. These remote sites include the carotid artery, renal artery, and abdominal aorta. Importantly, in mouse models that have various genetic deletions (knock-out models), targeted genetic, cytokine, and pharmacologic therapies that affect endothelial function need to be measured with precision and reproducibility, which may not be entirely representative at remote arterial sites while using the hind limb mouse model. In this study the authors design and validate a mouse model by studying the effects of femoral artery blood flow and the function of intact or injured endothelium. The authors utilize a transonic flow probe, using a laser flow detector around the left femoral artery to study changes in blood flow that are endothelial dependent by using acetylcholine, and for changes in blood flow that are endothelial independent by using sodium nitroprusside, which is infused as a bolus from the aortic bifurcation after an elaborate ligation of the pelvic arterial branches (Fig 1). To study the effects of endothelial dysfunction on arterial blood flow, the authors use rose bengal injection and subject the femoral artery to photo injury by applying a cold light-emitting diode at 532 nm for 5 minutes, which activates rose bengal, forming reactive oxygen species. Femoral artery blood flow was significantly decreased after

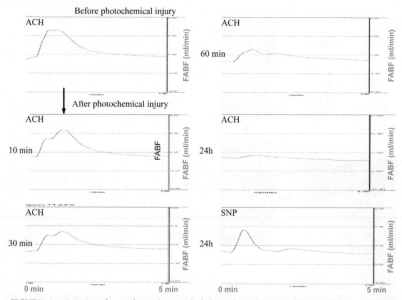

FIGURE 4.—A series of recordings show endothelium-dependent vasodilatation in the left femoral artery after 5 minutes of rose bengal-associated photochemical injury from 0 to 60 min and at 24 hours after the injury. Sodium nitroprusside (*SNP*)-induced vasodilatation is shown 24 hours after the photochemical injury. *ACH*, Acetylcholine; *FABF*, femoral artery blood flow. (Reprinted from the Journal of Vascular Surgery, Wang C-H, Chen K-T, Mei H-F, et al. Assessment of mouse hind limb endothelial function by measuring femoral artery blood flow responses. *J Vasc Surg*. 2011;53:1350-1358. Copyright 2011, with permission from The Society for Vascular Surgery.)

10 minutes and progressively deteriorated during endothelial-dependent vaso-dilatation with acetylcholine, while the integrity of the smooth muscle is maintained during relaxation via endothelial independent vasodilation with sodium nitroprusside, although diminished from baseline (Fig 4). In addition, the study also evaluated the use of a mechanical endothelial injury wire model of the femoral artery and measured endothelial dysfunction with the transonic laser flow probe. Because the wire is larger than the diameter of the mouse femoral and the iliac artery leading to arterial wall damage, there is significant reduction in femoral artery blood flow to both endothelial-dependent and endothelial-independent stimuli, indicating injury to both the endothelium and smooth muscle. This study is important because it is the first study to actually measure endothelial function with changes in arterial blood flow in the femoral artery that can be applied to a hind limb mouse model. By actually studying endothelial function in the hind limb of the mouse using different vascular pathologic models that utilize the transonic flow probe, we gain a better insight into endothelial changes directly related to the vascular bed injury as opposed to surrogate endothelial function in remote arterial sites, and we also gain a better understanding of the different therapies that may restore endothelial function.

J. D. Raffetto, MD

Association of Physical Activity With Vascular Endothelial Function and Intima-Media Thickness: A Longitudinal Study in Adolescents

Pahkala K, Heinonen OJ, Simell O, et al (Univ of Turku and Turku Univ Hosp, Finland)

Circulation 124:1956-1963, 2011

Background.—Impairment of vascular endothelial function and increased intima-media thickness (IMT) are important early steps in atherogenesis. Longitudinal data on the effect of physical activity on endothelial function and IMT in healthy adolescents are lacking. We investigated prospectively the association of leisure-time physical activity with endothelial function (brachial artery flow-mediated dilatation; FMD) and aortic IMT in adolescents.

Methods and Results.—FMD and IMT were measured with ultrasonography at 13 (n=553), 15 (n=531), and 17 (n=494) years of age in adolescents participating in a longitudinal atherosclerosis prevention study (Special Turku Coronary Risk Factor Intervention Project for Children). Mean aortic IMT, maximum FMD, and total FMD response (area under the dilatation curve 40 to 180 seconds after hyperemia) were calculated. Leisure-time physical activity was assessed with a questionnaire, and metabolic equivalent (MET) hours per week of leisure-time physical activity were calculated by multiplying weekly mean exercise intensity, duration, and frequency. Leisure-time physical activity was directly associated with endothelial function (P for maximum FMD=0.0021, P for total FMD response=0.0036) and inversely with IMT (P=0.011) after adjustment for age, sex, body mass index, high-density lipoprotein/total cholesterol, systolic blood pressure, and C-reactive protein and regarding FMD brachial artery diameter. Sedentary adolescents who increased their leisure-time physical activity from <5 to >5 (IMT) or >30 (maximum FMD) MET h/wk between 13 and 17 years of age had an increased maximum FMD (P=0.031) and decreased progression of IMT (P=0.047) compared with adolescents who remained sedentary. IMT progression was attenuated in persistently active adolescents compared with those who became sedentary (P=0.0072).

Conclusions.—Physical activity is favorably associated with endothelial function and IMT in adolescents.

Clinical Trial Registration.—URL: http://www.clinicaltrials.gov. Unique identifier: NCT00223600 (STRIP19902010).

▶ This is an important study on the effect of physical activity (leisure time physical activity [LTPA]) on brachial artery reactivity (as a marker of vascular dysfunction) and intimal medial thickness ([IMT] as a marker of arterial injury). It is a longitudinal study of adolescents (aged 13-17 years) that provides considerable support for more physical activity amongst young adults. There have been previous studies to show that physical activity enhances endothelial function in adults and a decrease in the progression of carotid and femoral medial thickness in healthy adults and in patients with coronary heart disease. Due to strains on the budgets of many school districts in the United States, many sports-related activities have been eliminated in secondary schools. Autopsy studies have shown the beginnings of atherosclerosis in young adolescents; therefore, this work is important for general consideration. In the studies, exercise training was able to induce regression of animal medial thickness. Longitudinal regression analyses showed a favorable effect of LTPA on aortic medial thickness. The strength of this study is its longitudinal design with repeated data assessment. This is unique and concerns physical activity and vascular function. Assessment of physical activity only during leisure time excluded the effects of physical education at school, which could bias the studies. Unfortunately, this article does little to provide information about the mechanisms that produce physical activity—associated improvements in IMT.

M. T. Watkins, MD

Cerium Oxide Nanoparticles Inhibit Oxidative Stress and Nuclear Factor-κB Activation in H9c2 Cardiomyocytes Exposed to Cigarette Smoke Extract
Niu J, Wang K, Kolattukudy PE (Univ of Central Florida, Orlando)
J Pharmacol Exp Ther 338:53-61, 2011

Cigarette smoke contains and generates a large amount of reactive oxygen species (ROS) that affect normal cellular function and have pathogenic consequences in the cardiovascular system. Increased oxidative stress and inflammation are considered to be an important mechanism of cardiovascular injury induced by cigarette smoke. Antioxidants may serve as effective therapeutic agents against smoke-related cardiovascular disease. Because of the presence of oxygen vacancies on its surface and self-regenerative cycle of its dual oxidation states, Ce^{3+} and Ce^{4+}, cerium oxide (CeO_2) nanoparticles offer a potential to quench ROS in biological systems. In this study, we determined the ability of CeO_2 nanoparticles to protect against cigarette smoke extract (CSE)-induced oxidative stress and inflammation in cultured rat H9c2 cardiomyocytes. CeO_2 nanoparticles pretreatment of H9c2 cells resulted in significant inhibition of CSE-induced ROS production and cell death. Pretreatment of H9c2 cells with CeO_2 nanoparticles suppressed CSE-induced phosphorylation of IκBα, nuclear translocation of p65 subunit of nuclear factor-κB (NF-κB), and NF-κB reporter activity in H9c2 cells. CeO_2 nanoparticles pretreatment also resulted in a significant down-regulation of NF-κB-regulated inflammatory genes tumor necrosis factor-α, interleukin (IL)-1β, IL-6, and inducible nitric-oxide synthase and further inhibited CSE-induced depletion of antioxidant enzymes, such as copper zinc superoxide dismutase, manganese superoxide dismutase, and intracellular glutathione content. These results indicate that CeO_2 nanoparticles can inhibit CSE-induced cell damage via inhibition of ROS generation, NF-κB activation, inflammatory gene expression, and antioxidant depletion and may have a great potential for treatment of smoking-related diseases.

▶ This is a curious article in the sense that the authors had already published data showing that these nanoparticles modulate injury in vitro in response to exogenously applied reactive oxygen species. In this article, the authors determined whether cigarette smoke extract modulated oxidant stress and cardiomyocytes and whether these nanoparticles could blunt or abrogate the oxidant response. Nanoparticle treatment resulted in significant downregulation of the inflammatory response as mediated by tumor necrosis factor, IL-1, and inducible nitric oxide synthase (iNOS). Furthermore, nanoparticles decreased the levels of endogenous antioxidant enzymes such as the superoxide dismutase and intracellular glutathione. Nanoparticles have received considerable attention in the literature as potential mechanisms for drug delivery. For the most part, they have very little toxicity and have extensive capability to penetrate cells. The article provides a complete road map for assessing cellular responses to oxidant stress and is exceptionally well written. The studies are particularly well done as the authors assess both messenger RNA and protein levels of iNOS. One must question what clinical scenario would be appropriate for these studies. Would they recommend this kind of treatment to decrease cardiovascular complications associated with smoking cessation? In other words, if a patient is going to smoke, he or she should go ahead but take the nanoparticles prior to lighting up. On a more serious note, the authors cite unpublished data that they have injected these particles into mice at high concentrations and found no overt systemic toxicity. This needs to be clarified and validated. I would keep an eye on these and similar agents, as they may be very useful for future studies of organ transplantation or ischemia reperfusion injury.

M. T. Watkins, MD

Inhibiting platelet-stimulated blood coagulation by inhibition of mitochondrial respiration
Barile CJ, Herrmann PC, Tyvoll DA, et al (Stanford Univ, CA; Loma Linda Univ School of Medicine, CA)
Proc Natl Acad Sci U S A 109:2539-2543, 2012

Platelets are important mediators of blood coagulation that lack nuclei, but contain mitochondria. Although the presence of mitochondria in platelets has long been recognized, platelet mitochondrial function remains largely unaddressed. On the basis of a small amount of literature that suggests platelet mitochondria are functional, we hypothesized that the inhibition of platelet mitochondria disrupts platelet function and platelet-activated blood coagulation. To test this hypothesis, members of the tetrazole, thiazole, and 1,2,3-triazole families of small molecule heterocycles were screened for the ability to inhibit isolated mitochondrial respiration and coagulation of whole blood. The families of heterocycles screened were chosen on the basis of the ability of the heterocycle family to inhibit a biomimetic model of cytochrome c oxidase (CcO). The strength of mitochondrial inhibition correlates with each compound's ability to deter platelet stimulation and platelet-activated blood clotting. These results suggest that for this class of molecules, inhibition of blood coagulation may be occurring through a mechanism involving mitochondrial inhibition.

▶ This article sheds light on the role of platelet mitochondria on platelet reactivity. The investigators show that a novel class of molecules that inhibit mitochondrial function is able to inhibit platelet activation. These investigations involve screening of substances that were found to inhibit the activity of cytochrome C oxidase in an in vitro model. Using this model for screening, they identified cyclic compounds that reversibly inhibited mitochondrial function. Once the compounds were identified, their effect on platelet function was tested using whole blood. The end points for platelet function were clumping, sticking, and clotting. All 3 were shortened in samples with activated platelets and correspondingly lengthened in samples with inhibited platelets. Some of the substances screened increased clumping and sticking by 10-fold and clotting time by 2-fold. This suggests a primary antiplatelet effect that may not result in frank bleeding or bruising in vivo. These heterocyclic compounds have the potential for clinical use because their effects are reversible. Irreversible inhibitors of mitochondrial function are universally toxic. Very little is known regarding the tissue distribution metabolism and binding affinities of these substances to other heme-based proteins such as cyclooxygenase and thromboxane A. Nevertheless, these unique substances may play a role in future clinical antiplatelet therapies.

M. T. Watkins, MD

Adventitial contributions of the extracellular signal—regulated kinase and Akt pathways to neointimal hyperplasia
Havelka GE, Hogg ME, Martinez J, et al (Northwestern Univ, Chicago, IL)
Am J Surg 202:515-519, 2011

Background.—We recently reported that the efficacy of nitric oxide (NO) appears to be based on both sex and hormone status. The mechanism responsible for this differential efficacy is unknown. The aim of this study was to characterize the effect of sex, hormones, and NO on the extracellular signal—regulated kinase (ERK) and Akt signaling pathways after arterial injury.

Methods.—Male and female Sprague—Dawley rats underwent castration or sham surgery. Two weeks later, they underwent carotid artery balloon injury. Treatment groups included the following: control, injury, and injury + 1-[2-(carboxylato)pyrrolidin-1-yl]diazen-1-ium-1,2-diolate (PROLI/NO) (n = 5 per group). Arteries were harvested 2 weeks after injury and assessed for phospho-ERK (pERK) and phospho-Akt (pAkt) expression.

Results.—After injury, more pERK and pAkt activity was seen in the adventitia than media in both sexes, regardless of hormone status (*P* < .05). In hormonally intact males, NO further increased pERK (44%) and pAkt (120%) after injury (*P* < .001). Castration attenuated the effects of NO. In hormonally intact females, NO caused the opposite pattern with pERK activity but did not affect pAkt activity.

Conclusions.—After arterial injury, ERK and Akt activity is significantly greater in the adventitia than the media, and depends on sex, hormone status, and NO. Understanding adventitial regulation of proliferative signaling pathways will allow the development of targeted therapies for neointimal hyperplasia.

▶ There is considerable work in the literature that suggests the extracellular signal—regulated kinase (ERK) and AKT signaling pathways are involved in the development of the vascular response to injury. Both pathways have been shown to regulate proliferation of vascular smooth muscle cells and adventitial tissue fibroblasts. This study involved a comparison of ERK and AKT activity in different parts of the arterial wall. This has considerable importance with respect to delivery of therapies that may modulate the vascular response to injury. Specifically there are a number of studies that suggest the best route of pharmacologic treatment might be through the lumen of the vessel. However, there are many experimental studies that suggest drug delivery at the adventitial surface might also prove beneficial. In this study, the Kibbe Lab has clearly and unambiguously shown that AKT and ERK activity was more predominant in the adventitia rather than the media. This activity was independent of gender or hormone status. Surprisingly when exogenous nitric oxide was administered, there were significant differences in the gender response. In men, there was an increase in ERK activity, whereas in women, exogenous nitric oxide decreased adventitial ERK activity. The study is an important biochemical analysis supporting anatomic data provided by other investigators who have shown that proliferation in the adventitia precedes proliferation in the media after arterial injury. It is interesting to note that the authors felt a limitation of this study was that it was performed 2 weeks after injury. In my mind, this is an important end point because it reflects a steady state component of the arterial injury. Moreover, it suggests that intervention at a time other than initial injury may be feasible.

M. T. Watkins, MD

Low molecular weight (LMW) heparin inhibits injury-induced femoral artery remodeling in mouse via upregulating CD44 expression
Zhao G, Shaik RS, Zhao H, et al (Massachusetts General Hosp, Boston)
J Vasc Surg 53:1359-1367, 2011

Objective.—The mechanism of postangioplasty restenosis remains poorly understood. Low molecular weight (LMW) heparin has been shown to inhibit the proliferation of vascular smooth muscle cells (VSMCs), which is the principal characteristic of restenosis. Studies have shown that LMW heparin could bind to CD44. We hypothesized that LMW heparin might modulate CD44 expression thereby decreasing vascular remodeling.

Methods.—Vascular remodeling was induced in CD44$^{+/+}$ and CD44$^{-/-}$ mice and treated with LMW heparin. The arteries were harvested for histologic assessment and determination of CD44 expression. Bone marrow transplantation was introduced to further explore the role and functional sites of CD44. Effects of LMW heparin on growth capacity, CD44 expression were further studied using the cultured mouse VSMCs.

Results.—Transluminal injury induced remarkable remodeling in mouse femoral artery (sham wall thickness percentage [WT%]: 3.4 ± 1.2% vs injury WT%: 31.8 ± 4.7%; $P < .001$). LMW heparin reduced the remodeling significantly (WT%: 17.8 ± 3.5%, $P < .005$). CD44$^{-/-}$ mice demonstrated considerably thicker arterial wall remodeling (WT%: 46.2 ± 7.6%, $P = .0035$), and CD44-chimeric mice exhibited equal contributions of the local and circulating CD44 signal to the neointima formation. LMW heparin markedly upregulated CD44 expression in the injured femoral arteries. In vitro, LMW heparin decreased mouse VSMC growth capacity and upregulated its CD44 expression simultaneously in a dose-dependent and time-dependent manner, which could be partially blocked by CD44 inhibitor.

Conclusions.—LMW heparin inhibits injury-induced femoral artery remodeling, at least partially, by upregulating CD44 expression.

▶ Neointimal hyperplasia is a significant problem that leads to graft failure, restenosis of grafts and stents, reinterventions, and reoperations. Significant basic science research has focused on mechanisms of smooth muscle activation and proliferation, endothelial—smooth muscle interactions, inflammatory pathways, and fibrosis. Currently, there are no clinical treatments that act as adjuncts to reduce neointimal hyperplasia; however, continued research is necessary to fully understand this problem that affects so many aspects of vascular surgery. In this interesting and well-designed study, the authors evaluate how low-molecular-weight heparin, which is known to inhibit smooth muscle proliferation, interacts with CD44 and modulates vascular remodeling. CD44 is a transmembrane glycoprotein and works as a principal cell receptor for hyaluronic acid, interacting with many extracellular matrix molecules and intracellular signaling molecules. The authors use a knockout (KO) mouse model that is deficient in CD44 (CD44$^{-/-}$) versus wild-type (WT) mice (CD44$^{+/+}$), and study vascular remodeling in the femoral artery spring coil injury model with and without low molecular weight heparin. The major findings of this study were the following: (1) CD44$^{+/+}$ mice had significant neointimal hyperplasia after injury that was significantly inhibited by low-molecular-weight heparin. (2) CD44$^{-/-}$ mice demonstrated significantly thicker femoral artery than CD44$^{+/+}$ following injury, indicating the involvement of CD44 gene in neointima formation. (3) In bone marrow chimeric mice, both groups of chimeric mice (WT-KO and KO-WT) had statistically thinner remodeling compared with KO-KO mice, demonstrating the contributions of both local and circulating CD44. (4) Low-molecular-weight heparin upregulated CD44 expression in remodeled femoral arteries. (5) Warfarin or saline-treated injured femoral arteries did not show any changes in remodeling thickness or CD44 expression. (6) Low-molecular-weight heparin did not inhibit the vascular remodeling in CD44$^{-/-}$ mice but significantly reduced remodeling in CD44$^{+/+}$ mice, suggesting that low-molecular-weight heparin exerts its antiproliferative effect on the vascular remodeling lesion, at least partially, via CD44 signal pathway. (7) In CD44$^{+/+}$ smooth muscle culture experiments, low-molecular-weight heparin inhibited vascular smooth muscle proliferation and increased the expression of CD44$^{+/+}$ but not in vascular smooth muscle from CD44$^{-/-}$. Likely, based on this study, targeted deficiency of the CD44 gene significantly enhances neointimal hyperplasia, suggesting that the CD44 gene has implications in the pathologic remodeling process and might play a protective role. Hopefully, future work in this very important field will provide therapeutic strategies that can be added to patients undergoing open, hybrid, or endovascular revascularization to reduce neointimal hyperplasia and graft/stent failures. Further understanding in how low-molecular-weight heparin upregulates CD44, and how CD44 regulates vascular smooth muscle is required before appropriate pharmacologic therapy can be considered.

J. D. Raffetto, MD

Inhibition of transforming growth factor-β restores endothelial thromboresistance in vein grafts

Kapur NK, Bian C, Lin E, et al (Johns Hopkins School of Medicine, Baltimore, MD)

J Vasc Surg 54:1117-1123, 2011

Background.—Thrombosis is a major cause of the early failure of vein grafts (VGs) implanted during peripheral and coronary arterial bypass surgeries. Endothelial expression of thrombomodulin (TM), a key constituent of the protein C anticoagulant pathway, is markedly suppressed in VGs after implantation and contributes to local thrombus formation. While stretch-induced paracrine release of transforming growth factor-β (TGF-β) is known to negatively regulate TM expression in heart tissue, its role in regulating TM expression in VGs remains unknown.

Methods.—Changes in relative mRNA expression of major TGF-β isoforms were measured by quantitative polymerase chain reaction (qPCR) in cultured human saphenous vein smooth muscle cells (HSVSMCs) subjected to cyclic stretch. To determine the effects of paracrine release of TGF-β on endothelial TM mRNA expression, human saphenous vein endothelial cells (HSVECs) were co-cultured with stretched HSVSMCs in the presence of 1D11, a pan-neutralizing TGF-β antibody, or 13C4, an isotype-control antibody. Groups of rabbits were then administered 1D11 or 13C4 and underwent interpositional grafting of jugular vein segments into the carotid circulation. The effect of TGF-β inhibition on TM gene expression was measured by qPCR; protein C activating capacity and local thrombus formation were measured by in situ chromogenic substrate assays; and VG remodeling was assessed by digital morphometry.

Results.—Cyclic stretch induced TGF-β_1 expression in HSVSMCs by 1.9 ± 0.2-fold ($P < .001$) without significant change in the expressions of TGF-β_2 and TGF-β_3. Paracrine release of TGF-β_1 by stretched HSVSMCs inhibited TM expression in stationary HSVECs placed in co-culture by 57 ± 12% ($P = .03$), an effect that was abolished in the presence of 1D11. Similarly, TGF-β_1 was the predominant isoform induced in rabbit VGs 7 days after implantation (3.5 ± 0.4-fold induction; $P < .001$). TGF-β_1 protein expression localized predominantly to the developing neointima and coincided with marked suppression of endothelial TM expression (16% ± 2% of vein controls; $P < .03$), a reduction in situ activated protein C (APC)-generating capacity (53% ± 9% of vein controls; $P = .001$) and increased local thrombus formation (3.7 ± 0.8-fold increase over vein controls; $P < .01$). External stenting of VGs to limit vessel distension significantly reduced TGF-β_1 induction and TM downregulation. Systemic administration of 1D11 also effectively prevented TM downregulation, preserved APC-generating capacity, and reduced local thrombus in rabbit VGs without observable effect on neointima formation and other morphometric parameters 6 weeks after implantation.

Conclusion.—TM downregulation in VGs is mediated by paracrine release of TGF-β_1 caused by pressure-induced vessel stretch. Systemic administration of an anti-TGF-β antibody effectively prevented TM downregulation and preserved local thromboresistance without negative effect on VG remodeling.

▶ The mechanism of thrombosis that occurs in vein grafts is a complex process. A major goal is to prevent early failure of infrainguinal bypass graft thrombosis in the postoperative period and within the first year. Vein grafts, unlike arterial grafts conduits, that are used in both the infrainguinal and coronary circulation can have between a 20% and 30% graft failure rate due to thrombus formation in the first year. Understanding the involved mechanisms in early vein graft failure is paramount to improving outcomes and quality of life. Thrombomodulin is a transmembrane protein that is essential in preventing vascular thrombosis. Thrombomodulin is expressed by endothelial cells, and its function is to bind to thrombin-active site, decreasing the formation of fibrin from thrombin-mediated cleavage of fibrinogen, and enable thrombin-mediated activation of the protein C anticoagulation pathway. Activated protein C deactivates factors Va and VIIIa of the coagulation cascade, thereby inhibiting further thrombin formation. It is known that in newly implanted saphenous graft, protein C pathway is suppressed and local thrombus formation ensues. Important in the regulation of thrombomodulin is transforming growth factor-beta (TGF-b); however, its function in vein grafts is not well defined. In this study, the authors study the effects of cyclic stretch on human saphenous vein smooth muscle cells and the expression of TGF-b, the effect of cocultured stretched human saphenous vein smooth muscle cells with human endothelial cells in the presence of TGF inhibitor (1D11), and in an animal model using rabbits the effects of administering 1D11 on rabbits that underwent interpositioned grafting of jugular vein segments into the carotid circulation. The study determined the following important findings: (1) In smooth muscle and endothelial cells from humans there was paracrine release of TGF-b1 caused by pressure-induced stretch with reduced thrombomodulin, and the effects were reversed by inhibition of TGF-b with 1D11. (2) In rabbit vein graft interposed into the carotid circulation at 7 days there was increased expression of TGF-b1, which localized to the developing neointima, with a loss of thrombomodulin in the overlying endothelial cells. (3) Stretch, and not the direct effect of pressure, is the critical hemodynamic stimulus responsible for TGF-b1 upregulation. (4) Inhibition of TGF-b1 in vivo effectively prevented stretch-induced downregulation of thrombomodulin gene and protein expression as well as restored activated protein C activity. (5) Inhibition of TGF-b1 by 1D11 caused the suppression of thrombus formation as measured by bound thrombin activity on the graft luminal surface. (6) In vivo inhibition of TGF-b1 with 1D11 had no discernable effects on vein graft remodeling including neointima formation. Clearly this study has elucidated the importance of TGF-b1 in vein graft thrombogenecity and the importance of stretch on smooth muscle being the inciting factor for TGF-b1 induction. Hopefully, there will be application of this information into the clinical setting. The overwhelming concerns are always unwanted side effects that can occur when systemically inhibiting important growth factors such as TGF-b that has many essential functions that occur during physiologic and injury processes, including inflammation, wound repair, angiogenesis, and tissue remodeling. Possibility of inhibiting TGF-b1 locally in vein grafts without systemic influences would be ideal, but the challenges will be to define timing and vehicle for delivery. In addition, as has been seen in other animal studies that have translated to human clinical trials, the desired effects that occurred in experimental models do not occur consistently when applied clinically.

J. D. Raffetto, MD

Aortic Medial Elastic Fiber Loss in Acute Ascending Aortic Dissection
Roberts WC, Vowels TJ, Kitchens BL, et al (Baylor Univ Med Ctr, Dallas, TX; Univ of Texas School of Medicine at San Antonio)
Am J Cardiol 108:1639-1644, 2011

The cause of acute aortic dissection continues to be debated. One school of thought suggests that underlying aortic medial cystic necrosis is the common denominator. The purpose of the present study was to determine if there was loss and, if so, how much loss of medial elastic fibers in the ascending aorta in patients with acute aortic dissection with the entrance tear in the ascending aorta. We examined operatively excised ascending aortas in 69 patients having acute dissection with tears in the ascending aorta. Patients with previous aortotomy, healed dissection, and connective tissue disorders were excluded. The 69 patients' ages ranged from 31 to 88 years (mean 56); 49 were men and 20 were women. Loss of aortic medial elastic fibers was graded as 0 (no loss), 1+ (trace), 2+ (mild), 3+ (moderate), and 4+ (full thickness loss). Of these 69 patients, 56 (82%) had 0 or 1+ elastic fiber loss; 13 patients (18%), 2+ to 4+ loss including 4 with 2+, 6 with 3+, and 2 with 4+. Nearly all patients (97%) had a history of systemic hypertension and/or had received antihypertensive drug therapy. In conclusion, most patients (82% in this study) having acute aortic dissection with entrance tears in the ascending aorta have normal numbers or only trace loss of aortic medial elastic fibers. Thus, underlying abnormal ascending aortic structure uncommonly precedes acute dissection.

▶ The purpose of this study was to use human tissue to determine whether there was evidence of aortic medial cystic necrosis in patients with acute aortic dissection. Not surprisingly, most of the patients had a history of hypertension and had received antihypertensive drug therapy. The authors were careful to exclude patients who had had previous aortotomy, healed dissection, or connective tissue disorders. The authors created a reproducible grading system to analyze the tissue sections. The ascending aorta from 19 necropsy cases were used as controls for the study, and this is possibly the weak link in this study because the age of the control patients was between 20 and 82 years. The mean age of the patients with aortic dissection tears was much greater. Another weakness is that there is no specific knowledge as to whether there is a history of drug use among the patients in this article. Despite these deficiencies, the authors found little evidence of significant loss of aortic medial elastic fibers, casting some doubt on the central dogma that the underlying aortic medial cystic necrosis is a common denominator for dissection. These data put more emphasis on the role of hypertension rather than a structural weakness in the vascular wall. This work is an important reference, as the number of tissues available for necropsy is steadily decreasing.

M. T. Watkins, MD

Elevation of hemopexin-like fragment of matrix metalloproteinase-2 tissue levels inhibits ischemic wound healing and angiogenesis
Nedeau AE, Gallagher KA, Liu Z-J, et al (Univ of Miami, FL)
J Vasc Surg 54:1430-1438, 2011

Objective.—Matrix metalloproteinase-2 (MMP-2) degrades type IV collagen and enables endothelial cell (EC) migration during angiogenesis and wound healing. Peroxisomal biogenesis factor 2 (PEX2), a by-product of activated MMP-2 autocatalysis, competitively inhibits newly activated MMP-2 from EC surface binding and migration. We hypothesize that PEX2 is elevated during limb ischemia and contributes to poor wound healing, with decreased capillary density.

Methods.—Western blot was used to identify PEX2 in the hind limbs of FVB/NJ mice with surgically induced ischemia. The PEX2 effect on healing was evaluated by calculating the area of exposed muscle after wounding the dorsum of mice and administering daily injections with human recombinant PEX2 (hrPEX2). Wounds were also injected with lentivirus-expressing PEX2 (PEX2-LV), harvested on postoperative day 7 and processed for staining. Epithelial gap was assessed with light microscopy. Capillary density was evaluated after wounding *Tie2*-green fluorescent protein (GFP)⁺ transgenic FVB mice (ECs labeled green) and viral transduction with PEX2-LV. Wounds were harvested on postoperative day (POD) 7, frozen in liquid nitrogen, sectioned, and stained with Hoechst. Vessel density was assessed via fluorescence microscopy as the average number of capillaries/10 high-powered fields. Paired t test was used to assess differences between the groups.

Results.—PEX2 was elevated 5.5 ± 2.0-fold ($P = .005$) on POD 2 and 2.9 ± 0.69-fold ($P = .004$) on POD 4 in gastrocnemius muscles of ischemic hind limbs. The wound surface area, or lack of granulation tissue and exposed muscle, decreased daily in all mice but was greater in the hrPEX2-treated mice by 12% to 16% ($P < .004$). Wounds in the control group were completely covered with granulation tissue by POD 3. Wounds injected with hrPEX2 were not completely covered by POD 7 but continued to have exposed muscle. Microscopic examination of wounds after PEX2-LV viral transduction demonstrated an average epithelial gap of 1.6 ± 0.3 vs 0.64 ± 0.3 μm in control wounds ($P < .04$). Wounds from *Tie2*-GFP mice had an average number of 3.8 ± 1.1 capillaries vs 6.9 ± 1.2 in control wounds ($P < .007$).

Conclusions.—Our study links elevated PEX2 to ischemia and poor wound healing. We demonstrate comparative PEX2 elevation in ischemic murine hind limbs. Less granulation tissue is produced and healing is retarded in wounds subjected to hrPEX2 or viral transduction with PEX2-LV. Microscopic examination shows the wounds exhibit fewer capillaries, supporting the hypothesis that PEX2 decreases angiogenesis.

▶ Ischemic wounds require normalization of blood flow to begin the healing process. However, the basic science of acute and chronic wounds has been extensively studied and involves inflammatory cells, a variety of cytokines and growth factors, vascular growth factors, neovascularization/angiogenesis, fibro-blasts, collagen turnover, and remodeling. Matrix metalloproteinases (MMP) are zinc-dependent endopeptidases with a zinc-binding motif bound by 3 histidine molecules with the conserved sequence HEXGHXXGXXH located in the catalytic domain and are very important in both acute and chronic wounds. Matrix metal-loproteinases main function is modulation of the extracellular matrix, collagen turnover, and gelatin degradation. Matrix metalloproteinases have been studied extensively in tumorigenesis and their role in angiogenesis. In this study, the authors evaluate a mouse hind-limb ischemia model and wounding. The authors hypothesize that peroxisomal biogenesis factor 2 (PEX2), a by-product of acti-vated MMP-2 autocatalysis that competitively inhibits newly activated MMP-2 from endothelial cell surface binding and migration, is elevated during limb ischemia and contributes to poor wound healing and decreased angiogenesis. In the mouse hind-limb ischemic model (induced by femoral artery and vein ligation/resection) and wounding (using a 6-mm punch biopsy to expose muscle), the authors found the following: (1) PEX2 was increased after day 2 and 4 in the ischemic hind-limb gastrocnemius muscle. (2) Direct injection of human recombinant PEX2 into the wound caused delay of granulation tissue formation compared with control. (3) Wounds treated with PEX2 had increased epithelial gap (large gaps with less intervening granulation tissue) and decreased capillaries into the wounded area. It appears that PEX2 is important to inhibiting angiogenesis. Its potential role in human chronic ischemic limbs needs to be determined before pharmacologic therapies directed at PEX2 or other antiangiogenic molecules (tumstatin and thrombospondin-2) can be implemented. Continued basic scientific research will be needed to fully elucidate the importance of these antiangiogenic molecules in chronic ischemia and to determine whether inhibitors of PEX2 are able to reverse the ischemic effects resulting from increased angiogenesis.

J. D. Raffetto, MD

Does Endovenous Laser Ablation Induce Endothelial Damage at the Saphenofemoral Junction?

Heere-Ress E, Veensalu M, Wacheck V, et al (Erasmus Univ Med Ctr, Rotterdam, The Netherlands; Med Univ of Vienna, Austria)
Dermatol Surg 37:1456-1463, 2011

Background and Objective.—One of the possible complications of endovenous laser ablation (EVLA) is thrombus progression into the common femoral vein or popliteal vein with the potential risk of pulmonary embolism or stroke. We set out to investigate the effect of laser energy applied under standardized treatment conditions on biomarkers of platelet and endothelial activation and on the hemostatic system.

Methods.—Twenty patients with incompetence of the great saphenous vein were included in this prospective study. Blood samples of the iliofemoral and anticubital veins were collected before, during, and after EVLA. Plasma levels of soluble (s) P-selectin, soluble thrombomodulin (sTM), prothrombin fragment F1 + 2 (F1 + 2), and D-dimer were measured. (s) P-selectin and sTM were analyzed as surrogate markers of endothelial and platelet activation. F1 + 2 and D-dimer were monitored to quantify the degree of surgical trauma.

Results.—Whereas there was no immediate rise of (s) P-selectin and sTM plasma concentrations in iliofemoral or anticubital blood, plasma levels of F1 + 2 and D-dimer increased significantly after EVLA.

Conclusion.—Pulsed mode laser ablation with an 810-nm fiber does not induce measurable platelet and endothelium activation in the iliofemoral or systemic blood. Furthermore, the immediate surgical trauma associated with EVLA appears to be modest.

▶ This is a very simple yet important analysis of the effects of endovenous laser ablation (EVLA) on systemic markers of thrombosis. The authors sought to determine whether the progression of thrombosis into the common femoral or popliteal vein might be due to induction of a systemic thrombolytic response. They evaluated samples of blood through central venous catheters placed in the ipsilateral femoral vein of the leg being treated. The authors use commercially available kits to measure plasma levels of P-selectin, D-dimer, and thrombomo-dulin. This study showed no evidence of systemic thrombosis as measured with these assays. There was no difference in the levels of thrombotic markers when levels in the iliofemoral vein were compared with samples from the antecubital vein. There was evidence of increased plasma levels of the D-dimer in iliofemoral blood as compared to the antecubital blood. The authors make the case that it is possible that thrombotic complications after EVLA likely represent inadvertent application errors rather than the thrombotic burden of the procedure itself. I think this is a big leap of faith, since there is a distinct incidence of popliteal vein and tibial vein thrombosis following EVLA and the laser is never anywhere near those of structures. The authors should have measured plasma levels of tissue factor, which is the most potent mediator of thrombosis.

M. T. Watkins, MD

In vivo three-dimensional blood velocity profile shapes in the human common, internal, and external carotid arteries
Kamenskiy AV, Dzenis YA, MacTaggart JN, et al (Univ of Nebraska-Lincoln; Univ of Nebraska-Med Ctr, Omaha)
J Vasc Surg 54:1011-1020, 2011

Objective.—True understanding of carotid bifurcation pathophysiology requires a detailed knowledge of the hemodynamic conditions within the arteries. Data on carotid artery hemodynamics are usually based on simplified, computer-based, or in vitro experimental models, most of which assume that the velocity profiles are axially symmetric away from the carotid bulb. Modeling accuracy and, more importantly, our understanding of the pathophysiology of carotid bifurcation disease could be considerably improved by more precise knowledge of the in vivo flow properties within the human carotid artery. The purpose of this work was to determine the three-dimensional pulsatile velocity profiles of human carotid arteries.

Methods.—Flow velocities were measured over the cardiac cycle using duplex ultrasonography, before and after endarterectomy, in the surgically exposed common (CCA), internal (ICA), and external (ECA) carotid arteries (n = 16) proximal and distal to the stenosis/endarterectomy zone. These measurements were linked to a standardized grid across the flow lumina of the CCA, ICA, and ECA. The individual velocities were then used to build mean three-dimensional pulsatile velocity profiles for each of the carotid artery branches.

Results.—Pulsatile velocity profiles in all arteries were asymmetric about the arterial centerline. Posterior velocities were higher than anterior velocities in all arteries. In the CCA and ECA, velocities were higher laterally, while in the ICA, velocities were higher medially. Pre- and postendarterectomy velocity profiles were significantly different. After endarterectomy, velocity values increased in the common and internal and decreased in the external carotid artery.

Conclusions.—The in vivo hemodynamics of the human carotid artery are different from those used in most current computer-based and in vitro models. The new information on three-dimensional blood velocity profiles can be used to design models that more closely replicate the actual hemodynamic conditions within the carotid bifurcation. Such models can be used to further improve our understanding of the pathophysiologic processes leading to stroke and for the rational design of medical and interventional therapies.

▶ The authors present an interesting approach to further investigate the difficult-to-study world of dynamic blood flow and how anatomy and cardiac cycle affect it. As the authors pointed out, the main difficulty with their technique was the use of duplex ultrasound scan to measure "instantaneous" velocities at preset locations. Overall, the error/standard deviations of their measurements do not allow any definitive conclusions with regard to spatial flow resolution, but they do show some interesting effects of carotid endarterectomy (CAE) on pre- and postprocedure changes. Interestingly, their series of patients had primary closure of their CAE rather than patch angioplasty, which would have intuitively changed the hemodynamic results they measured. My thought for them would be to use their duplex measurements as input and output boundary conditions for computational fluid dynamics analysis of the carotid bifurcation recreated from the patient-specific CT scans. This would provide a good comparison on which to reference their results. Overall, this is a good study but needs different modality than duplex and should provide some other method of flow assessment.

A. Chandra, MD

2 Epidemiology

Is the Incidence of Abdominal Aortic Aneurysm Declining in the 21st Century? Mortality and Hospital Admissions for England & Wales and Scotland

Anjum A, Powell JT (Imperial College, London, UK)

Eur J Vasc Endovasc Surg 43:161-166, 2012

Background.—Between 1951 and 1995 there was a steady increase in age-standardised deaths from all aortic aneurysms in men, from 2 to 56 per 100,000 population in England & Wales, supporting an increase in incidence. More recently, evidence from Sweden and elsewhere suggests that now the incidence of abdominal aortic aneurysm (AAA) may be declining.

Methods.—National statistics for hospital admissions and deaths from AAA, after population age-standardisation, were used to investigate current trends in England & Wales and Scotland.

Results.—Between 1997 and 2009 there has been a reduction in age-adjusted mortality from AAA from 40.4 to 25.7 per 100,000 population for England & Wales and from 30.1 to 20.8 per 100,000 population in Scotland. The decrease in mortality was more marked for men than women. Mortality decreased more than 2-fold in those <75 years versus 25% only in those >75 years. During this same time period the elective hospital admissions for AAA repair have only increased in the population >75 years.

Conclusions.—These data suggest that the age at which clinically-relevant aneurysms present has increased by 5–10 years and that incidence of clinically-relevant AAA in men in England & Wales and Scotland is declining rapidly. The reasons for this are unclear (Figs 1 and 7).

▶ In the past decade, mortality associated with abdominal aortic aneurysm has declined rapidly in the United Kingdom (Fig 1). One might automatically conclude that this is because of a rise in the number of elective aneurysm repairs. Not true, according to the data in this study. The more likely explanation is epidemiological. The rates of cigarette smoking and carbon monoxide emissions have steadily declined since the 1970s, commensurate with an increase in the use of antihypertensive and lipid-lowering medications (Fig 7).

The authors pose an important question: If the age of the population at greatest risk of aortic aneurysm has shifted to greater than 75 years, is 65 years too young for population screening? After all, the Multicentre Aneurysm Screening Study Group's trial has shown an increase in aneurysm ruptures in the screened

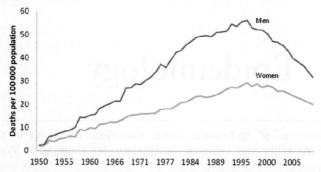

FIGURE 1.—Age-standardised mortality from aortic aneurysm (including thoracic and dissections) in England and Wales 1950–2009 by gender. Men shown by solid blue line, women shown by solid red line. To enable comparison with earlier work,[1] data were standardised from above the age of 40 years for total deaths of ICD 6/7/8/9/10 codes; 1950–1967 (451), 1968–1973 (441), 1975–1978 (441.0,1,2,9), 1979–2000 (441.0–6), 2001–2009 (I71.0–9). *Editor's Note*: Please refer to original journal article for full references. For interpretation of the references to color in this figure legend, the reader is referred to web version of this article. (Reprinted from European Journal of Vascular and Endovascular Surgery, Anjum A, Powell JT. Is the incidence of abdominal aortic aneurysm declining in the 21st century? Mortality and hospital admissions for England & Wales and Scotland. *Eur J Vasc Endovasc Surg.* 2012;43:161-166. Copyright 2012, with permission from the European Society for Vascular Surgery.)

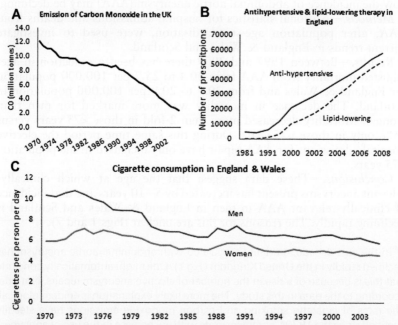

FIGURE 7.—Public health changes since 1970. Emission of Carbon Monoxide in the UK 1970–2005, shown by solid black line. Anti-hypertensive and lipid-lowering therapy in England 1981–2008; anti-hypertensives (solid grey line), lipid-lowering drugs (dotted grey line). Cigarette consumption in England and Wales 1970–2005, men (solid blue line) and women (solid red line). For interpretation of the references to color in this figure legend, the reader is referred to web version of this article. (Reprinted from European Journal of Vascular and Endovascular Surgery, Anjum A, Powell JT. Is the incidence of abdominal aortic aneurysm declining in the 21st century? Mortality and hospital admissions for England & Wales and Scotland. *Eur J Vasc Endovasc Surg.* 2012;43:161-166. Copyright 2012, with permission from the European Society for Vascular Surgery.)

group at 8 years after screening.[1] This would suggest that some aortic aneurysms may have developed after the age of 65 years.

B. W. Starnes, MD

Reference

1. Thompson SG, Ashton HA, Gao L, Scott RA; Multicentre Aneurysm Screening Study Group. Screening men for abdominal aortic aneurysm: 10 year mortality and cost effectiveness results from the randomised Multicentre Aneurysm Screening Study. Multicentre Aneurysm Screening Study Group. *BMJ*. 2009;338:b2307.

Association of Body Mass Index with Peripheral Arterial Disease in Older Adults: The Cardiovascular Health Study

Ix JH, Biggs ML, Kizer JR, et al (Veterans Affairs San Diego Healthcare System, CA; Univ of Washington, Seattle; Weill Med College of Cornell Univ, NY)
Am J Epidemiol 174:1036-1043, 2011

The authors hypothesized that the absence of cross-sectional associations of body mass index (BMI; weight (kg)/height $(m)^2$) with peripheral arterial disease (PAD) in prior studies may reflect lower weight among persons who smoke or have poor health status. They conducted an observational study among 5,419 noninstitutionalized residents of 4 US communities aged ≥ 65 years at baseline (1989–1990 or 1992–1993). Ankle brachial index was measured, and participants reported their history of PAD procedures. Participants were followed longitudinally for adjudicated incident PAD events. At baseline, mean BMI was 26.6 (standard deviation, 4.6), and 776 participants (14%) had prevalent PAD. During 13.2 (median) years of follow-up through June 30, 2007, 276 incident PAD events occurred. In cross-sectional analysis, each 5-unit increase in BMI was inversely associated with PAD (prevalence ratio (PR) = 0.92, 95% confidence interval (CI): 0.85, 1.00). However, among persons in good health who had never smoked, the direction of association was opposite (PR = 1.20, 95% CI: 0.94, 1.52). Similar results were observed between BMI calculated using weight at age 50 years and PAD prevalence (PR = 1.30, 95% CI: 1.11, 1.51) and between BMI at baseline and incident PAD events occurring during follow-up (hazard ratio = 1.32, 95% CI: 1.00, 1.76) among never smokers in good health. Greater BMI is associated with PAD in older persons who remain healthy and have never smoked. Normal weight maintenance may decrease PAD incidence and associated comorbidity in older age (Fig 2).

▶ Peripheral arterial disease (PAD) is a manifestation of atherosclerosis. As such, novel and traditional cardiovascular disease risk factors are associated with PAD. One important cardiovascular risk factor that has not been associated with PAD is body mass index (BMI). Large-scale epidemiologic studies have either not demonstrated a relationship between PAD and BMI[1,2] or have demonstrated an inverse association between BMI and PAD prevalence.[3] Most such

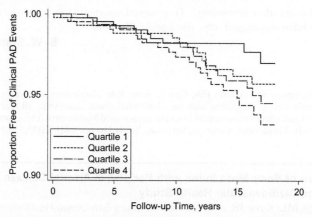

FIGURE 2.—Kaplan-Meier curve for time to first clinical peripheral arterial disease (PAD) event by sex-specific quartile of body mass index (weight (kg)/height (m)^2) in participants who had never smoked and reported good health status, Cardiovascular Health Study, 1989—2007. For women, body mass index quartiles 1—4 were defined as <23.1, 23.1—25.9, 26.0—29.4, and ≥29.5; for men, they were defined as <23.9, 23.9—26.0, 26.1—28.3, and ≥28.4. (Reprinted from Ix JH, Biggs ML, Kizer JR, et al. Association of body mass index with peripheral arterial disease in older adults: the cardiovascular health study. *Am J Epidemiol.* 2011;174:1036-1043, by permission from Oxford University Press on behalf of the Johns Hopkins Bloomberg School of Public Health.)

studies have been cross-sectional studies, and the authors have hypothesized that poor health and smoking status might simultaneously be associated with a lower BMI and greater PAD prevalence. This would obscure a positive association that might exist if adiposity itself either indirectly or directly leads to development of PAD. For this study, the authors evaluated the association of BMI and PAD cross-sectionally in adults age greater than 65 years at baseline who are participating in The Cardiovascular Health Study (a community based study of older adults with the goal to evaluate risk factors for development and progression of vascular disease). Basically, this study indicates that the previous lack of relationship between BMI and PAD was because of the design of previous studies. Although these studies showed inverse, U-shaped, or absent association of BMI with PAD prevalence, they did not evaluate association stratified according to health status or smoking status. This is the first major epidemiologic study to indicate an independent association between BMI and the prevalence of PAD (Fig 2). The study provides yet another reason to avoid weight gain as one grows older.

G. L. Moneta, MD

References

1. Murabito JM, Evans JC, Nieto K, Larson MG, Levy D, Wilson PW. Prevalence and clinical correlates of peripheral arterial disease in the Framingham Offspring Study. *Am Heart J.* 2002;143:961-965.
2. Meijer WT, Grobbee DE, Hunink MG, Hofman A, Hoes AW. Determinants of peripheral arterial disease in the elderly: the Rotterdam study. *Arch Intern Med.* 2000;160:2934-2938.
3. Criqui MH, Vargas V, Denenberg JO, et al. Ethnicity and peripheral arterial disease: the San Diego Population Study. *Circulation.* 2005;112:2703-2707.

Alcohol consumption and outcome in stable outpatients with peripheral artery disease

Garcia-Diaz AM, Marchena PJ, Toril J, et al (Primary Healthcare, Barcelona, Spain; Hosp Sant Boi, Barcelona, Spain; Centro Médico y de Rehabilitación, Castelldefels, Barcelona, Spain; et al)
J Vasc Surg 54:1081-1087, 2011

Background.—The influence of alcohol consumption on outcome in patients with peripheral artery disease (PAD) has not been thoroughly studied.

Methods.—Factores de Riesgo y ENfermedad Arterial (FRENA) is an ongoing, multicenter, observational registry of consecutive stable outpatients with arterial disease. We compared the mortality rate and the incidence of subsequent ischemic events in patients with PAD, according to their alcohol habits.

Results.—As of August 2010, 1073 patients with PAD were recruited, of whom 863 (80%) had intermittent claudication (Fontaine stage II), 102 (9.5%) had rest pain (Fontaine stage III), and 108 (10%) had ischemic skin lesions (Fontaine stage IV). In all, 422 patients (39%) consumed alcohol during the study period. Over a mean follow-up of 13 months, 150 patients (14%) developed subsequent ischemic events (myocardial infarction 28, stroke 30, disabling claudication/critical limb ischemia 100), and 70 patients (6.5%) died. The incidence of subsequent events was the same in both subgroups: 11.8 events per 100 patient-years (rate ratio: 1.00; 95% confidence interval [CI], 0.72-1.41), but the mortality rate was significantly lower in alcohol consumers than in non-consumers: 2.78 vs 6.58 deaths per 100 patient-years (rate ratio: 0.42; 95% CI, 0.23-0.74; $P = .002$). This better outcome was consistently found in patients with Fontaine stages II and III or IV, and persisted after multivariate adjustment (relative risk: 0.49; 95% CI, 0.28-0.88).

Conclusions.—In patients with PAD, moderate alcohol consumption was associated with lower cardiovascular mortality and overall mortality than abstention. These patients should be informed that low to moderate alcohol consumption may not be harmful to their health.

▶ Anyone who drinks in moderation, however that is defined, may initially be encouraged by the results of this study. The article adds to a significant body of literature stating that moderate alcohol consumption is somewhat protective for cardiovascular disease. In this case, that conclusion is extended to those patients who are known to have peripheral arterial disease. However, before you have a glass of wine to celebrate the results, it is important to recognize the limitations of the study as pointed out by the authors. First, alcohol consumers were 4 years younger with fewer comorbidities. Also they were less likely to be taking diuretic medications, β-blockers, anticoagulants, or insulin than nonalcohol consumers in this study. Better outcomes in the moderate drinkers may therefore reflect unrecognized preexisting disease despite the authors' attempts to adjust for these confounders. It is also possible that moderate drinkers have a different overall lifestyle than those who do not drink. Finally, data on levels of alcohol consumption were based exclusively on patient testimony without objective confirmation, and there was no information on the length of alcohol consumption prior to entering this study. It may be that patients with peripheral arterial disease had modified their drinking in response to their diagnosis. In light of this, the registry is useful in that it provides some insight into the natural history of arterial disease in an unselected patient population. It should be considered a hypothesis-seeking study. A randomized trial would clearly be of interest, but given social and ethical limitations, it is difficult to imagine conducting a randomized trial of alcohol consumption in patients with peripheral arterial disease.

G. L. Moneta, MD

Insights on the Role of Diabetes and Geographic Variation in Patients with Criticial Limb Ischaemia

Van Belle E, Nikol S, Norgren L, et al (Univ Lille-Nord de France, Lille Cedex; Asklepios Clinic St Georg, Hamburg, Germany; Orebro Univ Hosp, Sweden; et al)
Eur J Vasc Endovasc Surg 42:365-373, 2011

Background.—Patients with critical limb ischaemia (CLI) unsuitable for revascularisation have a high rate of amputation and mortality (30% and 25% at 1 year, respectively). Localised gene therapy using plasmid DNA encoding acidic fibroblast growth factor (NV1FGF, riferminogene pecaplasmid) has showed an increased amputation-free survival in a phase II trial. This article provides the rationale, design and baseline characteristics of CLI patients enrolled in the pivotal phase III trial (EFC6145/TAMARIS).

Methods.—An international, double-blind, placebo-controlled, randomised study composed of 525 CLI patients recruited from 170 sites worldwide who were unsuitable for revascularisation and had non-healing skin lesions was carried out to evaluate the potential benefit of repeated intramuscular administration of NV1FGF. Randomisation was stratified by country and by diabetic status.

Results.—The mean age of the study cohort was 70 ± 10 years, and included 70% males and 53% diabetic patients. Fifty-four percent of the patients had previous lower-extremity revascularisation and 22% had previous minor amputation of the index leg. In 94% of the patients, the index leg had distal occlusive disease affecting arteries below the knee. Statins were prescribed for 54% of the patients, and anti-platelet drugs for 80%. Variation in region of origin resulted in only minor demographic imbalance. Similarly, while diabetic status was associated with a frequent history of coronary artery disease, it had little impact on limb haemodynamics and vascular lesions.

Conclusions.—Clinical characteristics and vascular anatomy of CLI patients with ischaemic skin lesions who were unsuitable for revascularisation therapy show little variations by region of origin and diabetic status.

The findings from this large CLI cohort will contribute to our understanding of this disease process.

This study is registered with ClinicalTrials.gov, number NCT00566657.

▶ Disease patterns are often felt to have geographic variations in relation to the respective populations; for example, the incidence of gastric cancer is higher in Japan than the United States. Some countries have fairly homogenous populations, whereas others have a fairly heterogenous population; thus, the authors of this study found that patients with critical limb ischemia from different regions (North America, Latin America, Western Europe, Eastern Europe, and Asia) are very similar. The current study describes the characteristics of critical limb ischaemia (CLI) patients who were unsuitable for vascular reconstruction and were part of the cohort that was randomized for the TAMARIS trial. This large, international, placebo-controlled, double-blind, randomized phase III trial was designed to demonstrate the benefit of NVIFGF (riferminogene pecaplasmid). This recombinant DNA plasmid has been demonstrated to increase local expression of FGF1 for up to several weeks and increase tissue perfusion in animal models of hind-limb ischemia.

Patients from 170 sites around the world were recruited, and 525 patients met enrollment criteria. All patients had CLI with ischemic lesions (Fontaine stage IV). Because no a priori hypothesis regarding the baseline data were specified, no statistical analysis was performed, and only the numerical differences were presented. The majority of patients were 70 years old, and 70% were males. As would be expected, 61% of patients had a history of smoking, 53% had diabetes, 18% were obese, 80% had hypertension, and 60% had hypercholesterolemia. Other atherosclerotic processes such as coronary artery disease (CAD) were present in 44% of patients and history of stroke in 15%. Regional variation was noted within some of these baseline demographic characteristics such as CAD in 70% of the North American patients versus only 16% of the Latin American patients. Regarding the previous management and clinical and functional status of the index leg, 50% had undergone previous revascularization, and 20% had prior minor amputation. North American patients had a higher frequency (31%) of previous amputations versus the overall average (21%). Medications taken by the patients were notable for 80% taking cardiovascular medications (41% beta-blockers) and 60% taking lipid-lowering medications (56% statins). Antiplatelet drugs were taken by 80% of patients and hypoglycemic drugs in 50.7% of the sample.

This worldwide cohort of patients reveals that the baseline characteristics of this group have only modest variation from various regions. It is likely that once the disease progresses to this state of CLI, most of these patients are very similar in terms of the baseline characteristics and procedures they have undergone.

N. Singh, MD

Differential Effect of Low-Dose Aspirin for Primary Prevention of Atherosclerotic Events in Diabetes Management: A subanalysis of the JPAD trial

Okada S, for the Japanese Primary Prevention of Atherosclerosis with Aspirin for Diabetes (JPAD) Trial Investigators (Nara Med Univ, Japan; et al)

Diabetes Care 34:1277-1283, 2011

Objective.—Recent reports showed that low-dose aspirin was ineffective in the primary prevention of cardiovascular events in diabetic patients overall. We hypothesized that low-dose aspirin would be beneficial in patients receiving insulin therapy, as a high-risk group.

Research Design and Methods.—This study is a subanalysis of the Japanese Primary Prevention of Atherosclerosis With Aspirin for Diabetes (JPAD) trial—a randomized, controlled, open-label trial. We randomly assigned 2,539 patients with type 2 diabetes and no previous cardiovascular disease to the low-dose aspirin group (81 or 100 mg daily) or to the no-aspirin group. The median follow-up period was 4.4 years. We investigated the effect of low-dose aspirin on preventing atherosclerotic events in groups receiving different diabetes management.

Results.—At baseline, 326 patients were treated with insulin, 1,750 with oral hypoglycemic agents (OHAs), and 463 with diet alone. The insulin group had the longest history of diabetes, the worst glycemic control, and the highest prevalence of diabetic microangiopathies. The diet-alone group had the opposite characteristics. The incidence of atherosclerotic events was 26.6, 14.6, and 10.4 cases per 1,000 person-years in the insulin, OHA, and diet-alone groups, respectively. In the insulin and OHA groups, low-dose aspirin did not affect atherosclerotic events (insulin: hazard ratio [HR] 1.19 [95% CI 0.60−2.40]; OHA: HR 0.84 [0.57−1.24]). In the diet-alone group, low-dose aspirin significantly reduced atherosclerotic events, despite the lowest event rates (HR 0.21 [0.05−0.64]).

Conclusions.—Low-dose aspirin reduced atherosclerotic events predominantly in the diet-alone group and not in the insulin or OHA groups.

▶ There have been 2 recent large clinical trials investigating the effects of low-dose aspirin in reducing cardiovascular events in patients with diabetes but without known cardiovascular disease. Both were unable to demonstrate a benefit of aspirin, but both trials had methodological flaws. The Prevention of Progression of Arterial Disease and Diabetes (POPADAD) trial failed to document a benefit of aspirin in Scottish patients with either type 1 or type 2 diabetes. However, there were fewer than anticipated cardiovascular events and low compliance with aspirin therapy in the trial.[1] The second trial, Japanese Primary Prevention of Atherosclerosis with Aspirin for Diabetes (JPAD), did demonstrate a reduction in atherosclerotic events of 20% with the use of aspirin, but the numbers were insufficient to reach statistical significance.[2] There have also been epidemiologic studies that suggest patients with diabetes treated with insulin have increased mortality compared with those who receive therapy with oral hypoglycemic agents or through diet alone.[3] It follows that patients with diabetes treated with insulin may be most likely to benefit from low-dose aspirin therapy. The authors therefore performed a subanalysis of the JPAD trial, with the hypothesis that low-dose aspirin would be most beneficial for primary prevention in patients with diabetes who are receiving insulin. The findings of this study that aspirin was not effective in preventing atherosclerotic events in patients with diabetes treated with insulin and oral hypoglycemic agents is compatible with recent literature. However, the finding that aspirin was effective in reducing atherosclerotic events in patients treated with diet alone is new and somewhat surprising (Fig 1 in the original article). It may be that in patients with advanced diabetes the burden of atherosclerosis is such that new events are unpreventable with aspirin therapy or that these patients have relative aspirin resistance. The clinical decision to use aspirin to prevent cardiovascular events in patients with diabetes should probably consider not only conventional cardiovascular risk factors of the patients but also the stage of the diabetes.

G. L. Moneta, MD

References

1. Belch J, MacCuish A, Campbell I, et al. The prevention of progression of arterial disease and diabetes (POPADAD) trial: factorial randomised placebo controlled trial of aspirin and antioxidants in patients with diabetes and asymptomatic peripheral arterial disease. *BMJ.* 2008;337:a1840.
2. Ogawa H, Nakayama M, Morimoto T, et al. Low-dose aspirin for primary prevention of atherosclerotic events in patients with type 2 diabetes: a randomized controlled trial. *JAMA.* 2008;300:2134-2141.
3. Muggeo M, Verlato G, Bonora E, et al. The Verona diabetes study: a population-based survey on known diabetes mellitus prevalence and 5-year all-cause mortality. *Diabetologia.* 1995;38:318-325.

Secondary Prevention and Mortality in Peripheral Artery Disease: National Health and Nutrition Examination Study, 1999 to 2004

Pande RL, Perlstein TS, Beckman JA, et al (Brigham and Women's Hosp, Boston, MA)

Circulation 124:17-23, 2011

Background.—Whether individuals with peripheral artery disease (PAD) identified by screening ankle-brachial index benefit from preventive therapies to reduce cardiovascular risk is unknown. We aimed to determine the number of US adults with PAD who are not receiving preventive therapies and whether treatment is associated with reduced mortality in PAD subjects without known cardiovascular disease.

Methods and Results.—We analyzed data from the National Health and Nutrition Examination Survey (NHANES) 1999 to 2004 with mortality follow-up through December 31, 2006. We defined PAD as an ankle-brachial index ≤0.90. Of 7458 eligible participants ≥40 years, weighted PAD prevalence was $5.9 \pm 0.3\%$ (mean ± SE), corresponding to ≈7.1 million US adults with PAD. Statin use was reported in only $30.5 \pm 2.5\%$, angiotensin-converting enzyme inhibitor/angiotensin receptor blocker use in $24.9 \pm 1.9\%$, and aspirin use in $35.8 \pm 2.9\%$, corresponding to 5.0 million adults with PAD not taking statins, 5.4 million not taking angiotensin-converting enzyme inhibitors/angiotensin receptor blockers, and 4.5 million not receiving aspirin. After adjustment for age, sex, and race/ethnicity, PAD was associated with all-cause mortality (hazard ratio, 2.4; 95% confidence interval, 1.9 to 2.9; $P<0.0001$). Even after exclusion of individuals with known cardiovascular disease, subjects with PAD had higher mortality rates $(16.1 \pm 2.1\%)$ than subjects without PAD or cardiovascular disease $(4.1 \pm 0.3\%)$, with an adjusted hazard ratio of 1.9 (95% confidence interval, 1.3 to 2.8; $P=0.001$). Among PAD subjects without cardiovascular disease, use of multiple preventive therapies was associated with 65% lower all-cause mortality (hazard ratio, 0.35; 95% confidence interval, 0.20 to 0.86; $P=0.02$).

Conclusions.—Millions of US adults with PAD are not receiving secondary prevention therapies. Treatment with multiple therapies is associated with reduced all-cause mortality.

▶ A lack of evidence for screening-guided treatment in patients with peripheral artery disease (PAD) has led the US Preventative Services Task Force to recommend against screening for PAD with ankle-brachial index (ABI).[1] This stance has been strengthened by recent studies that have called into question preventive therapies, particularly aspirin, in patients with PAD.[2,3] However, guidelines for management of patients with PAD recommend lipid-lowering therapy with a statin; antihypertensive therapy to achieve a systolic blood pressure less than 140 mmHg, particularly angiotensin-converting enzyme inhibitors; and antiplatelet therapy.[4,5] Because of the inconsistencies regarding use and recommendations for secondary prevention in patients with PAD, the authors sought to determine whether treatment with multiple risk factor—modifying therapies was associated with reduced all-cause mortality in adults identified with PAD who otherwise had no established cardiovascular disease. The authors analyzed data from the National Health and Nutrition Examination survey (NHANES) from 1999 to 2004. NHANES is an ongoing series of surveys conducted by the National Center for Health Statistics. These surveys began in the early 1960s, and from 1999 to 2004, ABI measurements were obtained as part of the NHANES lower extremity examination. The data here are consistent with those of other studies in that PAD was associated with increased mortality independent of other cardiovascular risk factors. If these data truly can be extrapolated to the US population, potentially thousands of deaths could be avoided if secondary prevention therapies were universally applied and adhered to in patients with PAD. However, the literature regarding secondary prevention in PAD, particularly with respect to aspirin, is seriously conflicting. The authors call for a large-scale clinical trial to determine whether implementation of secondary preventative therapies in patients with PAD identified by low ABI can indeed reduce cardiovascular morbidity and mortality. Given the data presented here, this seems like a very reasonable idea.

G. L. Moneta, MD

References

1. U.S. Preventive Services Task Force. Using nontraditional risk factors in coronary heart disease risk assessment: U.S. Preventive Services Task Force recommendation statement. *Ann Intern Med.* 2009;151:474-482.
2. Berger JS, Krantz MJ, Kittelson JM, Hiatt WR. Aspirin for the prevention of cardiovascular events in patients with peripheral artery disease: a meta-analysis of randomized trials. *JAMA.* 2009;301:1909-1919.
3. Fowkes FG, Price JF, Stewart MC, et al. Aspirin for prevention of cardiovascular events in a general population screened for a low ankle brachial index: a randomized controlled trial. *JAMA.* 2010;303:841-848.
4. Yusuf S, Sleight P, Pogue J, Bosch J, Davies R, Dagenais G. Effects of an angiotensin-converting-enzyme inhibitor, ramipril, on cardiovascular events in high-risk patients. The Heart Outcomes Prevention Evaluation Study Investigators. *N Engl J Med.* 2000;342:145-153.
5. Heart Protection Study Collaborative Group. MRC/BHF Heart Protection Study of cholesterol lowering with simvastatin in 20,536 high-risk individuals: a randomised placebo-controlled trial. *Lancet.* 2002;360:7-22.

3 Vascular Laboratory and Imaging

Optimizing Protocols for Risk Prediction in Asymptomatic Carotid Stenosis Using Embolic Signal Detection: The Asymptomatic Carotid Emboli Study
King A, for the ACES Investigators (St. Georges Univ of London, UK; et al)
Stroke 42:2819-2824, 2011

Background and Purpose.—Improved methods are required to identify patients with asymptomatic carotid stenosis at high risk for stroke. The Asymptomatic Carotid Emboli Study recently showed embolic signals (ES) detected by transcranial Doppler on 2 recordings that lasted 1-hour independently predict 2-year stroke risk. ES detection is time-consuming, and whether similar predictive information could be obtained from simpler recording protocols is unknown.

Methods.—In a predefined secondary analysis of Asymptomatic Carotid Emboli Study, we looked at the temporal variation of ES. We determined the predictive yield associated with different recording protocols and with the use of a higher threshold to indicate increased risk (≥ 2 ES). To compare the different recording protocols, sensitivity and specificity analyses were performed using analysis of receiver-operator characteristic curves.

Results.—Of 477 patients, 467 had baseline recordings adequate for analysis; 77 of these had ES on 1 or both of the 2 recordings. ES status on the 2 recordings was significantly associated ($P<0.0001$), but there was poor agreement between ES positivity on the 2 recordings ($\kappa=0.266$). For the primary outcome of ipsilateral stroke or transient ischemic attack, the use of 2 baseline recordings lasting 1 hour had greater predictive accuracy than either the first baseline recording alone ($P=0.0005$), a single 30-minute ($P<0.0001$) recording, or 2 recordings lasting 30 minutes ($P<0.0001$). For the outcome of ipsilateral stroke alone, two recordings lasting 1 hour had greater predictive accuracy when compared to all other recording protocols (all $P<0.0001$).

Conclusions.—Our analysis demonstrates the relative predictive yield of different recording protocols that can be used in application of the technique in clinical practice. Two baseline recordings lasting 1 hour as used in Asymptomatic Carotid Emboli Study gave the best risk prediction (Fig 1).

▶ Strokes related to carotid stenosis are often not associated with previous transient ischemic attack or stroke. Randomized clinical trials have demonstrated that

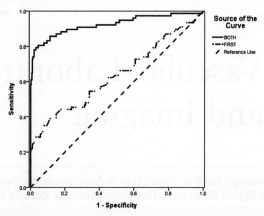

FIGURE 1.—Receiver-operator characteristic curves for ipsilateral stroke comparing 2 recordings lasting 1 hour (solid line) vs the first 1-hour recording alone (dashed line). The diagonal line indicates the shape if the test is no better at predicting the outcome than chance alone. (Reprinted from King A, for the ACES Investigators. Optimizing protocols for risk prediction in asymptomatic carotid stenosis using embolic signal detection: the asymptomatic carotid emboli study. *Stroke.* 2011;42:2819-2824.)

stroke risk can be reduced with prophylactic carotid endarterectomy (CEA). However, benefit is small, and it has been calculated that to prevent 1 disabling stroke over a 5-year period, approximately 32 CEAs need to be performed. Current estimates are that with the best medical treatment, stroke risk can be reduced from approximately 2% per year, as found in the randomized trials of CEA for asymptomatic disease, to 1% or less per year with current best medical management.[1,2] The implication is that CEA for asymptomatic carotid stenosis is of little benefit unless it is possible to identify a group with asymptomatic carotid stenosis at higher overall stroke risk. The Asymptomatic Carotid Emboli Study (ACES) found that embolic signals detected with transcranial Doppler on baseline recordings of 1 hour predicted stroke risk over a 2-year follow-up time.[3] The current study acknowledges that embolic signal detection is time-consuming and therefore sought to determine whether similar predictive information could be attained from a simpler recording protocol. This was a predefined secondary analysis of the ACES. Unfortunately, simpler protocols were not that effective. Shorter recording periods and/or increasing the requirement to more than 2 embolic signals as an indicator of stroke risk reduced the predictive power of TCD monitoring (Fig 1) because most subjects with embolic signals only had 1 embolic signal on their recording. The practical point is that if one wishes to use TCD embolic signal detection to predict stroke in patients with asymptomatic carotid disease, application of the technique will be labor intensive and will require experienced operators and validation of commercially available embolic signal detection symptoms. Nevertheless, given the low therapeutic index for CEA for patients with asymptomatic stenosis the time, effort, and cost may be worth it. Whether anyone will pay for it is a different but equally important question.

G. L. Moneta, MD

References

1. Abbott AL. Medical (nonsurgical) intervention alone is now best for prevention of stroke associated with asymptomatic severe carotid stenosis: results of a systematic review and analysis. *Stroke.* 2009;40:e573-e583.
2. Marquardt L, Geraghty OC, Mehta Z, Rothwell PM. Low risk of ipsilateral stroke in patients with asymptomatic carotid stenosis on best medical treatment: a prospective, population-based study. *Stroke.* 2010;41:e11-e17.
3. Markus HS, King A, Shipley M, et al. Asymptomatic embolisation for prediction of stroke in the Asymptomatic Carotid Emboli Study (ACES): a prospective observational study. *Lancet Neurol.* 2010;9:663-671.

Ultrasonic plaque echolucency and emboli signals predict stroke in asymptomatic carotid stenosis

Topakian R, For the ACES Investigators (St Georges Univ of London, UK; et al)
Neurology 77:751-758, 2011

Objectives.—Better methods are required to identify patients with asymptomatic carotid stenosis (ACS) at risk of future stroke. Two potential markers of high risk are echolucent plaque morphology on carotid ultrasound and embolic signals (ES) in the ipsilateral middle cerebral artery on transcranial Doppler ultrasound (TCD). We explored the predictive value of a score based on these 2 measures in the prospective, observational, international multicenter Asymptomatic Carotid Emboli Study.

Methods.—A total of 435 recruited subjects with ACS $\geq70\%$ had baseline ultrasound images and TCD data available. Subjects were prospectively followed up for 2 years.

Results.—A total of 164 (37.7%) plaques were graded as echolucent. Plaque echolucency at baseline was associated with an increased risk of ipsilateral stroke alone (hazard ratio [HR] 6.43, 95% confidence interval [CI] 1.36–30.44, $p = 0.019$). A combined variable of plaque echolucency and ES positivity at baseline was associated with a markedly increased risk of ipsilateral stroke alone (HR 10.61, 95% CI 2.98–37.82, $p = 0.0003$). This association remained significant after controlling for risk factors, degree of carotid stenosis, and antiplatelet medication.

Conclusions.—Plaque morphology assessed using a simple, and clinically applicable, visual rating scale predicts ipsilateral stroke risk in ACS. The combination of ES detection and plaque morphology allows a greater prediction than either measure alone and identifies a high-risk group with an annual stroke risk of 8%, and a low-risk group with a risk of <1% per annum. This risk stratification may prove useful in the selection of patients with ACS for endarterectomy (Fig).

▶ There is currently a debate on how to treat patients with asymptomatic carotid stenosis (ACS). Those favoring operative treatment of patients with ACS identify results from 2 large randomized controlled trials suggesting benefit from carotid endarterectomy plus medical management over medical management alone for

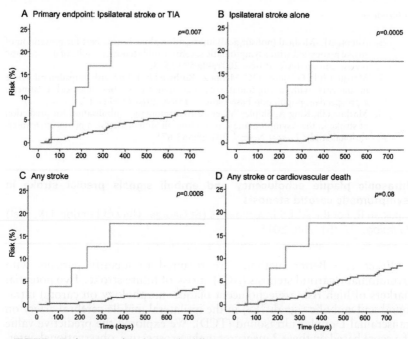

FIGURE.—Kaplan-Meier plots showing the difference in endpoints between the groups with (green) and without (blue) both echolucent plaque and embolic signals. (A) Ipsilateral stroke and TIA, (B) ipsilateral stroke, (C) any stroke, and (D) any stroke and cardiovascular death. For interpretation of the references to color in this figure legend, the reader is referred to web version of this article. (Reprinted from Topakian R, For the ACES Investigators. Ultrasonic plaque echolucency and emboli signals predict stroke in asymptomatic carotid stenosis. *Neurology.* 2011;77:751-758.)

prevention of stroke in patients with high-grade ACS. Those who question the benefit of surgical intervention in patients with ACS cite evidence that over the past decade stroke rates in ACS have fallen with medical intervention alone.[1,2] Nevertheless, while the percentage of patients with ACS who actually have had a stroke is small, the majority of ipsilateral strokes in patients with carotid stenosis are unheralded.[3] There is therefore a pressing need to identify patients with ACS who are at the highest risk of stroke to provide better selection for carotid intervention for ACS. Potential markers of high-risk plaques are those with echolucent plaque morphology on carotid ultrasound and those that produce embolic symbols (ES) in the ipsilateral middle cerebral artery as detected with transcranial Doppler ultrasound. Thus far the use of plaque morphology for subselect patients with ACS for carotid intervention, while theoretically attractive, has not been widely used, despite the fact that the classification system proposed by Geroulakos et al[4] has been available for almost 20 years. Clearly clinicians do not regard this subjective system as adding substantially to risk stratification of patients with ACS. Intuitively one would like to think that a high-grade stenotic, but echogenic, plaque not associated with ES and present in a patient who is not smoking and is on optimal medical management would present a low risk of stroke. However, for many surgeons, the risk of stroke following carotid endarterectomy for high-grade ACS in their patients is 1% or less. Given randomized data, despite the fact that they are old, supporting endarterectomy in patients with high grade ACS, data such as those shown in the Figure, while interesting, are not likely to change most surgeons' clinical practice.

G. L. Moneta, MD

References

1. Abbott AL. Medical (nonsurgical) intervention alone is now best for prevention of stroke associated with asymptomatic severe carotid stenosis: results of a systematic review and analysis. *Stroke.* 2009;40:e573-e583.
2. Marquardt L, Geraghty OC, Mehta Z, Rothwell PM. Low risk of ipsilateral stroke in patients with asymptomatic carotid stenosis on best medical treatment: a prospective, population-based study. *Stroke.* 2010;41:e11-e17.
3. Inzitari D, Eliasziw M, Gates P, et al. The causes and risk of stroke in patients with asymptomatic internal-carotid-artery stenosis. North American Symptomatic Carotid Endarterectomy Trial Collaborators. *N Engl J Med.* 2000;342:1693-1700.
4. Geroulakos G, Ramaswami G, Nicolaides A, et al. Characterization of symptomatic and asymptomatic carotid plaques using high-resolution real-time ultrasonography. *Br J Surg.* 1993;80:1274-1277.

The Value of a Carotid Duplex Surveillance Program for Stroke Prevention
Cull DL, Cole T, Miller B, et al (Greenville Hosp System-Univ Med Ctr, SC; Univ of South Carolina School of Medicine-Greenville Campus)
Ann Vasc Surg 25:887-894, 2011

Background.—Although duplex ultrasonography (DU) can readily identify progression of carotid stenosis, controversy regarding the natural history of asymptomatic carotid stenosis as well as the need and appropriate interval for carotid DU surveillance still exists. Furthermore, consensus has not yet been made in the surgical literature regarding the usefulness, cost-effectiveness, or timing of DU surveillance after carotid endarterectomy (CEA). The purpose of this study was to determine how often DU surveillance for asymptomatic carotid disease or postintervention stenosis resulted in any change in the patient's clinical management, how many strokes were prevented by DU surveillance, and the cost of such a DU surveillance program per stroke prevented.

Methods.—We reviewed a 9-year vascular surgical database to identify all patients enrolled in a carotid DU surveillance program for asymptomatic carotid stenosis or following CEA between January 1, 2000, and December 31, 2008. The number of duplex scans and CEAs performed in those patients through March 2010 was also determined. The results of the Asymptomatic Carotid Atherosclerosis Study were then used to estimate the number of strokes prevented by CEA in the study population. Reimbursement data were assessed to calculate the average cost of each DU and the cost of the DU surveillance program for each stroke prevented.

Results.—During the study period, there were 11,531 carotid duplex scans performed on 3,003 patients (mean: 3.84 scans per patient) who had been enrolled in the DU surveillance program. CEA for asymptomatic carotid stenosis was performed on 225 (7.5%) patients. The DU surveillance program prevented approximately 13 strokes (871 carotid duplex scans per stroke prevented). The mean cost of each duplex scan was $332 ± 170. The total cost of the DU surveillance program was approximately $3,830,000 or $290,000 per stroke prevented.

Conclusions.—Although a carotid DU surveillance program generates substantial revenue for a vascular surgery practice, it is costly and inefficient. A reappraisal of the "value" of carotid DU surveillance in stroke prevention is warranted. Consideration should be given to eliminating routine surveillance of postendarterectomy carotids in the absence of contralateral disease and limiting the number of DU surveillance studies for asymptomatic carotid disease.

▶ There is considerable controversy as to the effectiveness of carotid duplex surveillance programs. Timing of surveillance and potential cost effectiveness must be justified by clear documentation of rates of progression of carotid stenosis, rates of development of postintervention restenosis, and clinical consequences of progression of stenosis in native arteries, postendarterectomy arteries, or those that have been stented. Reported progression rates of carotid disease in native vessels are variable, ranging from 0% to 15%. Postendarterectomy restenosis rates over the first 5 years after surgery range from 4% to 25%. The Asymptomatic Carotid Surgery trial and the Asymptomatic Carotid Atherosclerosis Study indicate benefit for the combination of endarterectomy and best medical management versus best medical management alone in patients with high-grade asymptomatic carotid stenosis. That benefit, however, is relatively small and now under considerable question given current availability and penetrance of the use of better antiplatelet agents and statin medications to prevent neurologic events in patients with asymptomatic carotid stenosis. Given all this controversy, the authors decided to investigate the effectiveness of their surveillance program for patients with asymptomatic carotid stenosis greater than 50% or who have undergone carotid intervention. They wished to determine whether their surveillance program resulted in changes in clinical management or prevented stroke and what the cost was of the surveillance program per stroke prevented. The results of this study challenge perceived effectiveness and cost effectiveness of a carotid duplex ultrasound surveillance program and raise a significant question as to whether a carotid duplex surveillance program primarily benefits physicians and vascular laboratories but not patients. This study is limited by the fact that for about 40% of the patients, only 2 duplex ultrasound scans were performed during the surveillance period. Follow-up was, however, comparable to other studies in the literature and therefore the results can likely be generally applied to other practices as well. Clearly, although the cost of stroke is huge and morbidity of a stroke can be huge, this report calls into serious question the use of limited health care resources to fund carotid duplex surveillance programs.

G. L. Moneta, MD

Doppler Criteria for Identifying Proximal Vertebral Artery Stenosis of 50% or More

Yurdakul M, Tola M (Turkiye Yüksek Ihtisas Hosp, Ankara, Turkey)
J Ultrasound Med 30:163-168, 2011

Objectives.—The proximal segment of the vertebral artery is a frequent site of obstructive atherosclerosis. The purpose of this study was to determine Doppler criteria for identifying proximal vertebral artery stenosis of 50% or more by comparison with digital subtraction angiography.

Methods.—Forty-eight patients with vertebral artery stenosis were examined prospectively with color Doppler sonography and digital subtraction angiography. The peak systolic velocity (PSV), end-diastolic velocity (EDV), peak systolic velocity ratio (PSVr), and end-diastolic velocity ratio (EDVr) were evaluated by receiver operating characteristic curve analysis for their ability to detect vertebral artery stenosis of 50% or more. The optimal criteria for identifying proximal vertebral artery stenosis of 50% or more were determined.

Results.—For identifying vertebral artery stenosis, the parameter with the highest accuracy was the PSVr (area under the receiver operating characteristic curve, 0.967 [95% confidence interval, 0.899—0.994]). A PSVr of greater than 2.2 was found to be the optimal criterion for identifying proximal vertebral artery stenosis of 50% or more, with sensitivity and specificity of 96% and 89%, respectively. The optimal thresholds for the other Doppler parameters in identifying proximal vertebral artery stenosis of 50% or more were as follows: PSV, greater than 108 cm/s; EDV, greater than 36 cm/s; and EDVr, greater than 1.7.

Conclusions.—Color Doppler sonography is an accurate method for identifying proximal vertebral artery stenosis. The PSVr is superior to other Doppler parameters for detecting vertebral artery stenosis.

▶ Stroke in the vertebral basilar distribution has a mortality of 20% to 30%; considerably higher than that of stroke in the carotid circulation distribution.[1] About 20% of patients with posterior circulation ischemia have occlusive disease in the proximal vertebral artery.[2] The V1 segment of the vertebral artery is that portion of the artery extending from its origin to the entry to the transverse foramen of C6. It is a common site for atherosclerotic occlusive disease of the vertebral artery. Most carotid artery duplex scans by protocol include insonation of the vertebral artery, but very few studies have been performed to determine Doppler criteria to identify proximal vertebral artery stenosis. In this study, the authors sought to determine criteria for Doppler identification for proximal greater than 50% vertebral artery stenosis through comparisons of duplex scanning with digital subtraction angiography. In general, peak systolic velocity has proven to be the most useful Doppler parameter in the evaluation of carotid artery stenosis. However, it makes sense that a velocity ratio may be more accurate in evaluation of vertebral artery stenosis. The authors point out vertebral artery asymmetry is common, and flow in a dominant vertebral artery may be relatively high. Also, vertebral arteries ending in a posterioinferior cerebellar artery may have relatively low flow, and tandem lesions in vertebral or basilar arteries can result in low flow. These particular conditions, which do not exist for the carotid circulation, are common in the vertebral artery and thus may result in improved accuracy of velocity ratios over other Doppler parameters for determining vertebral artery stenosis.

G. L. Moneta, MD

References

1. Moufarrij NA, Little JR, Furlan AJ, Williams G, Marzewski DJ. Vertebral artery stenosis: long-term follow-up. *Stroke.* 1984;15:260-263.
2. Caplan LR, Wityk RJ, Glass TA, et al. New England medical center posterior circulation registry. *Ann Neurol.* 2004;56:389-398.

Transcranial Doppler Ultrasonography for Diagnosis of Cerebral Vasospasm After Aneurysmal Subarachnoid Hemorrhage: Mean Blood Flow Velocity Ratio of the Ipsilateral and Contralateral Middle Cerebral Arteries
Nakae R, Yokota H, Yoshida D, et al (Nippon Med School, Tokyo, Japan)
Neurosurgery 69:876-883, 2011

Background.—Transcranial Doppler (TCD) is widely accepted to monitor cerebral vasospasm after subarachnoid hemorrhage (SAH); however, its predictive value remains controversial.

Objective.—To investigate the predictive reliability of an increase in the mean blood flow velocity (mBFV) ratio of the ipsilateral to contralateral middle cerebral arteries (I/C mBFV) compared with the conventional absolute flow velocity.

Methods.—We retrospectively investigated the clinical and radiologic data of consecutive patients with SAH admitted from July 2003 to August 2009 who underwent TCD ultrasonography. The highest mBFV value in bilateral middle cerebral arteries was recorded, while delayed cerebral ischemia (DCI) was defined as neurological deficits or computed tomographic evidence of cerebral infarction caused by vasospasm. The ipsilateral side was defined as the side with higher mBFV value when evaluating the I/C mBFV. We thus elucidated the reliability of this rate in comparison with the conventional method for predicting DCI with receiver operating characteristic (ROC) analysis.

Results.—One hundred and forty-two patients were retrospectively analyzed with specific data from 1262 TCD studies. The ROC curve showed that the overall predictive value for DCI had an area under the curve of 0.86 (95% confidence interval: 0.76-0.96) when the I/C mBFV was used vs 0.80 (0.71-0.88) when the absolute flow velocity was used. The threshold value that best discriminated between patients with and without DCI was I/C mBFV of 1.5.

Conclusion.—In patients with SAH, the I/C mBFV demonstrated a more significant correlation to vasospasm than the absolute mean flow velocity (Fig 2).

▶ Transcranial Doppler (TCD) is one type of noninvasive testing available for accreditation by the Intersocietal Commission for Accreditation of Vascular Laboratories. A key component of this accreditation process is establishment of diagnostic criteria for clinically meaningful endpoints. Perhaps the most frequent use of TCD is monitoring for cerebral vasospasm. Current diagnostic criteria for cerebral vasospasm focus on analysis of absolute mean velocity in the middle cerebral artery or a comparison of mean velocities in the ipsilateral middle cerebral artery versus the ipsilateral extracranial internal carotid artery—the so-called hemispheric or Lindegaard ratio. A recent meta-analysis of 26 trials comparing TCD with cerebral angiography concluded that TCD of the middle cerebral artery has high specificity (99%) and a high positive predictive value (97%) but low sensitivity in detecting vasospasm of the middle cerebral artery. TCD of other arteries was not accurate in detecting vasospasm.[1] In an effort to review the sensitivity of TCD parameters in detecting cerebral vasospasm, the authors reviewed their patients with subarachnoid hemorrhage. In this study, TCD had a higher sensitivity (77%) and specificity (80%) for detecting delayed cerebral ischemia when the ipsilateral to contralateral (I/C) ratio of mean blood flow velocities in the middle cerebral was used (Fig 2). This ratio was more closely related to clinically

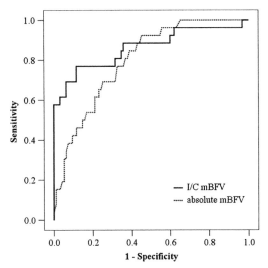

FIGURE 2.—Receiver operating characteristic curves comparing the absolute mean mBFV and the I/C mBFV for prediction of DCI. The area under the ROC curve for the I/C mBFV was 0.86 (95% confidence interval: 0.76-0.96), while that for the absolute mBFV was 0.80 (0.71-0.88). mBFV, mean blood flow velocity; I/C mBFV, mBFV of the ipsilateral to contralateral middle cerebral artery; ROC, receiver operating characteristic; DCI, delayed cerebral ischemia. (Reprinted from Nakae R, Yokota H, Yoshida D, et al. Transcranial Doppler ultrasonography for diagnosis of cerebral vasospasm after aneurysmal subarachnoid hemorrhage: mean blood flow velocity ratio of the ipsilateral and contralateral middle cerebral arteries. *Neurosurgery.* 2011;69:876-883, with permission from the Congress of Neurological Surgeons.)

significant vasospasm than absolute mean blood flow velocities in patients with subarachnoid hemorrhage. The data indicate that it may be possible to improve the low sensitivity of TCD for detection of delayed cerebral infarction. It would have been interesting if the authors had also compared the proposed I/C middle cerebral artery mean blood flow velocity ratio with the more commonly used Lindegaard ratio. Actual documentation of vasospasm by angiography by the proposed new ratio would also have contributed positively to the robustness of the data. Nevertheless, the article serves a valuable purpose in pointing out the inaccuracies of TCD in monitoring for cerebral vasospasm and the possibility of a new TCD parameter that may have increased sensitivity in detection of vasospasm than parameters that are currently widely used.

G. L. Moneta, MD

Reference

1. Lysakowski C, Walder B, Costanza MC, Tramèr MR. Transcranial Doppler versus angiography in patients with vasospasm due to a ruptured cerebral aneurysm: a systematic review. *Stroke.* 2001;32:2292-2298.

Ultrasound Measurement of Aortic Diameter in a National Screening Programme
Hartshorne TC, McCollum CN, Earnshaw JJ, et al (Leicester Royal Infirmary, UK; Univ of Manchester, UK; Gloucestershire Royal Hosp, UK)
Eur J Vasc Endovasc Surg 42:195-199, 2011

Objective.—Currently there is no universally accepted standard for ultrasound measurement of abdominal aortic aneurysm (AAA). The aim was to investigate the reliability and reproducibility of inner to inner (ITI) versus outer to outer (OTO) ultrasound measurement of AAA diameter.

Methods.—A prospective study design was used to collect 60 random images of aorta (1.4—7.1 cm). Inner and outer wall diameter measurements were then performed by 13 qualified AAA screening technicians and 11 vascular sonographers.

Results.—The mean (range) diameter for all 60 aortas by ITI was 3.91 cm (1.39—6.80) and by OTO was 4.18 cm (1.63—7.09), a significant mean difference of 0.27 cm (95% CI:0.23—0.32 cm). The reproducibility coefficients for differences between technicians were 0.30 cm (95% CI:0.24—0.36) for ITI and 0.42 cm (95% CI:0.35—0.49) for OTO indicating significantly better repeatability using ITI. Finally, 15 images were measured twice in random order by all screeners and sonographers. For AAAs >5 cm, repeatability was significantly better with ITI than OTO (0.14 vs. 0.21; $p = 0.016$).

Conclusion.—There was the expected difference in AAA diameter between the two methods (0.27 cm). However, ITI wall method was measurably more reproducible.

▶ The authors present a well-designed analysis of 2 ultrasound methods, inner versus outer wall measurements, for aortic aneurysm screening. Interobserver variability was statistically better for inner wall measurements (0.3 cm) versus outer wall measurement (0.42 cm). Intraobserver variability was similar (0.2 cm) for both measurement techniques. The limits of axial resolution at typical scanning depths were 1 to 2 mm in this study.

Similar studies have found both conflicting and similar results. Determining the limits of the outer aneurysmal wall can be subjective, which lends to this measurement some level of variation typically reported at 3 to 8 mm. The inner wall tends to be more distinct. The clinical impact 3 to 8 mm of variation should be considered in the context of a screening study. Although axial imaging is considered the gold standard, both surgeon and patient should consider axial imaging based on patient risk tolerance and planning for aneurysm repair.

Z. M. Arthurs, MD

The Cardiac Cycle is a Major Contributor to Variability in Size Measurements of Abdominal Aortic Aneurysms by Ultrasound
Grøndal N, Bramsen MB, Thomsen MD, et al (Viborg Hosp, Denmark)
Eur J Vasc Endovasc Surg 43:30-33, 2012

Aim.—The objective of the study was to evaluate the impact of the cardiac cycle on ultrasound measurements of abdominal aortic aneurysm (AAA) diameters.

Methods.—In total, 603 AAAs detected by screening were investigated with respect to the maximal systolic and diastolic anterior—posterior aortic diameters during the cardiac cycle using recorded ultrasound video sequences.

Results.—On average, the systolic AAA diameter was 41.60 mm, and the diastolic AAA diameter was 39.63 mm with a paired mean difference at 1.94 mm ($p < 0.0001$). No association between aneurysmal size and difference in systolic and diastolic size was noted.

The mean difference and variability between two observers, one measured during peak-systole and the other measured during end-diastole, was 2.65 and 2.21 mm, respectively, as compared with 0.86 and 1.52 mm, respectively, when both were measured during the peak of systole. The intraobserver variability was 0.94 during systole, 1.18 during diastole and 1.94 mm when systole and diastole measurements were combined.

Conclusion.—The lack of a standardised measurement of the AAA diameter during the cardiac cycle is a potential major contributor to the variability in ultrasonography measurements.

▶ Ultrasound variability in determining abdominal aortic aneurysm (AAA) diameter is generally reported to be about 5 mm and can reach as high as 8 mm in some studies.[1,2] This study quantifies for the first time the magnitude of differences in abdominal aortic size during the cardiac cycle. This, combined with previous data, suggests that the 2-mm variability in the ultrasound measurement, secondary to when the measurement is taken during the cardiac cycle, may account for up to 40% of the variability in ultrasound-determined

AAA diameter. It is important to remember that the measurements of variability determined in the study were observed under use of a strict protocol measuring maximal diameter during systole and diastole with only 2 observers. In clinical practice where multiple individuals may perform the ultrasound examinations and multiple individuals may interpret the ultrasound examinations, variability due to the cardiac cycle may actually be larger than that reported here. Practical implications of this study are that in ultrasound screening programs where additional follow-up is defined by detection of an aneurysm 30 mm in diameter, patients who have borderline aortas for additional follow-up may be denied this follow-up if their aneurysms were measured in diastole rather than systole. Similarly, there may be patients whose aneurysms, when measured in diastole, are slightly lower than 55 mm and are not offered aneurysm repair, whereas they may have been if their aneurysms had been measured during systole. These are, of course, small differences and the true clinical significance may be minimal.

G. L. Moneta, MD

References

1. Singh K, Bønaa KH, Solberg S, Sørlie DG, Bjørk L. Intra- and interobserver variability in ultrasound measurements of abdominal aortic diameter. The Tromsø Study. *Eur J Vasc Endovasc Surg.* 1998;15:497-504.
2. Lederle FA, Wilson SE, Johnson GR, et al. Variability in measurement of abdominal aortic aneurysms. Abdominal Aortic Aneurysm Detection and Management Veterans Administration Cooperative Study Group. *J Vasc Surg.* 1995;21:945-952.

Agreement between Computed Tomography and Ultrasound on Abdominal Aortic Aneurysms and Implications on Clinical Decisions
Foo FJ, Hammond CJ, Goldstone AR, et al (Leeds Teaching Hosps NHS Trust, UK; et al)
Eur J Vasc Endovasc Surg 42:608-614, 2011

Objectives.—The United Kingdom abdominal aortic aneurysm (AAA) screening programme refers aneurysms with ultrasound (US) diameters of ≥5.5 cm to vascular services for consideration of computed tomography (CT) and intervention. We investigated the discrepancy between US and CT, implications on clinical decisions and question at which stage CT be used.

Design/Methods.—AAA USs over 5 years were retrospectively analysed. Patients included had aneurysms measuring ≥5 cm on US with subsequent CT within 2 months ($n = 123$). Based on maximum US diameters, 44 patients had aneurysms between 5 and 5.4 cm (group I) and 79 patients ≥5.5 cm (group II). Results were cross-referenced. Correlation and limits of agreement were calculated. Two radiologists re-measured 44 pairs of CT/US scans and the inter-observer bias in determining discrepancies between imaging modalities calculated.

Results.—Mean difference between imaging modalities was 0.21 cm (± 0.39 cm, $p < 0.001$). Limits of agreement were −0.55 to 0.96 cm, exceeding clinical acceptability. Mean difference was higher and significant in group I (0.39 cm, $p < 0.001$) compared to group II (0.10 cm, $p > 0.05$). Seventy-percent of group I patients had CT scans revealing diameters of ≥ 5.5 cm. Inter-observer bias was not significant.

Conclusion.—Significant differences between imaging modalities, more in US diameters of below 5.5 cm, exist. We recommend AAAs measuring ≥ 5 cm on US should undergo earlier referral to a vascular service and CT.

▶ Duplex ultrasound has become the primary modality for abdominal aortic aneurysm (AAA) screening and surveillance. Several studies have compared ultrasound measurements with computed tomographic arteriography (CTA) measurements and found significant variance between the two imaging modalities. This study retrospectively reviewed 123 aneurysms that underwent both ultrasound examination and CTA. The study was limited to aneurysms larger than 5 cm by ultrasound examination. Overall, ultrasound measurements correlate well with CTA measurements, but the variation was ±0.39 cm for AAAs sized between 5.0 and 5.4 cm compared with ±0.1 cm for AAAs sized 5.5 cm and more.

The authors conclude that patients who have AAAs larger than 5 cm by ultrasound measurement should be referred for vascular surgery consultation. The limitations of this study are readily apparent; ultrasound examinations such as these demand internal validation. The authors' results are applicable to their institution but are not necessarily transferable to individual practices. The study highlights the limits of variation inherent to ultrasound measurements of AAAs and should prompt individual vascular laboratories to validate their results for clinical practice.

Z. M. Arthurs, MD

Assessment of the Accuracy of AortaScan for Detection of Abdominal Aortic Aneurysm (AAA)

Abbas A, Smith A, Cecelja M, et al (King's College London British Heart Foundation Centre of Res Excellence, London, UK)
Eur J Vasc Endovasc Surg 43:167-170, 2012

Background.—AortaScan AMI 9700 is a portable 3D ultrasound device that automatically measures the maximum diameter of the abdominal aorta without the need for a trained sonographer. It is designed to rapidly diagnose or exclude an AAA and may have particular use in screening programs. Our objective was to determine its accuracy to detect AAA.

Methods.—Subjects from our AAA screening and surveillance programs were examined. The aorta was scanned using the AortaScan and computed tomography (CT).

Results.—Ninety-one subjects underwent imaging (44 AAA on conventional ultrasound surveillance and 47 controls). The largest measurement obtained by AortaScan was compared against the CT-aortic measurement. The mean aortic diameter was 2.8 cm. The CT scan confirmed the diagnosis of AAA in 43 subjects. There was one false positive measurement on conventional ultrasound. AortaScan missed the diagnosis of AAA in eight subjects. There were thirteen false positive measurements. The sensitivity, specificity, positive and negative predictive values were 81%, 72%, 72% and 81% respectively.

Conclusion.—A device to detect AAA without the need for a trained operator would have potential in a community-based screening programme. The AortaScan, however, lacks adequate sensitivity and significant technical improvement is necessary before it could be considered a replacement for trained screening personnel (Figs 1 and 4, Table 2).

▶ A few years ago, Kirk Beach, the inventor of duplex ultrasonography, along with Gene Strandness at the University of Washington, walked into my clinic with a funny looking machine and said to me, "Lift up your shirt!" I said, "Excuse me?" Long story short, he placed the AortaScan probe (Fig 1) on my epigastrium and pulled the trigger. A few seconds later, a gleam came into his eyes as he immediately printed out an image and said, "Nope! No aneurysm. Your aorta is less than 3 cm in diameter."

This simple study compares measurements on patients with a body mass index (BMI) less than 35 kg/m^2 who harbored known abdominal aortic aneurysm (AAA) (n = 43) with normal control patients (n = 48). AortaScan missed the diagnosis of AAA in 8 patients. Sensitivity, specificity, and positive and negative predictive values are listed in Table 2.

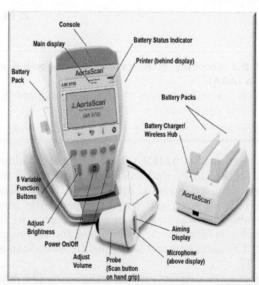

FIGURE 1.—AortaScan AMI 9700.[7] *Editor's Note*: Please refer to original journal article for full references. (Reprinted from European Journal of Vascular and Endovascular Surgery, Abbas A, Smith A, Cecelja M, et al. Assessment of the accuracy of AortaScan for detection of abdominal aortic aneurysm (AAA). *Eur J Vasc Endovasc Surg.* 2012;43:167-170. Copyright 2012, with permission from the European Society for Vascular Surgery.)

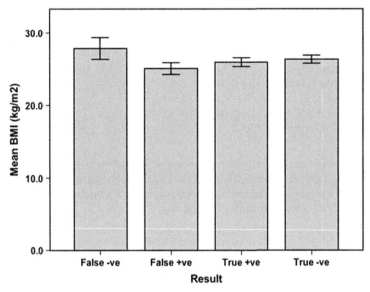

Error Bars: +/- 1 SE

FIGURE 4.—Comparison of body mass index (BMI ≤ 35 kg/m²) between different groups did not show any effect of BMI on AortaScan results. (Reprinted from European Journal of Vascular and Endovascular Surgery, Abbas A, Smith A, Cecelja M, et al. Assessment of the accuracy of AortaScan for detection of abdominal aortic aneurysm (AAA). *Eur J Vasc Endovasc Surg.* 2012;43:167-170. Copyright 2012, with permission from the European Society for Vascular Surgery.)

TABLE 2.—Contingency Table Showing Accuracy of AortaScan vs CT-Scan. Green Represents False Positive Results and Orange Shows False Negative Results in the Below Table

AortaScan BVI 9700	CT Scan		
	AAA (yes)	AAA (no)	
AAA (yes)	35	13	Positive predictive value 72%
AAA (no)	8	35	Negative predictive value 81%
	Sensitivity 81%	Specificity 72%	

For interpretation of the references to color in this figure legend, the reader is referred to web version of this article.

The overall conclusions of this comparison are that AortaScan, in its current form, does not have adequate sensitivity to be considered for a national screening program. One might think that BMI had an effect on the performance of the device. Unfortunately, this is not true. Although there was a trend toward greater BMI in those subjects with false-negative results, there was no relationship between incorrect results and BMI (Fig 4).

Regardless, this device represents one step closer to an effective screening tool for AAA. Remember the days before smart phones?

B. W. Starnes, MD

Prospective Comparative Analysis of Colour-Doppler Ultrasound, Contrast-enhanced Ultrasound, Computed Tomography and Magnetic Resonance in Detecting Endoleak after Endovascular Abdominal Aortic Aneurysm Repair
Cantisani V, Ricci P, Grazhdani H, et al (Univ 'La Sapienza', Rome, Italy; et al)
Eur J Vasc Endovasc Surg 41:186-192, 2011

Objectives.—To assess the accuracy of colour-Doppler ultrasound (CDUS), contrast-enhanced ultrasonography (CEUS), computed tomography angiography (CTA) and magnetic resonance angiography (MRA) in detecting endoleaks after endovascular abdominal aortic aneurysm repair (EVAR).

Design.—Prospective, observational study.

Materials and Methods.—From December 2007 to April 2009, 108 consecutive patients who underwent EVAR were evaluated with CDUS, CEUS, CTA and MRA as well as angiography, if further treatment was necessary. Sensitivity, specificity, accuracy and negative predictive value of ultrasound examinations were compared with CTA and MRA as the reference standards, or with angiography when available.

Results.—Twenty-four endoleaks (22%, type II: 22 cases, type III: two cases) were documented. Sensitivity and specificity of CDUS, CEUS, CTA, and MRA were 58% and 93%, 96% and 100%, 83% and 100% and 96% and 100% respectively. CEUS allowed better classification of endoleaks in 10, two and one patients compared with CDUS, CTA and MRA, respectively.

Conclusions.—The accuracy of CEUS in detecting endoleaks after EVAR is markedly better than CDUS and is similar to CTA and MRA. CEUS seems to be a feasible tool in the long-term surveillance after EVAR, and it may better classify endoleaks missed by other imaging techniques (Fig).

▶ Lifelong surveillance is recommended after stent graft placement to treat abdominal aortic aneurysm. Computed tomography angiography (CTA) is to date the preferred imaging modality to follow endovascular abdominal aortic aneurysm repair (EVAR) in patients. However, there is intense interest in using ultrasound as an imaging follow-up technique for EVAR patients. Ultrasound is less expensive and does not carry the risks of iodinated contrast administration or radiation. Nevertheless, reports to evaluate the accuracy of duplex ultrasound

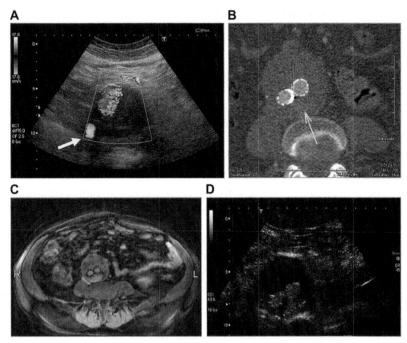

FIGURE.—Figures summarizing the findings according to four different imaging methods of a type II endoleak after endovascular repair of an abdominal aortic aneurysm: A) Colour-Doppler ultrasound: no flow signal is detected within the aneurysm sac (arrow indicates a hypertrophic lumbar artery); B) computed tomography angiography: no focal contrast-enhancement within the aneurysm sac (arrow indicates the place where the endoleak is not evident due to artefacts; C) magnetic resonance angiography and D) contrast-enhanced ultrasound: focal contrast-enhancement behind the iliac branches during arterial phase consistent with endoleak. (Reprinted from European Journal of Vascular and Endovascular Surgery, Cantisani V, Ricci P, Grazhdani H, et al. Prospective comparative analysis of colour-doppler ultrasound, contrast-enhanced ultrasound, computed tomography and magnetic resonance in detecting endoleak after endovascular abdominal aortic aneurysm repair. *Eur J Vasc Endovasc Surg.* 2011;41:186-192. Copyright 2011, with permission from the European Society for Vascular Surgery.)

following EVAR have shown mixed results in detection of endoleaks in comparison to CT scanning. In this study the authors compared CTA, magnetic resonance angiography, and ultrasound with and without contrast enhancement in the detection of endoleak following EVAR. Of particular interest is that ultrasound with contrast enhancement showed results for detection of endoleak equivalent to those of CTA. The authors used a second-generation contrast agent (SonoVue, Bracco, Milan, Italy). This agent consists of sulphur, hexafluoride gas microbubbles, and a phospholipid liquid membrane. It was administered by a single bolus of 2.4 mL and in an antecubital vein followed by 5 mL of saline (Fig). The results of this study would suggest that contrast-enhanced ultrasound is significantly more sensitive and specific than colored duplex ultrasound for detection of endoleak ($P < .001$) and approaches the accuracy of CTA for detection of endoleak. Unfortunately, contrast-enhanced ultrasound is limited by reimbursement issues (ie, many insurance companies will not pay for it).

G. L. Moneta, MD

Utility of duplex ultrasound in detecting and grading de novo femoropopliteal lesions

Khan SZ, Khan MA, Bradley B, et al (Columbia Univ College of Physicians and Surgeons, NY)
J Vasc Surg 54:1067-1073, 2011

Background.—Digital subtraction angiography (DSA) is the gold standard for diagnosing lower extremity (LE) arterial lesions. However, duplex ultrasound (DUS) is a widely used, safe, and noninvasive method of detecting LE lesions. The purpose of this study was to establish DUS criteria for detecting and grading de novo stenotic lesions in the femoropopliteal arterial segment.

Methods.—A prospective database was established including all patients who underwent LE endovascular interventions between 2004 and 2009. Patients with de novo stenotic lesions in the femoropopliteal segment were selected. DUS and DSA data pairs ≤ 30 days apart were analyzed. Peak systolic velocity (PSV; cm/s), velocity ratio (Vr), and DSA stenosis were noted. Linear regression and receiver operator characteristic (ROC) curves were used.

Results.—Two hundred seventy-five lesions in 200 patients were analyzed. Indications were claudication (50.5%), rest pain (12.5%), and tissue loss (37.0%). Mean time interval between DUS and DSA was 24 days. Both PSV ($R = .80$, $R^2 = .641$; $P < .001$) and Vr ($R = .73$, $R^2 = .546$; $P < .001$) showed strong correlation with the degree of angiographic stenosis. ROC analysis showed that to detect $\geq 70\%$ stenosis, a PSV of 200 cm/s had 89.2% sensitivity and 89.7% specificity, and a Vr of 2.0 had 88.7% sensitivity and 90.2% specificity. Similarly, to differentiate between <50% and $\geq 50\%$ stenosis, PSV of 150 cm/s and Vr of 1.5 were highly specific and predictive. Combining PSV 200 cm/s and Vr 2.0 for $\geq 70\%$ stenosis gave 79.0% sensitivity, 99.0% specificity, 99.0% positive predictive value, and 85.0% negative predictive value.

Conclusion.—DUS shows a strong agreement with angiography and has good accuracy in detecting femoropopliteal lesions. We propose DUS criteria of PSV 200 cm/s and Vr 2.0 to differentiate between <70% and $\geq 70\%$ de novo stenosis in the femoropopliteal arterial segment.

▶ This is a nicely structured study with a design based on those prior duplex ultrasound studies validating criteria for other vascular beds, such as the mesenteric and carotid circulations. These criteria provide a nice guideline by which to evaluate peripheral lesions without angiography. The key problems with the study are that (1) before these results can be generalized, a prospective evaluation must be performed to confirm the retrospective results the authors present, and (2) with digital subtraction angiography and intervention being more common, most of the time the decision to intervene for lower extremity disease is based on symptomatology and ankle-brachial index. That being said, a noninvasive method of grading stenoses can be useful to determine the optimal intervention method and potentially decrease procedural complications.

A. Chandra, MD

Evaluation of hyperspectral technology for assessing the presence and severity of peripheral artery disease

Chin JA, Wang EC, Kibbe MR (Northwestern Univ, Chicago, IL)
J Vasc Surg 54:1679-1688, 2011

Background.—Hyperspectral imaging is a novel technology that can noninvasively measure oxyhemoglobin and deoxyhemoglobin concentrations to create an anatomic oxygenation map. It has predicted healing of diabetic foot ulcers; however, its ability to assess peripheral arterial disease (PAD) has not been studied. The aims of this study were to determine if hyperspectral imaging could accurately assess the presence or absence of PAD and accurately predict PAD severity.

Methods.—This prospective study included consecutive consenting patients presenting to the vascular laboratory at the Jesse Brown VA Medical Center during a 10-week period for a lower extremity arterial study, including ankle-brachial index (ABI) and Doppler waveforms. Patients with lower extremity edema were excluded. Patients underwent hyperspectral imaging at nine angiosomes on each extremity. Additional sites were imaged when tissue loss was present. Medical records of enrolled patients were reviewed for demographic data, active medications, surgical history, and other information pertinent to PAD. Patients were separated into no-PAD and PAD groups. Differences in hyperspectral values between the groups were evaluated using the two-tailed t test. Analysis for differences in values over varying severities of PAD, as defined by triphasic, biphasic, or monophasic Doppler waveforms, was conducted using one-way analysis of variance. Hyperspectral values were correlated with the ABI using a Pearson bivariate linear correlation test.

Results.—The study enrolled 126 patients (252 limbs). After exclusion of 15 patients, 111 patients were left for analysis, including 46 (92 limbs) no-PAD patients and 65 (130 limbs) PAD patients. Groups differed in age, diabetes, coronary artery disease, congestive heart failure, tobacco use, and insulin use. Deoxyhemoglobin values for the plantar metatarsal, arch, and heel angiosomes were significantly different between patients with and without PAD ($P < .005$). Mean deoxyhemoglobin values for the same three angiosomes showed significant differences between patients with monophasic, biphasic, and triphasic waveforms ($P < .05$). In patients with PAD, there was also significant correlation between deoxyhemoglobin values and ABI for the same three angiosomes ($P = .001$). Oxyhemoglobin values did not predict the presence or absence of PAD, did not correlate with PAD severity, and did not correlate with the ABI.

Conclusions.—These results suggest the ability of hyperspectral imaging to detect the presence of PAD. Hyperspectral measurements can also evaluate different severities of PAD.

▶ The authors present a proof-of-concept study on the ability of hyperspectral imaging to predict presence and severity of peripheral arterial disease. The area of perfusion assessment in patients with critical limb ischemia is of vital importance to improve predictability of limb salvage; however, based on these results, it seems that hyperspectral imaging may not be accurate enough. Several limitations to this technology, including superficial depth of imaging, measurement of hemoglobin status as a surrogate of perfusion, and reproducibility of results, are the likely causes of the statistically significant but numerically overlapping results. This study should serve as a great example of a physician-initiated clinical trial with an industry partner to critically evaluate technology prior to marketing for clinical application. This type of evaluation is desperately needed for many new technologies seeking financial compensation from increasingly limited health care budgets.

A. Chandra, MD

Completion duplex ultrasound predicts early graft thrombosis after crural bypass in patients with critical limb ischemia
Scali ST, Beck AW, Nolan BW, et al (Univ of Florida, Gainesville; Dartmouth-Hitchcock Med Ctr, Lebanon, NH)
J Vasc Surg 54:1006-1010, 2011

Objective.—To determine if intraoperative distal graft end-diastolic velocity (EDV) using completion duplex ultrasound (CDU) predicts patency of crural bypass in patients with critical limb ischemia (CLI).

Methods.—Records of 116 non-consecutive patients who underwent crural revascularization with vein conduit and CDU between 1998 and 2008 were reviewed. Bypass grafts were performed for rest pain (34%) or tissue loss (66%), while 56% of the reported cases were categorized as "disadvantaged" because of compromised vein quality or diseased arterial outflow. A 10-MHz low-profile transducer was used to image the entire bypass at case completion. Technical adequacy of the grafts was verified by absence of retained valves, arteriovenous fistulas, or localized velocity increases and presence of bypass-dependent distal pulses. Modified Rutherford scores were calculated as surrogate markers of runoff resistance and compared to distal graft EDV. The primary study end point was graft patency during a 1-year posttreatment period. Patency rates were determined using Kaplan-Meier life table methodology and compared using the log-rank test. Predictors of graft patency were determined by Cox proportional hazards.

Results.—Primary, primary-assisted, and secondary patency for all crural bypasses were 62%, 66%, and 70% at 1 year, respectively. When stratified by tertiles of distal graft EDV (0 - <5 cm/s, 5-15 cm/s, >15 cm/s), 1-year primary patency rates were 32%, 64%, and 84% (*P* =.001). Low (0 - < 5 cm/s) distal graft EDV (hazard ratio [HR], 3.3 confidence interval [CI], 1.74-6.41; $P < .001$), poor-quality conduit (HR, 2.5; CI, 1.19-5.21; $P = .016$), age <70 (HR, 2.08; CI, 1.06-4.00; $P = .031$), and lack of statin use (HR, 2.04; CI, 1.04-4.00; $P = .038$) were independent predictors of graft failure. While the modified Rutherford score correlated with distal graft EDV ($P = .05$), it was not an independent predictor of patency ($P = .58$). Predictors of low EDV (<5 cm/s) included single-vessel runoff (odds ratio [OR], 3.33; CI, 1.14-9.71; $P = .027$), poor conduit (OR, 2.94; CI, 1.16-7.41; $P = 0.024$), and diabetes (OR, 2.86; CI, 1.14-7.21; $P = .025$).

Conclusions.—Distal graft EDV predicts crural vein graft patency in patients with CLI. Grafts with EDV <5 cm/s remain at high risk for early failure. The impacts on patency of statins, age, and poor-quality conduit are, again, confirmed. These results highlight the value of EDV using intraoperative CDU for anticipating and, possibly, improving results of open crural revascularization.

▶ Intraoperative assessment of lower extremity bypass graft using duplex ultrasound scan as a predictor of graft performance and durability has been previously demonstrated but has been of variable utility in clinical practice because of lack of clear guidelines. Use of distal graft end diastolic velocity (EDV), which correlated with early graft failure after crural bypass in patients with critical limb ischemia as described in this study, may be a simple, readily obtainable intraoperative duplex criteria that may be of some predictive utility. While this correlation is clearly supported by the data set, there are some study limitations, including retrospective design, potential intraobserver variability, variable adjuvant measures for identified "disadvantaged" grafts, and low distribution of postoperative anticoagulation use even if crural bypass was considered "disadvantaged." Ultimately, what clinical or intraoperative factors are addressed based on a low EDV to prevent graft failure of these "disadvantaged" grafts becomes most important. Furthermore, while this study focuses on EDV, other hemodynamic variables like peak systolic velocity (PSV) and resistive indexes (RI = PSV-EDV/PSV) were collected but not reported. While low distal EDV is one indirect measurable parameter, graft failure is more complex, and whether or not these other intraoperative parameters at the distal anastomosis or elsewhere in the graft are helpful remains unclear. Furthermore, while this data set is limited to crural bypass, whether it also applies to more proximal bypass is uncertain.

M. A. Passman, MD

Evaluation of an Electromagnetic 3D Navigation System to Facilitate Endovascular Tasks: A Feasibility Study

Sidhu R, Weir-McCall J, Cochennec F, et al (Imperial College London, UK; Guy's and St Thomas' NHS Trust, London, UK)
Eur J Vasc Endovasc Surg 43:22-29, 2012

Introduction.—We describe a novel approach to arterial cannulation using the StealthStation® Guidance System (Medtronic, USA). This uses electromagnetic technology to track the guidewire, displaying a 3D image of the vessel and guidewire.

Methods.—The study was performed on a 'bench top' simulation model called the Cannulation Suite comprising of a silicone aortic arch model and simulated fluoroscopy. The accuracy of the StealthStation® was assessed. 16 participants of varying experience in performing endovascular procedures (novices: 6 participants, ≤5 procedures performed; intermediate: 5 participants, 6−50 procedures performed; experts: 5 participants, >50 procedures performed) underwent a standardised training session in cannulating the left subclavian artery on the model with the conventional method (i.e. with fluoroscopy) and with the StealthStation®. Each participant was then assessed on cannulating the left subclavian artery using the conventional method and

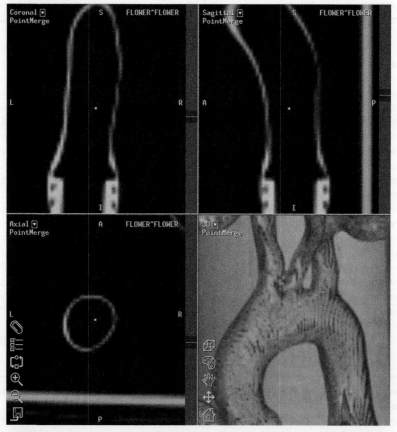

FIGURE 3.—Axial, coronal and saggital views of the descending aorta; the green dots correspond to the tip of the guidewire. 3D view of the aortic arch and proximal supra-aortic vessels; the tip of the blue arrow head corresponds to the tip of the guidewire. For interpretation of the references to color in this figure legend, the reader is referred to web version of this article. (Reprinted from European Journal of Vascular and Endovascular Surgery, Sidhu R, Weir-McCall J, Cochennec F, et al. Evaluation of an electromagnetic 3D navigation system to facilitate endovascular tasks: a feasibility study. *Eur J Vasc Endovasc Surg*. 2012;43:22-29. Copyright 2012, with permission from the European Society for Vascular Surgery.)

with the StealthStation®. Performance was video-recorded. The subjects then completed a structured questionnaire assessing the StealthStation®.

Results.—The StealthStation® was accurate to less than 1 mm [mean (SD) target registration error 0.56 mm (0.91)]. Every participant was able to complete the cannulation task with a significantly lower use of fluoroscopy with the navigation system compared with the conventional method [median 0 s (IQR 0–2) vs median 14 s (IQR 10–19), respectively; $p = <0.001$]. There was no significant difference between the StealthStation® and conventional method for: total procedure time [median 17 s (IQR 9–53) vs median 21 s (IQR 11–32), respectively; $p = 0.53$]; total guidewire hits to the vessel wall [median 0 (IQR 0–1) vs median 0 (IQR 0–1), respectively; $p = 0.86$]; catheter hits to the vessel wall [median 0.5 (IQR 0–2) vs median 0.5 (IQR 0–1), respectively; $p = 0.13$]; and cannulation performance on the global rating scale [median score, 39/40 (IQR 28–39) vs 38/40 (IQR 33–40), respectively; $p = 0.40$]. The intra-class correlation coefficient for agreement between video-assessors for all scores was 0.99. 88% strongly agreed that the StealthStation® can potentially decrease exposure of the patient to contrast and radiation.

Conclusion.—Arterial cannulation is feasible with the StealthStation® (Fig 3).

▶ Can you imagine a day when a 3-dimensional image can be superimposed on a human and an entire complex endovascular repair carried out without the use of fluoroscopy or contrast? This article would suggest this day is drawing near.

An estimated 43 000 to 47 000 people die annually in the United States from diseases of the aorta and its branches.[1] Endovascular procedures to treat these diseases are becoming more prevalent, and the downside to some of these more complex procedures has been the use of excessive radiation and contrast media. Navigation technology may help to counter some of these limitations.

Using a 3-D electromagnetic navigation system (ie, StealthStation; Fig 3), these authors compared three groups of endovascular interventionalists based on an arbitrary level of experience using conventional fluoroscopy and the Stealth-Station to cannulate the left subclavian artery. StealthStation had submillimeter accuracy and was associated with a highly significant reduction in fluoroscopy time when compared to conventional imaging.

This is further evidence of the increasing use of novel imaging modalities and potentially entirely robotic approaches to endovascular surgery. *Star Trek*, here we come!

B. W. Starnes, MD

Reference

1. Svensson LG, Kouchoukos NT, Miller DC, et al. Expert consensus document on the treatment of descending thoracic aortic disease using endovascular stent-grafts. *Ann Thorac Surg.* 2008;85:S1-S41.

4 Perioperative Considerations

The Predictive Ability of Pre-Operative B-Type Natriuretic Peptide in Vascular Patients for Major Adverse Cardiac Events: An Individual Patient Data Meta-Analysis

Rodseth RN, Lurati Buse GA, Bolliger D, et al (Univ of KwaZulu-Natal, Durban, South Africa; Univ Hosp Basel, Switzerland; et al)

J Am Coll Cardiol 58:522-529, 2011

Objectives.—The aims of this study were to perform an individual patient data meta-analysis of studies using B-type natriuretic peptides (BNPs) to predict the primary composite endpoint of cardiac death and nonfatal myocardial infarction (MI) within 30 days of vascular surgery and to determine: 1) the cut points for a natriuretic peptide (NP) diagnostic, optimal, and screening test; and 2) if pre-operative NPs improve the predictive accuracy of the revised cardiac risk index (RCRI).

Background.—NPs are independent predictors of cardiovascular events in noncardiac and vascular surgery. Their addition to clinical risk indexes may improve pre-operative risk stratification.

Methods.—Studies reporting the association of pre-operative NP concentrations and the primary study endpoint, post-operative major adverse cardiovascular events (defined as cardiovascular death and nonfatal MI) in vascular surgery, were identified by electronic database search. Secondary study endpoints included all-cause mortality, cardiac death, and nonfatal MI.

Results.—Six data sets were obtained, 5 for BNP (n = 632) and 1 for N-terminal pro-BNP (n = 218). An NP level higher than the optimal cut point was an independent predictor for the primary composite endpoint (odds ratio: 7.9; 95% confidence interval: 4.7 to 13.3). BNP cut points were 30 pg/ml for screening (95% sensitivity, 44% specificity), 116 pg/ml for optimal (highest accuracy point; 66% sensitivity, 82% specificity), and 372 pg/ml for diagnostic (32% sensitivity, 95% specificity). Subsequent to revised cardiac risk index stratification, reclassification using the optimal cut point significantly improved risk prediction in all groups (net reclassification improvement 58%, p < 0.000001), particularly in the intermediate-risk group (net reclassification improvement 84%, p < 0.001).

Conclusions.—Pre-operative NP levels can be used to independently predict cardiovascular events in the first 30 days after vascular surgery

Study	BNP above cut point n/N	BNP below cut point n/N	OR (random) 95%CI	Weight %	OR (random) 95% CI
Gibson	22/33	2/96		20.40	94.0 (19.43, 454.78)
Cuthbertson	2/57	0/13		10.14	1.22 (0.06, 26.84)
Mahla	14/85	5/133		25.31	5.05 (1.75, 14.59)
Bolliger	2/38	2/95		16.79	2.58 (0.35, 19.04)
Biccard	13/53	13/244		27.36	5.78 (2.50, 13.36)
Total (95% CI)	266	581		100.00	7.36 (2.23, 24.31)

Total events: 53 (BNP above cut point) 22 (BNP below cut point)
Test for heterogeneity, Chi²=13.37, df=4 (P=0.001), I²=70.1%
Test for overall effect: Z=3.27 (P=0.001)

0.001 0.01 0.1   1   10 100 1000

Below threshold   Above threshold

FIGURE 2.—Unadjusted ORs for a Pre-Operative BNP or NT-proBNP Concentration Above the Optimal General Cut Point (BNP 116 pg/ml, NT-proBNP 277.5 pg/ml) in Predicting Cardiovascular Outcomes 30 Days After Surgery. (Reprinted from the Journal of the American College of Cardiology, Rodseth RN, Lurati Buse GA, Bolliger D, et al. The predictive ability of pre-operative B-type natriuretic peptide in vascular patients for major adverse cardiac events: an individual patient data meta-analysis. J Am Coll Cardiol. 2011;58:522-529. Copyright 2011, with permission from the American College of Cardiology.)

and to significantly improve the predictive performance of the revised cardiac risk index (Fig 2).

▶ A recent randomized international control and study of 8351 patients from 190 hospitals and 23 countries found a 6.9 % incidence of cardiovascular events in patients 45 years of age or older undergoing noncardiac surgery.[1] There are even higher rates of preoperative mortality, adverse cardiovascular events, and rehospitalizations in patients presenting for vascular surgical procedures.[2,3] Current guidelines utilize clinical risk factors, type of surgery, and exercise tolerance to direct preoperative investigation.[4] Clinical factors include a history of compensated or prior heart failure, a history of ischemic heart disease, cerebral vascular events, renal insufficiency, and diabetes mellitus.[5] However, use of the revised cardiac risk index with performance of noninvasive tests and imaging studies has not provided good discrimination when applied to patients undergoing vascular surgery.[6]

Ventricular cardiomyocytes secrete B-type natriuretic peptide (BNP) in response to atrial or ventricular wall stress. Preoperative elevations of BNP or its prohormone have consistently and independently been associated with cardiovascular events following major vascular surgery.[7] The aim of this study was to determine optimal BNP cutoffs to predict cardiovascular events after vascular surgery and to determine whether the use of preoperative levels of BNP, or its prohormone, could improve current risk stratification prior to vascular surgery. The study was stimulated by the fact that cardiac risk stratification in vascular surgery has only been, at best, modestly successful in predicting preoperative events in the vascular surgical patient. Therefore, predicting cardiac risk in the vascular surgical patient has remained maddeningly frustrating for surgeons, anesthesiologists, and patients. The results here suggest that in patients risk stratified with the revised cardiac risk index, a BNP cut-off point can be used to reclassify these patients providing a more accurate risk assessment (Fig 2). By inference, this may help better identify patients who may benefit from further cardiac evaluation. Hopefully, this will work out to the betterment of the care of the vascular surgical patient. Importantly, it is also crucial to recognize that this meta-analysis and other studies in this area[8] raise serious concerns regarding the use of the revised cardiac risk index as a stand-alone tool in the preoperative cardiac evaluation of the vascular surgical patient.

G. L. Moneta, MD

References

1. Devereaux PJ, Yang H, Yusuf S, et al. Effects of extended-release metoprolol succinate in patients undergoing non-cardiac surgery (POISE trial): a randomised controlled trial. *Lancet.* 2008;371:1839-1847.
2. Noordzij PG, Poldermans D, Schouten O, Bax JJ, Schreiner FA, Boersma E. Postoperative mortality in The Netherlands: a population-based analysis of surgery-specific risk in adults. *Anesthesiology.* 2010;112:1105-1115.
3. Jencks SF, Williams MV, Coleman EA. Rehospitalizations among patients in the Medicare fee-for-service program. *N Engl J Med.* 2009;360:1418-1428.
4. Fleisher LA, Beckman JA, Brown KA, et al. ACC/AHA 2007 Guidelines on Perioperative Cardiovascular Evaluation and Care for Noncardiac Surgery: Executive Summary: A Report of the American College of Cardiology/American Heart Association Task Force on Practice Guidelines (Writing Committee to Revise the 2002 Guidelines on Perioperative Cardiovascular Evaluation for Noncardiac Surgery) Developed in Collaboration With the American Society of Echocardiography, American Society of Nuclear Cardiology, Heart Rhythm Society, Society of Cardiovascular Anesthesiologists, Society for Cardiovascular Angiography and Interventions, Society for Vascular Medicine and Biology, and Society for Vascular Surgery. *J Am Coll Cardiol.* 2007;50:1707-1732.
5. Lee TH, Marcantonio ER, Mangione CM, et al. Derivation and prospective validation of a simple index for prediction of cardiac risk of major noncardiac surgery. *Circulation.* 1999;100:1043-1049.
6. Kertai MD, Boersma E, Bax JJ, et al. A meta-analysis comparing the prognostic accuracy of six diagnostic tests for predicting perioperative cardiac risk in patients undergoing major vascular surgery. *Heart.* 2003;89:1327-1334.
7. Feringa HH, Schouten O, Dunkelgrun M, et al. Plasma N-terminal pro-B-type natriuretic peptide as long-term prognostic marker after major vascular surgery. *Heart.* 2007;93:226-231.
8. Ford MK, Beattie WS, Wijeysundera DN. Systematic review: prediction of perioperative cardiac complications and mortality by the revised cardiac risk index. *Ann Intern Med.* 2010;152:26-35.

Decreased Kidney Function: An Unrecognized and Often Untreated Risk Factor for Secondary Cardiovascular Events After Carotid Surgery
van Lammeren GW, Moll FL, Blankestijn PJ, et al (Univ Med Ctr Utrecht, The Netherlands; et al)
Stroke 42:307-312, 2011

Background and Purpose.—Chronic kidney disease is an important risk factor for development and progression of atherosclerosis. The objective of the current study was to investigate the contribution of moderate kidney failure to cardiovascular (CV) mortality and morbidity after carotid endarterectomy (CEA). In addition, we investigated which proportion received optimal medical treatment or underwent diagnostic workup of the kidneys prior to CEA.

Methods.—Between 2002 and 2009, 1085 patients undergoing CEA were included in this study. Estimated glomerular filtration rate (eGFR) was assessed at baseline. Moderate kidney failure was defined as an eGFR 30–59 and compared with normal or mildly reduced kidney function (eGFR ≥160). Primary endpoint was CV death, composed of fatal myocardial infarction, fatal stroke, and ruptured abdominal aneurysm. Secondary endpoints were CV morbidity.

Results.—Moderate kidney failure (eGFR 30–59) was observed in 26.5% (288/1085) of the patients. During a median follow-up of 2.95 years (0.0 to 3.0 years), the adjusted hazard ratio for CV death with an eGFR 30–59 was 2.22 (1.27 to 3.89). Adjusted hazard ratio for MI with an eGFR 30–59 was 1.90 (1.04 to 3.47). No higher risk for stroke and peripheral interventions was observed. Of all patients with an eGFR 30–59, 38.3% (105/274) received angiotensin-converting enzyme inhibitors, 74.5% (204/274) received statins, and 34.4% (99/288) visited a nephrologist.

Conclusions.—Patients with an eGFR 30–59 have a 2.2-fold increased risk for CV death and 1.9-fold increased risk for myocardial infarction the

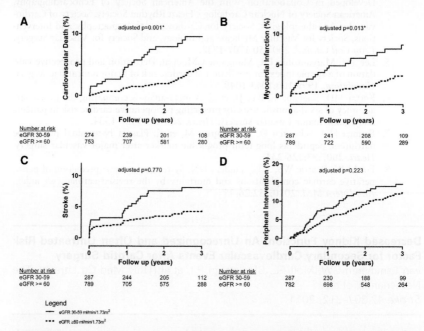

FIGURE 2.—Hazard functions for cardiovascular death (A), myocardial infarction (B), stroke (C), and peripheral interventions (D) after carotid endarterectomy. Probability values were corrected for cardiovascular risk factors and baseline differences. (Reprinted from van Lammeren GW, Moll FL, Blankestijn PJ, et al. Decreased kidney function: an unrecognized and often untreated risk factor for secondary cardiovascular events after carotid surgery. *Stroke.* 2011;42:307-312 American Heart Association, Inc.)

3 three years after CEA compared with patients with an eGFR ≥60, independent of other CV risk factors. A minority of these patients receive optimal medical treatment, which might explain the increased risk for progression of chronic kidney disease and CV morbidity and mortality (Fig 2).

▶ The prevalence of diabetes and hypertension is increasing and with it the presence of chronic kidney disease (CKD) is also likely to increase. It is known that impaired kidney function increases risk of death and hospitalization in the overall population, and that the prevalence of CKD in the United States is currently estimated to be 9.6% of the population.[1] The short-term risk of moderate kidney failure is largely unrecognized by many surgeons. CKD is irreversible but treatable. It is known that angiotensin converting enzyme (ACE) inhibitors and angiotensin II antagonists can delay progression of CKD.[2] The objective of this study was to assess cardiovascular mortality and morbidity following carotid endarterectomy in a population of patients with moderate kidney failure. The authors also sought to determine what proportion of patients with moderate kidney failure receive optimal medical treatment or undergo diagnostic workup of their renal failure prior to carotid endarterectomy (CEA). From the data presented (Fig 2) it does appear that moderate kidney failure does have an adverse prognosis following CEA. Currently there are no widespread formal screening programs for moderate kidney failure. However, all vascular surgery patients undergo basic metabolic testing and in essence are screened for underlying kidney disease. Based on these data, it would appear prudent for vascular surgeons to consider referral to a nephrologist for any patient they identify with even moderate renal insufficiency.

G. L. Moneta, MD

References

1. Coresh J, Byrd-Holt D, Astor BC, et al. Chronic kidney disease awareness, prevalence, and trends among U.S. adults, 1999 to 2000. *J Am Soc Nephrol*. 2005;16: 180-188.
2. Brenner BM, Cooper ME, de Zeeuw D, et al. Effects of losartan on renal and cardiovascular outcomes in patients with type 2 diabetes and nephropathy. *N Engl J Med*. 2001;345:861-869.

On-treatment Function Testing of Platelets and Long-term Outcome of Patients with Peripheral Arterial Disease Undergoing Transluminal Angioplasty

van der Loo B, Braun J, Koppensteiner R (Univ Hosp Zurich, Switzerland; Univ of Zurich, Switzerland)

Eur J Vasc Endovasc Surg 42:809-816, 2011

Objective.—To assess the clinical importance of on-treatment function testing of platelets in patients on aspirin after catheter-based vascular interventions.

Materials and Methods.—In 109 patients with symptomatic peripheral arterial disease (PAD) of the lower limbs, platelet function testing (adenosine diphosphate-, collagen- and epinephrine-induced aggregation using light transmission aggregometry) was performed before and at multiple time points up to 1 year after a percutaneous angioplasty. Using univariate mixture models and Box—Cox transformation to ensure normally distributed individual variances, we investigated if an intraindividual variability exists and if it has a consequence for clinical outcome.

Results.—Response to aspirin as measured by platelet aggregometry varies considerably over time in most patients. However, the intraindividual variance over time was not significantly correlated either with restenosis/ reocclusion after 1 year or with adverse long-term outcome (occurrence of death for cardiovascular cause, stroke or myocardial infarction in up to 8 years follow-up).

Conclusions.—Response to aspirin does not seem to have a role in determining long-term outcome in patients with symptomatic PAD. The fact that testing of platelet function at only one time point has reduced significance may have implications for all clinical settings in which aspirin is used for the prevention of thrombo-embolic events.

▶ Intraindividual platelet response to aspirin is variable.[1] Whereas aspirin is used routinely to prevent thromboembolic cardiovascular events, only about 25% of vascular complications are prevented with aspirin therapy.[2] The authors found intraindividual variation in response to aspirin did not correlate with restenosis or reocclusion of angioplasty sites after 1 year. Being a nonresponder to aspirin at one point in time, however, does not necessarily mean the individual would always be a nonresponder to aspirin. Indeed, in one study of patients undergoing coronary artery bypass surgery, patients were classified as aspirin resistant shortly after their operations, but the majority became aspirin responsive at 1-month follow-up.[3] There may be modifiable factors that influence response to aspirin. Testing patients for platelet-functional response to aspirin, or perhaps any antiplatelet agent, at a single point in time may not be clinically relevant. Additional work is required to determine whether tests of platelet responsiveness are sufficiently predictive of favorable or unfavorable cardiovascular effects and whether they can be advocated for routine clinical practice. The circumstances under which tests of platelet responsiveness to antiplatelet agents are most likely to produce clinically relevant results also need to be determined.

G. L. Moneta, MD

References

1. Storey RF. Variability of response to antiplatelet therapy. *Eur Heart J Suppl.* 2008; 10:A21-A27.
2. Patrono C, Rocca B. Drug insight: aspirin resistance—fact or fashion? *Nat Clin Pract Cardiovasc Med.* 2007;4:42-50.
3. Golański J, Chłopicki S, Golański R, Gresner P, Iwaszkiewicz A, Watala C. Resistance to aspirin in patients after coronary artery bypass grafting is transient: impact on the monitoring of aspirin antiplatelet therapy. *Ther Drug Monit.* 2005;27: 484-490.

Standardised Frailty Indicator as Predictor for Postoperative Delirium after Vascular Surgery: A Prospective Cohort Study
Pol RA, van Leeuwen BL, Visser L, et al (Univ of Groningen, The Netherlands)
Eur J Vasc Endovasc Surg 42:824-830, 2011

Objectives.—To determine whether the Groningen Frailty Indicator (GFI) has a positive predictive value for postoperative delirium (POD) after vascular surgery.

Methods.—Between March and August 2010, 142 consecutive vascular surgery patients were prospectively evaluated. Preoperatively, the GFI was obtained and postoperatively patients were screened with the Delirium Observation Scale (DOS). Patients with a DOS-score ≥ 3 points were assessed by a geriatrician. Delirium was defined by the DSM-IV-TR criteria. Primary outcome variable was the incidence of POD. Secondary outcome variables were any surgical complication and hospital length of stay (HLOS) (>7 days).

Results.—Ten patients (7%) developed POD. The highest incidence of POD was found after aortic surgery (17%) and amputation procedures (40%). Increased comorbidities ($p = 0.006$), GFI score ($p = 0.03$), renal insufficiency ($p = 0.04$), elevated C-reactive protein ($p = 0.008$), high American Society of Anaesthesiologists score ($p = 0.05$), a DOS-score of ≥ 3 points ($p = 0.001$), post-operative intensive care unit admittance ($p = 0.01$) and HLOS ≥ 7 days ($p = 0.005$) were risk factors for POD. The GFI score was not associated with a prolonged HLOS. A mean number of 2 ± 1 (range $0-5$) complications were registered. The receiver operator characteristics (ROC) area under the curve for the GFI was 0.70.

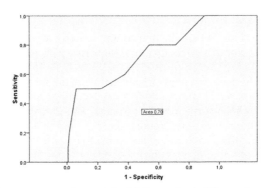

FIGURE 1.—Receiver operator characteristics (ROC) curve for the GFI as predictor for delirium in 142 patients undergoing elective vascular procedures. The area under the curve is 0.70 with the GFI set at ≥ 4 as indicative of an increased risk for POD (sensitivity 50%, specificity 78%). With a GFI cut-off point of ≥ 6 points, the area under the curve increased to 0.89 (sensitivity 50%, specificity 86%). (Reprinted from European Journal of Vascular and Endovascular Surgery, Pol RA, van Leeuwen BL, Visser L, et al. Standardised frailty indicator as predictor for postoperative delirium after vascular surgery: a prospective cohort study. *Eur J Vasc Endovasc Surg.* 2011;42:824-830. Copyright 2011, with permission from the European Society for Vascular Surgery.)

TABLE 1.—The Groningen Frailty Indicator (GFI)

	YES	NO	
Mobility			
Can the patient perform this task without any help? (using tools like walking sticks, wheelchairs or walker is regarded as independent)			
1. Go shopping	0	1	
2. Walk around outside (around the house or to neighbours)	0	1	
3. Dressing and undressing	0	1	
4. Toilet visit	0	1	
Vision			
5. Does the patient experience problems in daily life by poor vision?	1	0	
Hearing			
6. Does the patient experience problems in daily life by poor hearing?	1	0	
Nutrition			
7. Has the patient involuntarily lost weight (≥6 kg) in the past 6 months (or ≥3 kg in one month)	1	0	
Co-morbidity			
8. Does the patient currently use four or more different types of medication?	1	0	
	Yes	No	Sometimes
Cognition			
9. Does the patient currently has complaints about his memory (or has a history of dementia)	1	0	0
Psychosocial			
10. Does the patient sometimes experience emptiness around him?	1	0	1
11. Does the patient sometimes miss people around him?	1	0	1
12. Does the patient sometimes feel abandoned?	1	0	1
13. Has the patient recently felt sad or depressed?	1	0	1
14. Has the patient recently felt nervous or anxious?	1	0	1
Physical fitness			
15. Which grade would the patient give its physical fitness (0–10, ranging from very bad to good) 0–6 = 1 7–10 = 0	1	0	0
Total score GFI			

A score of four or more indicates a higher risk for frailty and possibly delirium.

Conclusions.—The GFI can be helpful in the early identification of POD after vascular surgery in a select group of high-risk patients (Fig 1, Table 1).

▶ Delirium is a frequently encountered complication in the elderly patient undergoing a major surgical procedure. It is disturbing to patients and their families, results in an increased length of stay, and can predispose to other medical complications. Vascular surgeons spend a great deal of time attempting to anticipate and predict cardiac complications following their surgical procedures. On the other hand, almost no time is spent trying to predict complications of cognition following vascular surgical procedures. Part of the problem is an inability to quantify risk for delirium. The Groningen Frailty Indicator (GFI) was developed to identify patients at risk for postoperative delirium[1] (Table 1). Data here indicate that a GFI index ≥ 4 (Fig 1) places patients at an increased risk for postoperative delirium with a sensitivity of 50% and a specificity of 78%. This study is useful in that it gives the vascular surgeon a basis from which to inform their patients about the risk of postoperative delirium.

More importantly, however, it allows the surgeon to inform the patient's family about such risks. By anticipating the occurrence of postoperative delirium, perhaps it will be possible to modify its severity and decrease the consequences of delirium, such as falls, aspiration, and medication noncompliance.

G. L. Moneta, MD

Reference

1. Steverink N, Slaets JPJ, Schuurmans H, van Lis M. Measuring frailty: developing and testing the GFI (Groningen Frailty Indicator). *Gerontologist.* 2001;41:236-237.

Asymptomatic carotid artery stenosis and cognitive outcomes after coronary artery bypass grafting
Norkienė I, Samalavičius R, Ivaškevičius J, et al (Vilnius Univ, Lithuania; et al)
Scand Cardiovasc J 45:169-173, 2011

Objective.—Cognitive decline has a negative impact on early postoperative morbidity and affects subjective quality of life. The role of asymptomatic cerebrovascular disease in developing postoperative neurocognitive damage remains controversial. The aim of our study was to evaluate the impact of asymptomatic carotid artery stenosis on postoperative cognitive decline.

Design.—We investigated 127 patients undergoing coronary artery bypass grafting. The neuropsychological examination, including a cognitive battery of seven tests and two scales for evaluation of mood disorders, was conducted the day before surgery and before the discharge from hospital.

Results.—Early postoperative cognitive decline (POCD) was detected in 46% of patients. POCD was associated with longer duration of surgery (p = 0.02), low cardiac output syndrome perioperatively (p < 0.05), postoperative bleeding (p = 0.03), longer postoperative mechanical ventilation time and intensive care unit stay (p < 0.05). Carotid artery lesion was detected in 42 (68.8%) patients. Multivariate regression analysis showed that carotid artery stenosis of more than 50% was an independant predictor of POCD (OR 26.89, CI 6.44—112.34).

Conclusions.—Asymptomatic carotid artery stenosis is a risk factor for cognitive decline after coronary artery bypass grafting.

▶ Most patients anticipate coronary artery bypass grafting (CABG) will improve their quality of life.[1] Psycho-emotional well being is an important quality to be preserved and improved for an enhanced quality of life. Neuropsychological disorders are now becoming more frequently addressed in the care of a variety of conditions, particularly postoperative states. Cerebrovascular disease and coronary artery disease potentially put patients at risk for cognitive decline. In this article, the authors sought to correlate the presence of asymptomatic carotid stenosis with possible cognitive decline following CABG. They sought to detect the incidence of cognitive decline following CABG, identify risk factors associated with cognitive decline following CABG, and investigate a possible link between cognitive performance and asymptomatic carotid stenosis. The striking finding in this study is a very strong statistical relationship between asymptomatic carotid stenosis and cognitive performance following CABG. It may be that carotid stenosis diminishes cerebral blood flow or somehow impairs autoregulation and thereby increases the susceptibility of the brain to unfavorable perioperative factors, such as microembolization or lowered cerebral blood flow. The authors used their data to suggest that screening for cervical carotid artery disease be performed in patients undergoing CABG, and this may help identify patients at risk of neurocognitive damage following CABG. Such information could possibly be of use in counseling of patients regarding their overall quality of life following CABG. It is, however, unclear whether correction of carotid stenosis, either before CABG, or concurrent with CABG, can serve as a mechanism to diminish cognitive decline associated with coronary artery bypassing grafting and carotid artery stenosis.

G. L. Moneta, MD

Reference

1. Koch CG, Khandwala F, Blackstone EH. Health-related quality of life after cardiac surgery. *Semin Cardiothorac Vasc Anesth.* 2008;12:203-217.

5 Grafts and Graft Complications

Infrainguinal Bypass for Peripheral Arterial Occlusive Disease: When Arms Save Legs
Vauclair F, Haller C, Marques-Vidal P, et al (Lausanne Univ Hosp, Switzerland)
Eur J Vasc Endovasc Surg 43:48-53, 2012

Objectives.—Determine if arm veins are good conduits for infrainguinal revascularisation and should be used when good quality saphenous vein is not available.

Design.—Retrospective study.

Materials and Methods.—We evaluated a consecutive series of infrainguinal bypass (IB) using arm vein conduits from March 2001 to December 2006. We selected arm vein by preoperative ultrasound mapping to identify suitable veins. We measured vein diameter and assessed vein wall quality. We followed patients with systematic duplex imaging at 1 week, 1, 3, 6 and 12 months, and annually thereafter. We treated significative stenoses found during the follow-up.

Results.—We performed 56 infrainguinal revascularisation using arm vein conduits in 56 patients. Primary patency rates at 1, 2 and 3 years were 65%, 51% and 47%. Primary assisted patencies at 1, 2 and 3 years were 96%, 96% and 82%. Secondary patency rates at 1, 2 and 3 years were 92%, 88% and 88%. The three-year limb salvage rate was 88%.

Conclusions.—We conclude that infrainguinal bypass using arm vein for conduits gives good patency rates, if selected by a preoperative US mapping to use the best autogenous conduit available (Figs 2 and 3).

▶ This article is a bit of déjà vu. For more than 20 years, vascular surgeons have been touting the use of arm veins for infrainguinal bypass in selected patients. While it is clear arm veins are never as good as a good-quality saphenous vein, the data here indicate that arm vein bypass (Fig 2) can provide excellent primary assisted patency rates (Fig 3) if the grafts are carefully followed with a regular program of duplex ultrasound surveillance. In this article, the authors remind us of a number of technical tips for using arm veins for infrainguinal bypass. These include avoiding thick-wall veins, veins less than 2.5 mm in diameter, and those with evidence of previous thrombosis. Again, there is really nothing new in this article. It is, however, refreshing to know that there are still some groups who still remember that the first rule of infrainguinal bypass is to secure a good conduit for the bypass.

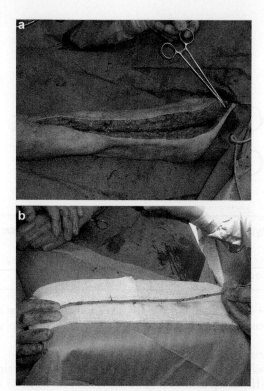

FIGURE 2.—Preparation of arm vein with ligation of collaterals. (Reprinted from European Journal of Vascular and Endovascular Surgery, Vauclair F, Haller C, Marques-Vidal P, et al. Infrainguinal bypass for peripheral arterial occlusive disease: when arms save legs. *Eur J Vasc Endovasc Surg*. 2012;43:48-53. Copyright 2012, with permission from the European Society for Vascular Surgery.)

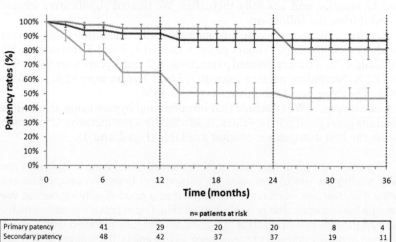

FIGURE 3.—Kaplan-Meier survival curves. (Reprinted from European Journal of Vascular and Endovascular Surgery, Vauclair F, Haller C, Marques-Vidal P, et al. Infrainguinal bypass for peripheral arterial occlusive disease: when arms save legs. *Eur J Vasc Endovasc Surg*. 2012;43:48-53. Copyright 2012, with permission from the European Society for Vascular Surgery.)

I tell my residents that lower-extremity bypass is not an artery operation but a vein procedure. The operating surgeon should use the best available vein for the bypass and choose inflow and outflow sites to maximize the quality of the venous conduit.

G. L. Moneta, MD

Use of ViaBahn Open Revascularisation Technique for Above-knee Femoro-popliteal Anastomosis: A Technical Note
Greenberg G, Szendro G, Mayzler O, et al (Ben-Gurion Univ of the Negev, Israel)
Eur J Vasc Endovasc Surg 42:202-205, 2011

We describe a ViaBahn Open Revascularization TEChnique (VORTEC) application in peripheral femoro-popliteal polytetrafluoroethylene (PTFE) graft bypass in 13 patients (Figs 1 and 2).

▶ The authors describe their technique and immediate results of the ViaBahn open revascularization technique in the femoral to above-knee bypass. The initial

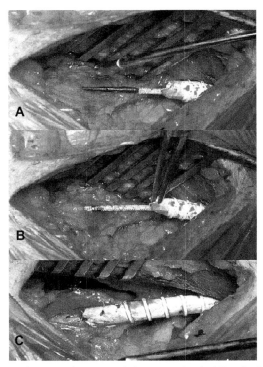

FIGURE 1.—A. ViaBahn on a guidewire in just before penetrating the AK popliteal artery. B. The distal portion of the ViaBahn stent graft desired to be lodged into the artery marked and introduced into the artery up to the mark. C. The stent graft is sutured to the artery and to the graft by one or two 5/0 Prolene stitches. (Reprinted from European Journal of Vascular and Endovascular Surgery, Greenberg G, Szendro G, Mayzler O, et al. Use of ViaBahn open revascularisation technique for above-knee femoro-popliteal anastomosis: a technical note. *Eur J Vasc Endovasc Surg.* 2011;42:202-205. Copyright 2011, with permission from the European Society for Vascular Surgery.)

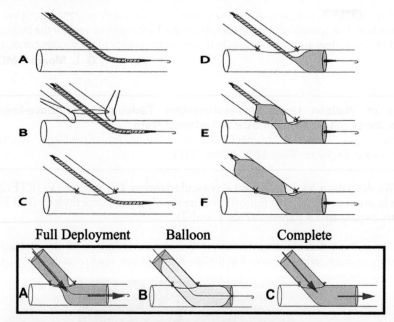

FIGURE 2.—Schematic drawing of VORTEC deployment in the AK popliteal artery. (Reproduced and modified from Mario Lachat's manuscript, with permission). (Reprinted from European Journal of Vascular and Endovascular Surgery, Greenberg G, Szendro G, Mayzler O, et al. Use of ViaBahn open revascularisation technique for above-knee femoro-popliteal anastomosis: a technical note. *Eur J Vasc Endovasc Surg.* 2011;42:202-205. Copyright 2011, with permission from the European Society for Vascular Surgery.)

technique described by Lachat et al[1] was performed in renal arteries to simplify the technical issues associated with thoracoabdominal aneurysms. This hybrid approach, although performed in a few specialized centers, is a novel and appealing technique in that situation.[2] The described technique involves an inguinal incision to expose the femoral artery and a standard medial thigh incision to expose the above-knee popliteal artery followed by tunneling of an externally supported polytetrafluoroethylene (PTFE) graft and introduction of a 5 mm or 6 mm ViaBahn stent graft that is 10 cm long through the graft from the femoral incision. The ViaBahn stent graft is then introduced into the artery and deployed and secured to the graft, completing the procedure with the proximal anastomosis (Figs 1 and 2).

One of the main issues in the infrainguinal region is that this technique still requires exposure of the femoral and above-knee popliteal artery. Although the authors state that one of the benefits is the limited dissection of the above-knee popliteal artery, most surgeons would find that this dissection can be accomplished with minimal morbidity. The main benefit of this technique is the elimination of the sutured distal anastomosis. The drawback of this technique is the loss of retrograde flow from the popliteal artery, which can improve outflow and maintain patency. Although the authors duly note these drawbacks in addition to cost of this bypass (an added 2500 euros), it remains to be seen if the long-term results will be better than the already known adequate results for standard femoral to above-knee bypass with PTFE.

N. Singh, MD

References

1. Lachat M, Mayer D, Criado FJ, et al. New technique to facilitate renal revascularization with use of telescoping self-expanding stent grafts: VORTEC. *Vascular.* 2008;16:69-72.
2. Donas KP, Lachat M, Rancic Z, et al. Early and midterm outcome of a novel technique to simplify the hybrid procedures in the treatment of thoracoabdominal and pararenal aortic aneurysms. *J Vasc Surg.* 2009;50:1280-1284.

Long-Term Results of Vascular Graft and Artery Preserving Treatment With Negative Pressure Wound Therapy in Szilagyi Grade III Infections Justify a Paradigm Shift
Mayer D, Hasse B, Koelliker J, et al (Univ Hosp of Zurich, Switzerland; et al)
Ann Surg 254:754-760, 2011

Objective.—To present the first long-term results of Szilagyi III vascular infections treated by negative pressure wound therapy (NPWT) with graft preservation.

Background Data.—Szilagyi III infections are usually treated by graft/artery excision and secondary vascular/plastic reconstruction. Small series treated with NPWT without graft removal are reported with good short-term to midterm results.

Methods.—The outcomes of 44 polymorbid patients (mean age = 62 years) with Szilagyi III infections from 2002 to 2009 were analyzed. Thirteen of forty-four required intensive care unit treatment. Forty grafts (prosthetic = 24, vein = 3, biological = 13) and 9 native arteries were involved. Negative pressure wound therapy (VAC; KCI International, Amstelveen, Netherlands) was applied directly on grafts/arteries (negative pressure = 50–125 mm Hg) after radical debridement of infected tissue. Antibiotic treatment was initiated and adapted according to microbiology.

Results.—Median duration of NPWT was 33 days (IQR: 20–78), of hospital stay 32 (IQR: 20–82) days. All patients survived 30 days. One-year mortality was 16% (7/44). Long-term mortality after a mean follow-up of 43 months (SD: 21) was 41% (18/44).

Complete wound healing was achieved in 91% (40/44). In 37 of 44 patients, grafts were preserved long-term without reinfection. There was no statistically significant difference in outcome between the various graft types involved.

Conclusions.—Vascular graft/arterial preserving treatment with NPWT in Szilagyi III infections was safe and effective with a very low short-term mortality. The majority of infected grafts were preserved without reinfection during a mean long-term follow-up of 4 years. This new treatment algorithm avoids major reconstructive surgery and should be used when dealing with Szilagyi III vascular infections (Fig 2).

▶ Wound infections with prosthetic graft or arterial involvement (Szilagyi grade III infections) can be associated with high morbidity and mortality.[1,2] Traditional treatment for Szilagyi type III infections is graft excision, radical debridement, and secondary vascular reconstruction. Negative pressure wound therapy (NPWT) was first introduced in 1997 by Argenta and Morykwas.[3] Recently there have been small series of patients with vascular graft infections treated by NPWT without graft excision. These series have reported good short-term and midterm results.[4,5] There remains, however, no universally accepted plan of management for infection of prosthetic grafts, vein grafts, or native arteries. The results presented here using VAC therapy for such infections are very encouraging (Fig 2) in that there was only 1 infected graft-related death. Because of its relative convenience for both the patient and the physician and widespread favorable clinical experience, VAC therapy has revolutionized care of open wounds in recent years. Through a combination of antimicrobial activity, stimulation of granulation tissue, and increased local perfusion, it appears VAC therapy can create an

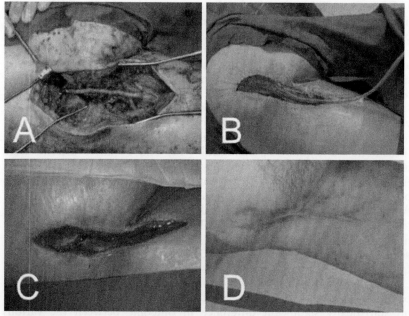

FIGURE 2.—Complete wound healing in Szilagyi grade III infection by NPWT. 41-year-old women after intravenous drug abuse with acute bleeding from infected pseudoaneurysm (coagulase-negative *Staphylococcus* and *Enterobacter*). A, The completely destroyed femoral artery was immediately reconstructed with a homograft at the first revision. B, A black openpore polyurethane foam was directly applied to the vascular reconstruction during the same operation. C, Situs 16 days after surgery. D, Healed wound at 28 months without reinfection 6 years postoperative. Intravenous drug abuse was suspended. (Reprinted from Mayer D, Hasse B, Koelliker J, et al. Long-term results of vascular graft and artery preserving treatment with negative pressure wound therapy in szilagyi grade III infections justify a paradigm shift. *Ann Surg.* 2011;254:754-760. © Southeastern Surgical Congress.)

environment suitable to combat infection. The authors' implication that the results of NPWT for Szilagyi III infections justify a paradigm shift in the management of vascular graft infections just may be true.

G. L. Moneta, MD

References

1. Liekweg WG Jr, Greenfield LJ. Vascular prosthetic infections: collected experience and results of treatment. *Surgery.* 1977;81:335-342.
2. Kikta MJ, Goodson SF, Bishara RA, Meyer JP, Schuler JJ, Flanigan DP. Mortality and limb loss with infected infrainguinal bypass grafts. *J Vasc Surg.* 1987;5:566-571.
3. Argenta LC, Morykwas MJ. Vacuum-assisted closure: a new method for wound control and treatment: clinical experience. *Ann Plast Surg.* 1997;38:563-576.
4. Demaria RG, Giovannini UM, Téot L, Frapier JM, Albat B. Topical negative pressure therapy. A very useful new method to treat severe infected vascular approaches in the groin. *J Cardiovasc Surg (Torino).* 2003;44:757-761.
5. Dosluoglu HH, Loghmanee C, Lall P, Cherr GS, Harris LM, Dryjski ML. Management of early (<30 day) vascular groin infections using vacuum-assisted closure alone without muscle flap coverage in a consecutive patient series. *J Vasc Surg.* 2010;51:1160-1166.

Knitted nitinol represents a new generation of constrictive external vein graft meshes
Zilla P, Moodley L, Wolf MF, et al (Univ of Cape Town, South Africa; Medtronic Inc, Minneapolis, MN)
J Vasc Surg 54:1439-1450, 2011

Objective.—Constriction of vein grafts with braided external nitinol meshes had previously led to the successful elimination of neointimal tissue formation. We investigated whether pulse compliance, smaller kink-free bending radius, and milder medial atrophy can be achieved by knitting the meshes rather than braiding, without losing the suppressive effect on intimal hyperplasia.

Methods.—Pulse compliance, bending stiffness, and bending radius, as well as longitudinal-radial deformation-coupling and radial compression, were compared in braided and knitted nitinol meshes. Identical to previous studies with braided mesh grafts, a senescent nonhuman primate model (Chacma baboons; bilateral femoral interposition grafts/6 months) mimicking the clinical size mismatch between vein grafts and runoff arteries was used to examine the effect of knitted external meshes on vein grafts: nitinol mesh-constricted (group 1); nitinol mesh-constricted and fibrin sealant (FS) spray-coated for mesh attachment (group 2); untreated control veins (group 3), and FS spray-coated control veins (group 4).

Results.—Compared with braided meshes, knitted meshes had 3.8-times higher pulse compliance (3.43 ± 0.53 vs $0.94 \pm 0.12\%/100$ mm Hg; $P = .00002$); 30-times lower bending stiffness (0.015 ± 0.002 vs 0.462 ± 0.077 Nmm^2; $P = .0006$); 9.2-times narrower kink-free bending radius (15.3 ± 0.4 vs 140.8 ± 22.4 mm; $P = .0006$), and 4.3-times lower radial narrowing caused by axial distension (18.0% ± 1.0% vs 77.0% ± 3.7%; $P = .00001$). Compared with mesh-supported grafts, neointimal tissue was 8.5-times thicker in group I (195 ± 45 μm) vs group III (23.0 ± 21.0 μm; $P < .001$) corresponding with a 14.3-times larger neointimal area in group I (4330 ± 957 × 103 μm^2) vs group III (303 ± 221 × 103 μm^2; $P < .00004$). FS had no significant influence. Medial muscle mass remained at 43.4% in knitted meshes vs the 28.1% previously observed in braided meshes.

Conclusion.—Combining the suppression of intimal hyperplasia with a more physiologic remodeling process of the media, manifold higher kink-resistance, and lower fraying than in braided meshes makes knitted nitinol an attractive concept in external vein graft protection.

▶ This study of nitinol external mesh supports of vein grafts brings up some interesting points but seems to be more applicable to future stent design than to a foreseeable application for graft support. First, these are only applicable to vein interposition grafts because the configuration would be hard to conceive for an end-to-side vein graft/artery anastomosis. What the authors have essentially created is a tissue-lined stent. The materials and mechanical engineering of the knitted versus braided designs should be considered relative to current stent design.

A. Chandra, MD

Early and Late Results of Contemporary Management of 37 Secondary Aortoenteric Fistulae

Batt M, Jean-Baptiste E, O'Connor S, et al (Univ of Nice Sophia-Antipolis, France; 4, The Green, Bromham, Bedfordshire, UK; et al)
Eur J Vasc Endovasc Surg 41:748-757, 2011

Purpose.—Evaluate the results of the two modalities used for the treatment of Secondary Aorto-Enteric Fistula (SAEF): *In situ* Reconstruction (ISR) and Extra-Anatomic Reconstruction (EAR). The primary endpoints of this study were early standard 30-day mortality and reinfection (RI). Secondary endpoints were perioperative morbidity, late mortality, primary graft patency, and major amputation rates.

Material & Method.—Diagnosis of SAEF was based on clinical examination and the results of pre-operative duplex or CT scans. Surgical management was performed according to local protocols at the participating institutions:

— Elective surgery: ISR or staged EAR
— Emergency surgery: aortic clamping followed by ISR or EAR
— Selected high-risk patients: endovascular repair.

Statistical analyses were performed using the actuarial method. Univariate analysis was used for analysis of categorical variables, and multivariate analysis was performed with a Cox proportional hazard regression.

Results.—A total of 37 patients were included in this retrospective multicentre study. Mean follow-up was 41 months. The majority of the patients (20, 54%) presented acutely. EAR was performed in 9 patients (24%), ISR in 25 (68%), and 3 patients underwent endovascular repair. Bacteriological cultures were negative in 3 patients (9%). The most frequent organisms identified were Candida species and *Escherichia coli*. The 30-day mortality was 43% (16 patients). Patient age (>75 years) was the sole predictive factor associated with operative mortality ($p = 0.02$); pre-operative shock was not statistically significant ($p = 0.08$). There were 2 graft thromboses and 1 femoral amputation. Primary graft patency was respectively 89% at 1 year and 86% at 5 years; limb salvage rates were 100% at 1 and 5 years and 86% at 6 years, with no difference between ISR and EAR. RI occurred after 9.3 ± 13 months in 8 of 17 surviving patients and was fatal in all cases. For all surviving patients, the RI rate at 1 and 2 years was 24% and 41% respectively. There was no significant difference in the rate of RI after ISR or EAR.

Conclusion.—EAR does not appear to be superior to ISR. The risk of RI increased with the length of follow-up, irrespective of the treatment modality. Life-long surveillance is mandatory. Our results with endovascular sealing of SAEF should be considered a bridge to open repair.

▶ The study highlights the difficulty of managing patients with secondary aortoenteric fistulas. The study was nonrandomized, and any conclusions as to the effectiveness of one form of therapy versus another for treatment of aortoenteric fistula must be somewhat circumspect. Nevertheless, review of these data suggest that it is possible to achieve equal morbidity and mortality rates using extra-anatomic or in situ repair of aortoenteric fistulas. Because the patients may not be equal with respect to characteristics influencing overall outcome, it is best to conclude that in situ and extra-anatomic repair of aortoenteric fistulas can provide equal results. Which technique to use will obviously depend on individual circumstances and individual patients.

The authors used endovascular repair in a few cases in this series. Because of the high reinfection rate of the endovascular repairs, the data here suggest endovascular repair of aortoenteric fistulae is best used as a bridge to more definitive in situ or extra-anatomic repair. Overall, aortoenteric fistula remains a highly lethal condition. Technique of repair can be individualized. This approach appears to lead to equal overall results with in situ versus extra-anatomic repair.

G. L. Moneta, MD

Comparison of straight and Venaflo-type cuffed arteriovenous ePTFE grafts in an animal study

Heise M, Husmann I, Grneberg A-K, et al (Friedrich-Schiller-Univ, Jena, Germany; et al)
J Vasc Surg 53:1661-1667, 2011

Background.—The long-term prognosis of arteriovenous (AV) polytetrafluoroethylene (PTFE) hemodialysis grafts is dissatisfying. Responsible for the poor outcome is a stenosis of the venous anastomosis. This originates from both pseudointimal (PI) and neointimal hyperplasia (IH) development. Although cuffed grafts have a better short-term prognosis than straight grafts, the late results of both types are poor. This current study aimed to compare both arteriovenous straight and Venaflo-type (Bard, Tempe, Ariz) prostheses in an animal study with regard to patency, PI, and IH development.

Methods.—Sixteen iliac arteriovenous expanded polytetrafluoroethylene (ePTFE) loops were inserted into 16 pigs. Animals were randomized into two groups. Group 1 animals received straight configured ePTFE grafts and group 2 animals received grafts with a Venaflo-type cuffed venous anastomosis. After insertion of the shunts and immediately before graft harvest, the shunt flows were measured. Six weeks after implantation, patency rates and development of pseudointima (PI) within the grafts were noted. The thickness of the venous intimal hyperplasia was measured using digital planimetry.

Results.—Patency rates after 6 weeks were 25% for straight and 62% for Venaflo-type grafts. In both groups a significant decrease of the graft blood flow compared with the preoperative levels was observed, which was attributed to the marked development of pseudointima. The reduction in flow at graft harvest was greater in the straight ePTFE group (658 ± 68 vs 260 ± 42 mL/min, $P < .05$) than for the Venaflo-type grafts (770 ± 107 vs 661 ± 284 mL/min, $P = $ ns), but the differences between the groups were statistically not significant. A marked pseudointima developed in the Venaflo cuff. The PI development was significantly higher in the graft hood (2.9 ± 0.6 mm) than in the heel (2.5 ± 0.4 mm, $P < .05$). In both groups, an intimal hyperplasia formed on the vein wall just opposite to the graft inflow. The intimal hyperplasia development was more pronounced in the straight configured shunts.

Conclusions.—The results of the present study confirm the inferior clinical results of ePTFE grafts used for hemodialysis access. Although the patency rates of cuffed grafts were superior, in both graft types a significant pseudointima leading to subtotal graft stenosis was observed in all grafts. Both straight and Venaflo-grafts. The Venaflo grafts have a slightly better-type cuffed ePTFE grafts have major hemodynamic drawbacks that have to be addressed in future graft design efforts (Fig 6).

▶ The optimal treatment for arteriovenous access in patients with chronic renal failure is autogenous arteriovenous fistulas. However, in patients with inadequate arm vein or exhausted previous arteriovenous fistulas, the treatment options are limited to prosthetic or biologic materials. Prosthetic materials are likely used initially because of availability and costs. The limiting factor of prosthetic materials used in arteriovenous fistula construction for dialysis use is early failure due to the development of both pseudointima hyperplasia (passive remodeling of expanded polytetrafluoroethylene [ePTFE]) and neointimal hyperplasia (active adaptation of the vein wall), usually at the venous anastomosis. In this study, the authors examine iliac arteriovenous fistulae ePTFE

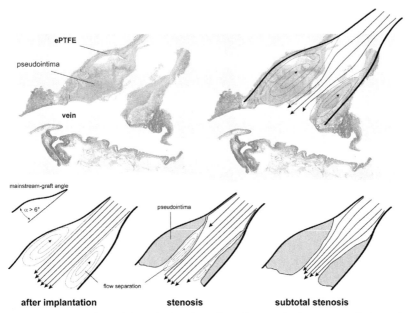

FIGURE 6.—Hypothesis of the pathophysiology of pseudointima development in cuffed expanded polytetrafluoroethylene (*ePTFE*) grafts. The sudden widening of the anastomosis in the cuff section leads to flow separation areas near the ePTFE wall. Comparable flow separations were previously found both in in vitro studies as well as in computational fluid dynamics calculations.[8,9] In the flow separation zones the flow recirculates forward and backward with a long contact time between blood and graft wall. Due to the high thrombogenicity of PTFE, eventually a pseudointima develops in the separation areas during the course of weeks and months after the implantation. *Editor's Note*: Please refer to original journal article for full references. (Reprinted from the Journal of Vascular Surgery, Heise M, Husmann I, Grneberg A-K, et al. Comparison of straight and Venaflo-type cuffed arteriovenous ePTFE grafts in an animal study. *J Vasc Surg*. 2011;53:1661-1667. Copyright 2011, with permission from The Society for Vascular Surgery.)

straight configuration in a pig model and compare it with an iliac arteriovenous fistulae using ePTFE Venaflo-type cuffed venous anastomosis. The main findings of this study were as follows: (1) Patency rates after 6 weeks were 25% for straight ePTFE and 62% for ePTFE Venaflo-type grafts. (2) In both groups a significant decrease of the graft blood flow compared with the preoperative levels was observed, which was attributed to the marked development of pseudointima. (3) The reduction in flow at graft harvest was greater in the straight ePTFE group (658 ± 68 vs 260 ± 42 mL/min; $P < .05$) than for the Venaflo-type grafts (770 ± 107 vs 661 ± 284 mL/min; $P =$ ns). (4) A marked pseudointima developed in the Venaflo cuff. (5) Both prosthetic grafts demonstrated neointimal hyperplasia in the vein wall opposite the graft inflow. The authors offer explanations for the pseudointima that develops in PTFE grafts and describe a complex of shear stress forces, velocity changes, flow separation, luminal diameters, graft thrombogenicity, and wall angle changes that reach 6° to 8° (Fig 6). The actual events that lead to the pseudointima, with the characteristic thick formation of fibrin and thrombus elements within the wall of prosthetic grafts in arteriovenous fistulas, are unknown, and pharmacologic treatments and anatomic changes in graft design have not been able to correct this significant problem, which leads to graft failure, hospital admissions, and increased health care costs. Future studies are required to find optimal material with low rates of thrombogenicity and can maintain adequate blood flows for patients requiring hemodialysis and do not have autogenous venous options.

J. D. Raffetto, MD

6 Aortic Aneurysm

The Strange Relationship between Diabetes and Abdominal Aortic Aneurysm

Lederle FA (Veterans Affairs Med Ctr, Minneapolis, MN)
Eur J Vasc Endovasc Surg 43:254-256, 2012

In a 1997 report of a large abdominal aortic aneurysm (AAA) screening study, we observed a negative association between diabetes and AAA. Although this was not previously described and negative associations between diseases are rare, the credibility of the finding was supported by consistent results in several previous studies and by the absence of an obvious artifactual explanation. Since that time, a variety of studies of AAA diagnosis, both by screening and prospective clinical follow-up, have confirmed the finding. Other studies have reported slower aneurysm enlargement and fewer repairs for rupture in diabetics. The seeming protective effect of diabetes for AAA contrasts with its causal role in

TABLE 1.—Odds Ratios for Diagnosis of AAA in Diabetics vs. Non-Diabetics

Cohort	Age (Years)	Gender	No. Subjects		No. AAA	Odds Ratio	95% CI
Ultrasound screening diagnosis of AAA							
Smith 1993[5]	65—75	men	2669		219	0.83[a]	NA (NS)
Pleumeekers 1995[6]	>55	both	5419		113	0.83[a]	NA (NS)
Kanagasabay 1996[7]	65—80	both	5392		218	0.80	0.41—1.58 (NS)
Lederle 1997[1]	50—79	97% men	73,451	3.0—3.9 cm:	2217	0.68	0.60—0.77
				≥4.0 cm:	985	0.54	0.44—0.65
Lederle 2000[10]	50—79	97% men	52,745	3.0—3.9 cm:	1237	0.60	0.50—0.71
				≥4.0 cm:	583	0.50	0.39—0.65
Le 2007[11]	65—83	men	12,203		933	0.79	0.63—0.98
Kent 2010[12]	<85	both	3,055,455		23,446	0.75	0.73—0.77
Svensjö 2011[13]	65	men	14,611		233	0.88[a]	NA (NS)
Prospective clinical diagnosis of AAA							
Törnwall 2001[14]	50	men	29,133		181	0.43[a]	0.16—1.15 (NS)
Rodin 2003[15]	>40	both	19,274		418	0.81[b]	NA (NS)
Wong 2007[16]	>40	men	39,352		376	0.55[b]	0.26—1.17 (NS)
Iribarren 2007[17]	>18	both	104,813		605	0.62[b]	0.36—1.05 (NS)
Baumgartner 2008[18]	>45	both	68,236		1722	0.59	0.54—0.66
Lederle 2008[19]	>50	women	161,808		184	0.29	0.13—0.68

AAA = abdominal aortic aneurysm, CI = confidence interval, NA = not available, NS = not statistically significant at 0.05 level.
Editor's Note: Please refer to original journal article for full references.
[a]Univariate relative risk calculated from numbers provided in article.
[b]Hazard ratio.

occlusive vascular disease and so provides a strong challenge to the traditional view of AAA as a manifestation of atherosclerosis. Research focused on a protective effect of diabetes has already increased our understanding of the etiology of AAA, and might eventually pave the way for new therapies to slow AAA progression (Table 1).

▶ The relationship between diabetes and abdominal aortic aneurysm (AAA) is indeed strange but nevertheless extremely interesting. The author, widely known for his work in this area, was one of the first investigators to demonstrate a negative correlation between diabetes and AAA (Table 1), namely, diabetic patients have lower rates of AAA development and less incidence of rupture. There is a growing body of literature that attempts to explain this association. For example, the group at Stanford has shown that hypoglycemia in mice is associated with slower AAA enlargement, and this effect is diminished with insulin therapy.[1] This brief report is worth reading as it emphasizes the improvements in our understanding of the pathophysiology of aneurysmal disease.

B. W. Starnes, MD

Reference

1. Miyama N, Dua MM, Yeung JJ, et al. Hyperglycemia limits experimental aortic aneurysm progression. *J Vasc Surg.* 2010;52:975-983.

Effects of Age on the Elastic Properties of the Intraluminal Thrombus and the Thrombus-covered Wall in Abdominal Aortic Aneurysms: Biaxial Extension Behaviour and Material Modelling
Tong J, Cohnert T, Regitnig P, et al (Graz Univ of Technology, Austria; Med Univ Graz, Austria)
Eur J Vasc Endovasc Surg 42:207-219, 2011

Objective.—The intraluminal thrombus (ILT) present in the majority of abdominal aortic aneurysms (AAAs) plays an important role in aneurysm wall weakening. Studying the age-dependent elastic properties of the ILT and the thrombus-covered wall provides a better understanding of the potential effect of ILT on AAA remodelling.

Materials and Methods.—A total of 43 AAA samples (mean age 67 ± 6 years) including ILT and AAA wall was harvested. Biaxial extension tests on the three individual ILT layers and the thrombus-covered wall were performed. Histological investigations of the thrombi were performed to determine four different age phases, and to correlate with the change in the mechanical properties. A three-dimensional material model was fitted to the experimental data.

Results.—The luminal layers of the ILT exhibit anisotropic stress responses, whereas the medial and the abluminal layers are isotropic materials. The stresses at failure in the equibiaxial protocol continuously decrease from the luminal to the abluminal side, whereby cracks, mainly oriented along the longitudinal direction, can be observed in the ruptured luminal layers. The thrombi in the third and fourth phases contribute to wall weakening and to an increase of the mechanical anisotropy of their covered walls. The material models for the thrombi and the thrombus-covered walls are in excellent agreement with the experimental data.

Conclusion.—Our results suggest that thrombus age might be a potential predictor for the strength of the wall underneath the ILT and AAA rupture.

▶ The authors performed a detailed analysis of intraluminal thrombus associated with abdominal aortic aneurysms. Intraluminal thrombus has been implicated in aneurysm size, aneurysm growth, and aneurysm rupture. In the current study, intraluminal thrombus was found to be heterogeneous, varied by location, and varied by organization. Luminal thrombus seemed to have stronger characteristics with both axial and longitudinal loads, whereas thrombus approximating the wall failed with lighter loads. At each location, samples were also heterogeneous. Some luminal samples were isotropic, while others were anisotropic; more importantly, they behaved differently in response to stress. In addition, aneurysm wall intimately associated with organized thrombus (assumed to be "older" thrombus) was found to fail at lower loads compared with aneurysm wall associated with fresh thrombus.

This study further implicates intraluminal thrombus as a potential marker for aneurysmal wall degeneration. At this stage, organized laminated thrombus is associated with an aneurysm wall that fatigues with less stress; more clinical research is needed to link types of intraluminal thrombus with aneurysm evolution.

Z. M. Arthurs, MD

Abdominal aortic aneurysm and abdominal wall hernia as manifestations of a connective tissue disorder

Antoniou GA, Georgiadis GS, Antoniou SA, et al (Democritus Univ of Thrace, Alexandroupolis, Greece; Hospital "Maria v. d. Aposteln" Neuwerk, Mönchengladbach, Germany)
J Vasc Surg 54:1175-1181, 2011

Background.—Abdominal aortic aneurysms (AAAs) and abdominal wall hernias represent chronic degenerative conditions. Both aortic aneurysms and inguinal hernias share common epidemiologic features, and several investigators have found an increased propensity for hernia development in patients treated for aortic aneurysms. Chronic inflammation and dysregulation in connective tissue metabolism constitute underlying biological processes, whereas genetic influences appear to be independently associated with both disease states. A literature review was conducted to identify all published evidence correlating aneurysms and hernias to a common pathology.

Methods.—PubMed/Medline was searched for studies investigating the clinical, biochemical, and genetic associations of AAAs and abdominal wall hernias. The literature was searched using the MeSH terms "aortic aneurysm, abdominal," "hernia, inguinal," "hernia, ventral," "collagen," "connective tissue," "matrix metalloproteinases," and "genetics" in all possible combinations. An evaluation, analysis, and critical overview of current clinical data and pathogenic mechanisms suggesting an association between aneurysms and hernias were undertaken.

Results.—Ample evidence lending support to the clinical correlation between AAAs and abdominal wall hernias exists. Pooled analysis demonstrated that patients undergoing aortic aneurysm repair through a midline abdominal incision have a 2.9-fold increased risk of developing a postoperative incisional hernia compared with patients treated for aortoiliac occlusive disease (odds ratio, 2.86; 95% confidence interval, 1.97-4.16; $P < .00001$), whereas the risk of inguinal hernia was 2.3 (odds ratio, 2.30; 95% confidence interval, 1.52-3.48; $P < .0001$). Emerging evidence has identified inguinal hernia as an independent risk factor for aneurysm development. Although mechanisms of extracellular matrix remodeling and the imbalance between connective tissue degrading enzymes and their inhibitors instigating inflammatory responses have separately been described for both disease states, comparative studies investigating these biological processes in aneurysm and hernia populations are scarce. A genetic predisposition has been documented in familial and observational segregation studies; however, the pertinent literature lacks sufficient supporting evidence for a common genetic basis for aneurysm and hernia.

Conclusions.—Insufficient data are currently available to support a systemic connective tissue defect affecting the structural integrity of the aortic and abdominal wall. Future investigations may elucidate obscure aspects of aneurysm and hernia pathophysiology and create novel targets for pharmaceutical and gene strategies for disease prevention and treatment (Figs 1 and 2).

▶ Abdominal aortic aneurysm pathophysiology is a complex process that involves risk factors, genetics, metabolic proteinase abnormalities, and collagen alterations. Abdominal wall hernias are a common disorder and share many of the same pathologic factors as abdominal aortic aneurysm. In this review, the

FIGURE 1.—Meta-analysis of studies comparing the incidence of incisional hernias in patients with abdominal aortic aneurysms (*AAAs*) and aortoiliac occlusive disease (*AOD*). CI, Confidence interval; *OR*, odds ratio. (Reprinted from the Journal of Vascular Surgery, Antoniou GA, Georgiadis GS, Antoniou SA, et al. Abdominal aortic aneurysm and abdominal wall hernia as manifestations of a connective tissue disorder. *J Vasc Surg*. 2011;54:1175-1181. Copyright 2011, with permission from The Society for Vascular Surgery.)

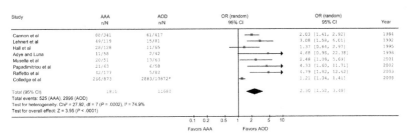

Study	AAA n/N	AOD n/N	OR (random) 95% CI	OR (random) 95% CI	Year
Cannon et al	88/341	61/417		2.03 [1.41, 2.92]	1984
Lehnert et al	49/119	15/81		3.08 [1.58, 6.01]	1992
Hall et al	28/128	11/65		1.37 [0.64, 2.97]	1995
Adye and Luna	11/58	2/42		4.68 [0.98, 22.38]	1998
Musella et al	20/51	13/63		2.48 [1.08, 5.69]	2001
Papadimitriou et al	21/63	6/58		4.33 [1.60, 11.71]	2002
Raffetto et al	42/177	5/82		4.79 [1.82, 12.62]	2003
Colledge et al	266/873	2883/10872		1.21 [1.04, 1.41]	2008
Total (95% CI)	**1810**	**11680**		**2.30 [1.52, 3.48]**	

Total events: 525 (AAA), 2996 (AOD)
Test for heterogeneity: Chi² = 27.92, df = 7 (P = .0002), I² = 74.9%
Test for overall effect: Z = 3.95 (P < .0001)

0.1 0.2 0.5 1 2 5 10
Favors AAA   Favors AOD

FIGURE 2.—Meta-analysis of studies reporting on the risk of inguinal hernia in patients with abdominal aortic aneurysms (*AAAs*) and controls. *AOD*, Aortoiliac occlusive disease; *CI*, confidence interval; *OR*, odds ratio. (Reprinted from the Journal of Vascular Surgery, Antoniou GA, Georgiadis GS, Antoniou SA, et al. Abdominal aortic aneurysm and abdominal wall hernia as manifestations of a connective tissue disorder. *J Vasc Surg*. 2011;54:1175-1181. Copyright 2011, with permission from The Society for Vascular Surgery.)

authors perform an exhaustive literature review to identify all published evidence correlating aneurysms and hernias to a common pathology. From a pathogenesis perspective, the major findings of this review are as follows: (1) In both abdominal aortic aneurysm and abdominal wall hernias, there exist mechanisms of extracellular matrix remodeling that involve the imbalance between connective tissue degrading enzymes and their inhibitors leading to a chronic state of inflammatory responses. (2) Comparative studies investigating these biological processes in aneurysm and hernia populations are scarce. A genetic predisposition has been documented in familial and observational segregation studies; however, the pertinent literature lacks sufficient supporting evidence for a common genetic basis for aneurysm and hernia. Both clinicians and vascular surgeons in their clinical practices have seen the association of patients with abdominal aortic aneurysms and abdominal wall hernias. The interesting fact is that evidence has identified inguinal hernia as an independent risk factor for aneurysm development, with male patients with inguinal hernia having a 4-fold increased prevalence of abdominal aortic aneurysms compared with control subjects without hernias. These findings have interesting considerations for screening and early treatment, especially with pharmacologic targets. In addition, an interesting finding is that patients undergoing aortic aneurysm repair through a midline abdominal incision have a 2.9-fold increased risk of developing a postoperative incisional hernia compared with patients treated for aortoiliac occlusive disease (odds ratio [OR], 2.86; 95% confidence interval [CI], 1.97—4.16; *P* < .00001) (Fig 1). The reported rates from comparative studies evaluating the incidence of postoperative incisional hernias range between 10% and 37% for patients treated for abdominal aortic aneurysms and 3% and 19% for those having aortoiliac occlusive disease. Patients treated for abdominal aortic aneurysm have a 2.3-fold increased risk of inguinal hernia development compared with aortoiliac occlusive disease reconstruction (OR, 2.30; 95% CI, 1.52—3.48; *P* < .0001; Fig 2). Reported prevalence of inguinal hernias range between 19% and 41% for patients with a history of abdominal aortic aneurysm repair, whereas values for nonaneurysm patients range between 5% and 27%. In this review, the authors provide a detailed analysis of the biochemical changes that take place with the structural proteins elastin and collagen, the importance of inflammatory infiltrate, the effects on smooth muscle function and oxidative stress, and the changes that occur in the extracellular matrix that are initiated by the imbalance of matrix metalloproteinases and their inhibitors. Commonalities between abdominal aortic aneurysms and abdominal wall hernias are an increased proteolytic activity and disruption of protease/ antiprotease balance. This results in an abnormal connective tissue remodeling process, with disorganized collagen synthesis and enhanced degradation. Inflammation is an important feature in the pathologic process of both conditions. This is a good review of the basic science changes that occur in abdominal aortic aneurysms and abdominal wall hernias. All of these findings would suggest a common pathophysiologic and genetic mechanism between abdominal aortic aneurysms and hernias. Although the evidence supports a clinical and basic science association between abdominal aortic aneurysms and abdominal wall hernias, there are no studies that have evaluated a common gene to explain the systemic effects in both conditions. As the authors state "Insufficient data are currently available to support a systemic connective tissue defect affecting the structural integrity of the aortic and abdominal wall." Hopefully in future research a unified biological theory will be discovered that links aneurysms and hernias to a common pathology through which potential directed therapy may be possible to treat this perplexing but fascinating set of conditions.

J. D. Raffetto, MD

Low Prevalence of Abdominal Aortic Aneurysm Among 65-Year-Old Swedish Men Indicates a Change in the Epidemiology of the Disease
Svensjö S, Björck M, Gürtelschmid M, et al (Uppsala Univ, Sweden)
Circulation 124:1118-1123, 2011

Background.—Screening elderly men with ultrasound is an established method to reduce mortality from ruptured abdominal aortic aneurysm (AAA; Evidence Level 1a). Such programs are being implemented and generally consist of a single scan at 65 years of age. We report the results from screening 65-year-old men for AAA in middle Sweden.

Methods and Results.—All 65-year-old men (n=26 256), identified through the National Population Registry, were invited to an ultrasound examination. An AAA was defined as a maximum infrarenal aortic diameter of ≥ 30 mm. In total, 22 187 (85%) accepted, and 373 AAAs were detected (1.7%; 95% confidence interval, 1.5 to 1.9). With 127 previously known AAAs (repaired/under surveillance) included, the total prevalence of the disease in the population was 2.2% (95% confidence interval, 2.0 to 2.4). Self-reported smoking (odds ratio, 3.4; $P<0.001$), coronary artery disease (odds ratio, 2.0; $P<0.001$), and hypertension (odds ratio, 1.6; $P=0.001$) were independently associated with AAA in a multivariate logistic regression model. Thirteen percent of the entire population reported to be current smokers, one third of the frequency reported in the 1980s. The observed low prevalence of AAA was explained mainly by this change in smoking habits.

Conclusions.—On the basis of the observed reduced exposure to risk factors, lower-than-expected prevalence of AAA among 65-year-old men, unchanged AAA repair rate, and significantly improved longevity of the elderly population, the current generally agreed-on AAA screening model can be questioned. Important issues to address are the threshold diameter for follow-up, the possible need for rescreening at a higher age, and selective screening among smokers (Fig 1).

▶ The most effective method to reduce mortality from abdominal aortic aneurysm (AAA) appears to be early detection of aneurysm by screening with ultrasound and prophylactic surgery in appropriately selected patients. A common recommendation for a screening model is one in which 65-year-old men are invited to a 1-time ultrasound screening. In Sweden, there has been a rapid introduction of such screening programs, and now there is practically nationwide coverage.[1] By 2009, screening programs had been implemented in 5 contiguous counties of central Sweden (Fig 1). The 65-year-old men in these counties are identified every 3 months through the national population registry. They are then invited to a 1-time ultrasound examination of the abdominal aorta. In 2009, these 5 counties comprised approximately 15% of Sweden's population (1 404 978 individuals). In this study, the authors report their results of screening 65-year-old men for AAA in middle Sweden. The population-based study design and the high participation in the screening program (85%) suggests the results presented here are generalizable, at least to the Swedish population. The

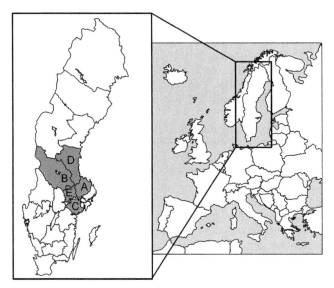

FIGURE 1.—The setting of the study. Five counties in middle Sweden—(A) Uppsala, population 331 898; (B) Dalarna, population 276 454; (C) Sörmland, population 269 053, (D) Gävleborg, population 276 220, and (E) Västmanland, population 251 353—constitute the uptake area. Population numbers from 2009. (Reprinted from Svensjö S, Björck M, Gürtelschmid M, et al. Low prevalence of abdominal aortic aneurysm among 65-year-old Swedish men indicates a change in the epidemiology of the disease. *Circulation.* 2011;124:1118-1123. © American Heart Association, Inc.)

prevalence of the AAA in this study is one-half to one-third of that reported elsewhere, and it seemed to parallel a dramatic reduction in the prevalence of smoking in the patients in the area screened. The authors point out that the decreased prevalence of smoking combined with the significant increase in life expectancy of the male population at the risk for AAA has implications for the methodology of screening programs. The effectiveness of screening programs depends on the prevalence of the disease and of the relevant risk factors. Based on what is apparently a decreased prevalence of disease and decreased risk factors, cost-effectiveness of current screening programs may need to be reevaluated considering current epidemiological data.

G. L. Moneta, MD

Reference

1. Wanhainen A, Björck M. The Swedish experience of screening for abdominal aortic aneurysm. *J Vas Surg.* 2011;53:1164-1165.

First-year results of a national abdominal aortic aneurysm screening programme in a single centre
Conway AM, Malkawi AH, Hinchliffe RJ, et al (St George's Healthcare NHS Trust, London, UK)
Br J Surg 99:73-77, 2012

Background.—The UK Multicentre Aneurysm Screening Study (MASS) demonstrated reduced mortality from screening for abdominal aortic aneurysm (AAA). As a result, the National Health Service AAA Screening Programme was introduced in England. This study reports the results from an early-implementation screening centre.

Methods.—Men aged 65 years were invited to attend an ultrasound assessment. Data were analysed for 15 months from the onset of the screening programme.

Results.—A total of 6091 men aged 65 years were invited between April 2009 and June 2010, of whom 2037 (33·4 per cent) failed to attend. There were 162 self-referrals (median age 71·3 years) so that 4216 men were screened. Of those scanned, 4146 (98·3 per cent) had an aortic diameter of less than 3·0 cm, 65 (1·5 per cent) had an aneurysm measuring 3·0—5·4 cm, and five (0·1 per cent) had an aneurysm with a diameter of 5·5 cm and above. The presence of an aneurysm was more common in those who self-referred than in the invited group (*P* < 0·001). All 70 screen-detected aneurysms were found in white men.

Conclusion.—The prevalence of AAA was lower than expected. This reflects the younger age of this cohort compared with those in published large multicentre studies and the diverse ethnic background of the local population.

▶ This is another article that has come out in the last year or 2 with significant implications for abdominal aortic aneurysm (AAA) screening programs. Several studies have found reduced mortality from AAA with screening programs. AAA screening is cheap and easy to do; therefore, AAA screening seems like a good idea. Even Bob Dole and the US congress and senate have bought into the concept! However, for screening programs to be worthwhile, ie, medically and cost effective, there must be reasonable yield, and this yield will depend on who is screened and when. This article points out that screening of AAA at age 65 does not find as many aneurysms as would have been expected based on the previous trials evaluating AAA screening. However, the epidemiology of AAA seems to be changing, and as the patient population ages, it may be necessary to reevaluate the concept of one-time screening of men at age 65 as the best approach. Age 65 may be too young for screening, and one-time screening may be too restrictive in an aging population in which there are minimally invasive methods of treating the AAA. We need data on how many patients negative for AAA at age 65 are found to have developed an AAA at age 80 and who are healthy enough to justify intervention at that age. We may have jumped the gun a bit in implementing AAA screening in its current form. Some "tweaking" of current protocols for AAA screening will likely be necessary as the population ages and the prevalence of smoking goes down.

G. L. Moneta, MD

Systematic review and meta-analysis of growth rates of small abdominal aortic aneurysms

Powell JT, Sweeting MJ, Brown LC, et al (Imperial College London, UK; Inst of Public Health, Cambridge, UK; et al)
Br J Surg 98:609-618, 2011

Background.—Small abdominal aortic aneurysms are usually asymptomatic and managed safely in ultrasound surveillance programmes until they grow to a diameter threshold where intervention is considered. The aim of this study was to synthesize systematically the published data on growth rates for small aneurysms to investigate the evidence basis for surveillance intervals.

Methods.—This was a systematic review of the literature published before January 2010, which identified 61 potentially eligible reports. Detailed review yielded 15 studies providing growth rates for aneurysms 3·0-5·5 cm in diameter (14 in millimetres per year, 1 as percentage change per year). These studies included 7630 people (predominantly men) enrolled during 1976—2005.

Results.—The pooled mean growth rate was 2·32 (95 per cent confidence interval 1·95 to 2·70) mm/year but there was very high heterogeneity between studies; the growth rate ranged from −0·33 to +3·95 mm/year. Six studies reported growth rates by 5-mm diameter bands, which showed the trend for growth rate to increase with aneurysm diameter. Simple methods to determine growth rate were associated with higher estimates. Meta-regression analysis showed that a 10-mm increase in aneurysm diameter was associated with a mean(s.e.m.) 1·62(0·20) mm/year increase in growth rate. Neither mean age nor percentage of women in each study had a significant effect. On average, a 3·5-cm aneurysm would take 6·2 years to reach 5·5 cm, whereas a 4·5-cm aneurysm would take only 2·3 years.

Conclusion.—There was considerable variation in the reported growth rates of small aneurysms beyond that explained by aneurysm diameter. Fuller evidence on which to base surveillance intervals for patients in screening programmes requires a meta-analysis based on individual patient data (Fig 2).

▶ Four population-based screening trials for abdominal aortic aneurysms (AAA) provide evidence in favor of population screening of older men for AAA. Based on these studies, many institutions and countries have adopted policies for screening for AAA in older men. However, although the screening process itself appears effective in reducing death from ruptured AAA, there is relatively little information on optimal surveillance protocols in patients whose AAA has been identified but does not meet size criteria for operative repair. In addition to the screening trials, there have been other observational studies that have reported growth rates of small AAAs. These have resulted in disparate recommendations for follow-up examinations for AAAs that do not meet threshold criteria for repair. Some of these recommendations have used simple linear regression methods to estimate growth rates.[1] However, such methods do not account for the fact that aneurysm growth rate may accelerate with increasing diameter. Additional questions include whether aneurysm growth rate is faster in smokers and slower in patients with diabetes, and whether there are any gender differences in growth rates. Given these considerations, the authors thought to synthesize the published data on growth rates for small AAA in a systematic review to provide an evidence basis for surveillance

Reference	Baseline (mm)	AAA growth (mm/year)
Brady et al.[10]	28–85	2·60 (2·54, 2·66)
Brown et al.[16]	30–49	3·82 (3·51, 4·14)
Karlsson et al.[9]	35–49	2·20 (1·93, 2·47)
PATI[13]	30–50	2·38 (2·13, 2·63)
Lederle et al.[17]	40–54	3·20 (3·04, 3·36)
Lindholt et al.[18]	30–49	2·80 (2·41, 3·19)
McCarthy et al.[8]	30–39	1·90 (1·72, 2·07)
Santilli et al.[19]	30–39	1·60 (1·46, 1·74)
Schlösser et al.[21]	30–55	2·50 (1·99, 3·01)
Schouten et al.[7]	25–53	2·95 (2·50, 3·40)
Solberg et al.[12]	30 to > 49	1·82 (1·55, 2·09)
Vardulaki et al.[22] Huntingdon	30–49	−0·33 (−0·79, 0·14)
Vardulaki et al.[22] Chichester	30–59	0·92 (0·64, 1·21)
Vega de Céniga et al.[11]	30–49	2·87 (2·42, 3·32)
Vega de Céniga et al.[23]	40–49	3·95 (3·11, 4·79)
Overall $I^2 = 97·9\%$, $P < 0·001$		2·32 (1·95, 2·70)

FIGURE 2.—Overall abdominal aortic aneurysm (AAA) growth rate estimate for each study, with baseline AAA diameter size range. Estimates were pooled using a random-effects model, owing to considerable heterogeneity ($I^2 = 97·9$ per cent). An estimate from Schewe and colleagues[20] could not be included as no standard error was available. AAA growth rates are shown with 95 per cent confidence intervals. PATI, Propranolol Aneurysm Trial Investigators. *Editor's Note*: Please refer to original journal article for full references. (Reprinted from Powell JT, Sweeting MJ, Brown LC, et al. Systematic review and meta-analysis of growth rates of small abdominal aortic aneurysms. *Br J Surg.* 2011;98:609-618. © British Journal of Surgery Society Ltd. Reproduced with permission. Permission is granted by John Wiley & Sons Ltd on behalf of the BJSS Ltd.)

intervals. This study provides reasonable evidence that growth rates of AAAs increase with aneurysm diameter. However, because of the marked heterogeneity of growth rates in individual studies (Fig 2), it cannot completely satisfy the other primary goal of the study, which was to determine optimal surveillance intervals. Whereas the data would indicate that larger aneurysms grow faster than smaller aneurysms, something most of us already suspected, it does not provide information on the influence of patient characteristics, including age, sex, smoking, diabetes, and other relevant factors on growth rates that would help optimize recommendations for surveillance intervals. Because the patient-specific data are not available, the data also cannot justify prophylactic repair of so-called borderline AAAs using the reasoning that the AAA will soon reach the threshold level for repair.

G. L. Moneta, MD

Reference

1. McCarthy RJ, Shaw E, Whyman MR, Earnshaw JJ, Poskitt KR, Heather BP. Recommendations for screening intervals for small aortic aneurysms. *Br J Surg.* 2003;90:821-826.

A Randomised Placebo-controlled Double-blind Trial to Evaluate Lipid-lowering Pharmacotherapy on Proteolysis and Inflammation in Abdominal Aortic Aneurysms

Dawson JA, Choke E, Loftus IM, et al (St George's Hosp, London, UK)
Eur J Vasc Endovasc Surg 41:28-35, 2011

Objectives.—Modulation of abdominal aortic aneurysm (AAA) expansion by HMG-CoA reductase inhibitors (statins) might be linked to reducing IL-6 and MMP-9, which may be consequent on reducing plasma cholesterol. Ezetimibe is a novel cholesterol absorption inhibitor used in combination with statins. This pilot study compared the biological effects of ezetimibe combination therapy with simvastatin alone on parameters relevant to aneurysm expansion including cytokines and proteolytic enzymes.

Design.—Randomised placebo-controlled double-blind trial.

Materials & Methods.—Eighteen patients scheduled for elective open AAA repair were randomised to simvastatin 40 mg plus ezetimibe 10 mg ($n = 9$), or simvastatin 40 mg plus placebo ($n = 9$), for 32.5 days (IQR 28−50.5) until the day of surgery. Total concentrations of TNF-α, IL-1β, IL-6, IL-8, IL-10, MMPs-1, -2, -3, -8, -9, -12, -13, TIMP-1 and -2 were measured in plasma, aortic wall homogenates and tissue culture explants.

Results.—Two patients in the placebo arm did not undergo open repair precluding aortic samples. Ezetimibe was associated with a significant reduction in aortic wall MMP-9 ($p = 0.02$) and aortic wall IL-6 ($p = 0.02$), associated with a reduction in plasma lipids.

Conclusions.—These results suggest that ezetimibe combination therapy reduces aortic wall proteolysis and inflammation, key processes that drive AAA expansion. A larger RCT is justified focussing on aneurysm growth rates in small AAA (Figs 2 and 3).

▶ Ezetimibe is a cholesterol absorption inhibitor. When combined with the statin simvastatin, ezetimibe has a synergistic effect on reducing cholesterol levels.[1] Thus far, despite 40 years of research, there is no pharmacologic agent unequivocally demonstrated to decrease or halt abdominal aortic aneurysm (AAA) expansion. It has, however, been suggested that statins, HMG-CoA (or 3-hydroxy-3-methyl-glutaryl-coenzyme A) reductase inhibitors, can reduce AAA growth both in animal models and human cohort studies. It is virtually impossible to perform a randomized trial of statin therapy in AAA patients because of near ubiquitous use of statins in patients with vascular risk factors. The authors therefore tested the hypothesis of adding ezetimibe to a statin agent to see if the additional cholesterol-lowering effects of ezetimibe would affect parameters likely relevant to aneurysm expansion, such as matrix metalloproteinases (MMPs), tissue inhibitor of matrix metalloproteinases (TIMPS), and cytokines. The research is particularly relevant in the ever expanding use of aneurysm screening programs likely to identify a large number of small AAAs for which there is currently no treatment. In samples taken directly from the aortic wall, the authors found that ezetimibe decreased aortic wall MMP-9 levels as well as interleukin-6 levels (Figs 2 and 3). The data are consistent

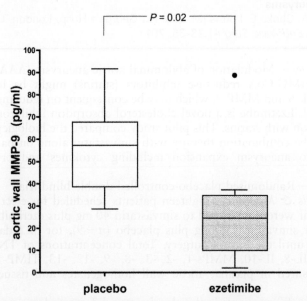

FIGURE 2.—Box and whisker plot representing aortic wall MMP-9 in the ezetimibe and placebo groups. Whiskers represent data within 1.5 IQR of the lower and upper quartiles. Mild outliers are represented by dots. (Reprinted from European Journal of Vascular and Endovascular Surgery, Dawson JA, Choke E, Loftus IM, et al. A randomised placebo-controlled double-blind trial to evaluate lipid-lowering pharmacotherapy on proteolysis and inflammation in abdominal aortic aneurysms. *Eur J Vasc Endovasc Surg.* 2011;41:28-35. Copyright 2011, with permission from the European Society for Vascular Surgery.)

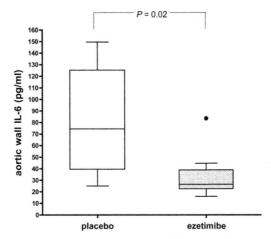

FIGURE 3.—Box and whisker plot representing aortic wall interleukin-6 in the ezetimibe and placebo groups. Whiskers represent data within 1.5 IQR of the lower and upper quartiles. Mild outliers are represented by dots. (Reprinted from European Journal of Vascular and Endovascular Surgery, Dawson JA, Choke E, Loftus IM, et al. A randomised placebo-controlled double-blind trial to evaluate lipid-lowering pharmacotherapy on proteolysis and inflammation in abdominal aortic aneurysms. *Eur J Vasc Endovasc Surg.* 2011;41:28-35. Copyright 2011, with permission from the European Society for Vascular Surgery.)

with human cohort studies that have reported a 50% reduction in aneurysm expansion associated with statin use.[2] The fact that statin inhibition of aneurysm growth may be greatest in small AAAs is an additional argument for widespread implementation of aortic aneurysm screening programs.

G. L. Moneta, MD

References

1. Bays HE, Ose L, Fraser N, et al. A multicenter, randomized, double-blind, placebo-controlled, factorial design study to evaluate the lipid-altering efficacy and safety profile of the ezetimibe/simvastatin tablet compared with ezetimibe and simvastatin monotherapy in patients with primary hypercholesterolemia. *Clin Ther.* 2004; 26:1758-1773.
2. Sukhija R, Aronow WS, Sandhu R, Kakar P, Babu S. Mortality and size of abdominal aortic aneurysm at long-term follow-up of patients not treated surgically and treated with and without statins. *Am J Cardiol.* 2006;97:279-280.

The influence of gender and aortic aneurysm size on eligibility for endovascular abdominal aortic aneurysm repair
Sweet MP, Fillinger MF, Morrison TM, et al (U.S. Food and Drug Administration, Rockville, MD; Dartmouth Hitchcock Med Ctr, Lebanon, NH)
J Vasc Surg 54:931-937, 2011

Objectives.—The purpose of this study was to compare the eligibility of men and women with infrarenal abdominal aortic aneurysms (AAAs) for on-label endovascular aneurysm repair (EVAR) as part of the clinician-Food & Drug Administration (FDA) collaborative effort, the Characterization of Human Aortic Anatomy Project (CHAP).

Methods.—Computed tomography (CT) scans with 3D reconstruction from a single institution obtained between July 1996 and December 2009, including standardized measurements by a blinded third-party (M2S, West Lebanon, NH) were examined. For inclusion, abdominal aortic aneurysm (AAA) had to be infrarenal, unrepaired, and >5 cm, or 4 cm to 5 cm if the orthogonal sac diameter was more than twice the aortic diameter at the renal level. Scans were included regardless of subsequent EVAR, open repair, or lack of treatment. One thousand sixty-three unique, unrepaired AAAs were analyzed.

Results.—Neck length, diameter, and angulation differ for women (P < .001) even after adjustment for patient age and AAA size. EVAR eligibility based on device Instructions for Use (IFU) criterion is affected by gender. Neck length <15 mm was found in 47% of men and 63% of women. Neck angulation exceeding 60 degrees was found in 12% of men and 26% of women. Minimum iliac diameter of 6 mm was found in 35% of men and 55% of women. Only 32% of men and 12% of women met all three neck criterion and had iliac lumen diameters >6 mm. Logistic regression modeling shows that older patient age (odds ratio [OR], 0.84 per decade), increased aneurysm diameter (OR, 0.70 per cm), and female gender (OR, 0.4) are each independently associated with decreased odds of meeting all device IFU neck criterion (P < .05). EVAR eligibility by neck criterion does not decline significantly until AAA size exceeds 5.5 cm in women and 6.5 cm in men.

Conclusion.—Women are significantly less likely to meet device IFU criterion for EVAR. Aortic neck criteria and iliac access are important for men and women, but more women than men fail to meet IFU criterion. Devices that accommodate shorter infrarenal AAA neck length will have the greatest impact on expanding on-label EVAR regardless of gender. Lower profile devices and those that accommodate higher neck angulation are expected to expand EVAR eligibility further for women. EVAR eligibility is unlikely to be lost as AAAs enlarge to 5.5 cm in women and 6.5 cm in men. Observation of small AAAs until they reach the standard threshold size for repair should not compromise EVAR eligibility.

▶ As part of the Characterization of Human Aortic Anatomy Project (CHAP), a collaboration between the US Food and Drug Administration (FDA) and clinicians to better characterize aortic anatomy in the context of endovascular aortic devices, this study quantitatively describes differences in abdominal aortic aneurysm (AAA) morphology between men and women using anatomic measurements made by blinded observers from high-quality 3-dimensional computed tomography imaging from M2S. While differences in aortic anatomic features based on gender have been previously observed, this large data set focuses on the relationship among gender, Instructions for Use (IFU) eligibility, and AAA size. While several differences are noted showing less likelihood for women to meet IFU criteria based on aortic neck length less than 15 mm, neck angulation greater than 60°, and iliac access diameter less than 6 mm, as well as decreased EVAR eligibility when AAA reach 5.5 cm in women and 6.5 in men, these anatomic observations should be qualified. First, as a single-center study from an academic regional tertiary referral center, distribution of the anatomic data is skewed, reflecting more complex cases. Second, as is the problem with other AAA studies looking at gender, frequency of AAA in these studies is lower for women than for men. A disparate gender distribution is also noted here (76% men [N = 812]; 24% women [N = 24]), which has some statistical implications. Lastly, AAA measurements are devoid of any clinical data, leaving any connection to clinically important factors short. Recalling that AAA anatomy and potential rupture risk based on gender and size may be different in men and women, this data set does not close the gap between these observations and clinically relevant information. While this study provides interesting anatomic information, even when placed in this context, extrapolation to a larger population awaits future planned CHAP directions. Ultimately, this information will be of use to clinicians, industry, and FDA in terms of new-generation devices directed at these anatomic challenges. However, whenever the FDA is involved in evaluation of use of FDA-approved devices within IFU criteria, there is always concern that these data can be used to limit options for use of these devices, so care needs to be taken in how these data are interpreted and implemented.

M. A. Passman, MD

DynaCT in Pre-treatment Evaluation of Aortic Aneurysm before EVAR

Eide KR, Ødegård A, Myhre HO, et al (Sør-Trøndelag Univ College, Trondheim, Norway; Univ Hosp of Trondheim, Norway)
Eur J Vasc Endovasc Surg 42:332-339, 2011

Objective.—DynaCT® is a method for obtaining computed tomography (CT)-like images using a C-arm system. Our aim was to compare the accuracy of these images to multidetector CT (MDCT) images prior to endovascular aortic repair (EVAR).

Methods.—A non-consecutive group of 20 elective patients were prospectively exposed to MDCT and one additional DynaCT before EVAR. Six arterial measurements and nine anatomical areas were chosen to: (1) visualise the peri-aortic soft tissue and assess the possibility to diagnose a potential haemorrhage from a ruptured aneurysm and (2) make the pre-treatment measurements before insertion of stent graft. Differences between modalities and readers were statistically compared using a linear mixed model.

Results.—For maximum aortic diameter, a significant difference of 1.3 mm was found between techniques ($p = 0.043$). Visibility scores were significantly better for all areas in MDCT data. Pre-treatment evaluation with DynaCT before EVAR was possible for all areas; evaluation of the iliac arteries were suboptimal due to a limited imaging volume size. Significant inter-reader differences were found for all anatomical areas.

Conclusion.—The result indicates that DynaCT gives sufficient information to determine the correct treatment and for selecting the proper stent graft before EVAR. A limited volume size reduces the evaluation of the iliac arteries.

▶ Two of the most common hybrid suite manufacturers, Siemens (Medical Solutions, Germany) and Philips (Philips Healthcare, The Netherlands), have packaged rotational computed tomography (CT) into their most current vascular software packages. This technology has been used in advanced neurosurgical and orthopedic surgeries, but its usefulness has yet to be defined for vascular surgery. The current article compares Siemens DynaCT with standard multidetector CT (MDCT).

Qualitative comparisons of anatomic structures outside of the vasculature are comparable to early-generation CT scanners. This study highlights that gross information regarding retroperitoneal structures can be obtained with DynaCT, but it is limited when compared with MDCT. However, DynaCT performed very well for discrete arterial measurements such as maximal aneurysm diameter, diameter of the neck, and length from the renal arteries to aortic bifurcation. The variation in measurements ranged from 0.4 to 1.5 mm, which is not clinically relevant for most aortic procedures. In addition, the authors' inter-reader variability was higher than the variability between imaging modalities; thus, the provider interpreting the examination is more important than the choice of imaging modality.

Z. M. Arthurs, MD

Triglyceride to HDL Ratio is a Reliable Predictor of Adverse Outcomes in Risk Stratification for Candidates Undergoing Abdominal Aortic Surgery
Gambardella I, Blair PH, McKinley A, et al (Royal Victoria Hosp, Belfast, UK)
Eur J Vasc Endovasc Surg 41:249-255, 2011

Introduction.—The aim of this study was to establish if an elevated triglyceride to high-density lipoprotein (HDL) ratio (THR) is not only a risk factor for cardiovascular and overall morbidity as the updated evidence shows, but could also be employed as a significant predictor for surgical adverse outcomes and hence be a valid tool for risk stratification of candidates undergoing abdominal aortic surgery.

Methods.—This is a single-centre retrospective analysis of 2224 patients who underwent open abdominal aortic surgery between January 1996 and 2009. This cohort was divided into quartiles of THR. A list of covariates has been entered with THR into a multiple logistic model with forwards stepwise selection. The obtained result is an adjusted model, conceived to establish the association between THR and perioperative adverse events. Discrimination of the model so obtained and comparison with vascular-specific risk stratification scoring systems were evaluated using the area under the receiver operating characteristic (AUROC).

Results.—THR had the highest predictive value for the outcomes of interest. The adjusted odds ratios (ORs) per every 0.1 augmentation of THR

TABLE 2.—Percentages of the Outcomes of Interest, in the Whole Population and Amongst THR Quartiles

Adverse Event	Overall %	THR Quartiles %				P for Trend
		Q1	Q2		Q3	
Morbidity:						
- Cardiac	1.3	0.4	0.7	1.2	2.6	<.005
- Respiratory	4.1	2.2	2.7	4.2	4.9	<.005
- Renal	1.1	0.6	0.9	1.3	2.5	< 005
Mortality	0.9	0.5	0.7	1.1	1.8	<.005

were 1.41 (1.08—1.88) for cardiac, 1.38 (1.09—1.84) for respiratory, 1.27 (1.06—1.54) for renal adverse events and 1.02 (0.84—1.23) for mortality.

Regarding mortality, either of the scoring systems Vascular Physiological and Operative Severity Score for the enUmeration of Mortality and morbidity (POSSUM) and customised probability index (CPI) and the THR ranked as moderate discriminators, with THR performing the worst (AUROC 0.71) compared with Vascular POSSUM (AUROC 0.76) and CPI (AUROC 0.78). THR performed as a very strong predictor of morbidity (AUROC 0.86), ranking above Vascular POSSUM (AUROC 0.72).

Conclusions.—THR is a significant predictor of perioperative morbidity and mortality. THR offers a broad outlook on the metabolic state of patients undergoing major abdominal aortic surgery and hence their propensity to adverse events, allowing us to risk-stratify the prognostic outcome of surgical intervention and possibly intervene preoperatively to optimise results (Table 2).

▶ An elevated triglyceride to high-density lipoprotein ratio (THR) is both a risk factor for cardiovascular morbidity and mortality and overall mortality (Table 2). Risk stratification in patients undergoing vascular surgery attracts the attention of many clinical researchers. However, effective risk stratification in vascular surgical patients with high sensitivities and specificities for cardiovascular morbidity and mortality following vascular surgery has not been achieved. Elevated THR is strongly related to hyperinsulinemia in the overall concept of metabolic syndrome. Elevated THR is also associated with relative hypercoagulable states as mediated through deficient fibrinolysis and higher levels of plasminogen activator inhibitor-1. Patients with elevated THRs also have evidence of an increased inflammatory state. Based on these and other determinations, the authors finding that an elevated THR is a significant predictor of perioperative morbidity and mortality following abdominal aortic aneurysm (AAA) repair makes sense. Triglyceride and high-density lipoprotein cholesterol levels are routinely available through testing. In the elective patient, improving the THR prior to AAA surgery should probably be considered.

G. L. Moneta, MD

Preoperative Spirometry Results as a Determinant for Long-term Mortality after EVAR for AAA

Ohrlander T, Dencker M, Acosta S (Eksjö County Hosp, Sweden; Skäne Univ Hosp, Malmö, Sweden)
Eur J Vasc Endovasc Surg 43:43-47, 2012

Objectives.—The aim of this study was to analyse lung function test determinants for long-term mortality after standard endovascular aneurysm repair (EVAR) for infrarenal abdominal aortic aneurysm (AAA).

Design.—Retrospective analysis.

Materials.—Three-hundred and four consecutive patients treated electively with EVAR (Zenith® stent grafts, Cook) between May 1998 and February 2006 were prospectively enrolled in a computerised database.

Methods.—The Global Initiative for Chronic Obstructive Lung Diseases (GOLD) guideline was used to grade the severity of obstructive lung disease. Mortality was checked until 1 December 2010. Median follow-up time was 68 (interquartile range (IQR) 40—94) months.

Results.—The percentage of patients with mild, moderate or severe (grade 3) chronic obstructive pulmonary disease (COPD) was 9.9%, 23.2% and 7.7%, respectively. In a combined medical severity assessment, arterial partial pressure of oxygen (PaO_2) <8.0 kPa or COPD, grade ≥ 3 (hazard ratio (HR) 2.06; 95% confidence interval (CI) (1.24—3.42)), anaemia (HR 1.72; 95% CI (1.21—2.44)), chronic kidney disease, stage ≥ 3 (HR 1.55; 95% CI (1.08—2.24)) and age ≥ 80 years (HR 1.55; 95% CI (1.04—2.31)) were independently associated with long-term mortality. Lower forced expiratory volume in 1 s (FEV_1) ($p = 0.002$) and lower forced vital capacity (FVC) ($p = 0.003$) were independently associated with long-term mortality.

Conclusions.—Our findings strengthen the need for formal evaluation of lung function with spirometry prior to proceeding to AAA repair.

▶ These authors suggest that chronic obstructive pulmonary disease (COPD) is underdiagnosed and under-reported in patients with abdominal aortic aneurysms. The purpose of this study was to analyze lung function test determinants for long-term mortality after standard endovascular aneurysm repair (EVAR). A total of 304 consecutive patients were evaluated over 8 years, of whom 233 underwent preoperative spirometry.

The authors suggest that severity of COPD or forced expiratory volume in the first second of expiration or forced vital capacity should be included in preoperative risk stratification models to identify high-risk patients with expected short-term survival. Even in large aneurysms exceeding 6 cm in diameter, elective EVAR in patients with severe COPD may seldom be indicated.

This article strengthens the argument for formal spirometry prior to proceeding to abdominal aortic aneurysm repair. Patients with COPD have an increased risk of mortality, which must be balanced against risk of rupture of the aneurysm.

B. W. Starnes, MD

Part One: All Major Arterial Interventions Should Now be Performed in High Volume Centres — Abdominal Aortic Aneurysms

Thompson M, Holt P, Loftus I (St George's Hosp NHS Trust, London, UK)
Eur J Vasc Endovasc Surg 42:411-418, 2011

Background.—Vascular professionals are still debating whether complex surgical interventions such as abdominal aortic aneurysm (AAA) treatment should be performed predominantly at centers with a greater caseload and experience or can be done safely at local, low-volume provider hospitals. Evidence supporting the premise that fewer patients die immediately after elective aneurysm repair if the procedure is done in a unit with a high case volume and record of safety was reviewed.

Evidence for Volume-Outcome Relationship.—A meta-analysis of studies covering 421,299 elective aneurysm repairs reported a weighted odds ratio of 0.66 in favor of higher volume centers. Meta-analyses can be subject to publication bias, heterogeneity, and data source criticisms, however. A review of national administrative data found that the mortality in low-caseload units was 8.5% whereas that at high-caseload units was 5.9%. Many small-volume centers had a mortality for elective AAA surgery exceeding 20%. Safety plots assess the individual hospital performance. Of 410 hospitals, 30 at the low end of the volume spectrum had an elective AAA surgery mortality significantly higher than the national average.

Objections to Centralization.—All patients should have access to high-quality services with a proven record of safety, making it somewhat irrelevant what difference in mortality is sufficient to support centralization. Between 2003 and 2008, data on ruptured AAA from the United Kingdom indicated an absolute mortality between hospitals in the lowest and highest volume quintiles of 24%. Focusing on case mix and patients deemed ineligible for surgery showed disparate practices for emergency patients between the highest and lowest quintile units. No surgical intervention is offered to over 50% of emergency patients in the lowest quintile units but only 20% in the highest volume centers. Data indicating low-volume units have an elective AAA mortality of 0% may not actually have good results but simply too few cases.

Endovascular approaches have altered elective aneurysm surgery. However, hospital volume is significantly related to elective aneurysm mortality for open repair, endovascular repair, and combined approaches. Higher volume hospitals are more likely to adopt endovascular therapy. Those that do both endovascular and open repair have better than average results from the open repairs.

Patients must consider added travel time as well as clinical issues. About 92% of persons have indicated a willingness to travel at least 1 hour beyond their nearest hospital to access services with lower perioperative mortality, lower nonfatal complication rate, high annual caseload of AAA repairs, and routine availability of endovascular repairs.

The institutional experience is the most important contributor to delivering good quality care. Ceasing to perform aneurysm surgery in a center does not imply the surgeons are performing poorly, since the surgery is just one aspect of treatment. Outcomes may be defined by facilities, protocols, and familiarity with the challenging management of complex interventions.

Conclusions.—The evidence indicates that aneurysm services should be centralized to high-quality, high-volume providers with a proven record of safety. The recommended volume is the performance of not fewer than 50 cases and optimally 150 cases annually.

▶ The debate rages on. Should aneurysm repair be centralized at high volume centers? Both Thompson et al and Forbes[1] present cogent arguments. Here are two excerpts:

DrThompson: "The brief review of evidence presented ... mandates the centralization of aneurysm services to high quality, high volume providers with a proven record of safety. There appear to be no convincing arguments for maintaining aneurysm repair in low volume hospitals. We have deliberately not discussed the financial implications of such centralization but these are likely to be neutral at worst with increased travel times balanced by increased quality and reduced hospital stay as units move toward national and international exemplars."

Dr Forbes: "I don't doubt that a volume-outcome relationship does exist in some instances involving aneurysm care. However, case volumes don't necessarily equate with care quality in as simple a linear fashion as we might hope. Therefore, it is too simplistic for important health care delivery decisions, such as centralization, to depend solely on case volumes, whether it be at the surgeon or the hospital level. Patient outcomes and other quality of care indices should drive such decisions and also serve to assess their effects, and need for revision, on an ongoing basis."[1]

B. W. Starnes, MD

Reference

1. Forbes TL. Part two: the case against centralisation of abdominal aortic aneurysm surgery in higher volume centers. *Eur J Vasc Endovasc Surg.* 2011;42:414-417.

Part Two: The Case Against Centralisation of Abdominal Aortic Aneurysm Surgery in Higher Volume Centers
Forbes TL (London Health Sciences Ctr and The Univ of Western Ontario, Ontario, Canada)
Eur J Vasc Endovasc Surg 42:414-417, 2011

Background.—The centerpiece for arguments favoring the centralization of abdominal aortic aneurysm (AAA) surgery is the volume-outcome relationship. The intricacies, challenges, and possible negative effects with centralization were reviewed.

Volume-Outcome Relationship.—Recent systematic reviews question the existence or at least the strength of the volume-outcome relationship based on methodological challenges. Some studies focus on the surgeon's experience whereas others consider hospital case volumes in determining the volume component. In addition, definitions of what constitutes a high or low volume are inconsistent. An alternative method is to consider quality of care indices, since a higher case volume may not necessarily cause better patient outcomes. A California study found a 51% reduction in mortality in hospitals with a policy of perioperative beta-blocker use but no difference between hospitals based on case volume threshold. Achieving quality of care indices improves patient outcomes more successfully than performing a certain number of repairs. Positive volume-outcome relationships may reflect certain best practices and quality of care standards accompanying experience.

Other Considerations.—If aneurysm repair is centralized, regional centers must be equipped to meet the increased demands for emergency surgery in terms of human resources and infrastructure. Centralization will be unsuccessful without these measures.

Ruptured aneurysms present a time-sensitive, life-threatening problem requiring immediate attention. Three North American studies found that although transferring patients to the regional center delayed definitive surgical repair, it did not adversely affect patients' chances of survival. However, these studies only considered patients who survived transfer, a preselection that excludes unstable patients who died before or during transfer. No attempt was made to determine if such patients would have survived if offered repair at the local hospital. Centralization may therefore produce low operative and survival rates in patients not transferred to regional vascular units. Also, the actual aneurysm repair is just one component of treatment, with expert anesthesia and intensive care unit experiences also needed to ensure survival.

Patients may see local care as offering benefits not available with a regional center. These benefits include convenience, proximity to personal support systems, and continuity of care with familiar physicians. Forty-five percent of American patients indicated they would prefer local surgery for pancreatic cancer even if mortality was double that at a regional center. The specific patient population being considered must also be assessed. North American patients must travel farther distances to obtain tertiary and quaternary surgical care compared with European patients.

The impact of centralization on the provision of general vascular care must also be considered. Hospitals that no longer offer AAA repairs may also lose most vascular surgery coverage because vascular surgeons will shift practices to the centers where AAA surgery is done. Financial and budgetary benefits are additional concerns.

Conclusions.—It is simplistic to depend only on case volumes to determine if AAA surgery should be limited to regional centers that perform a high volume of cases. Service consolidations must consider patient outcomes and other quality of care indices, special clinical scenarios, specific patient populations, and vascular surgeon issues.

▶ The debate rages on. Should aneurysm repair be centralized at high-volume centers? Both Forbes and Thompson et al[1] present cogent arguments. Here are two excerpts:

Dr Thompson: "The brief review of evidence presented ... mandates the central-ization of aneurysm services to high quality, high volume providers with a proven record of safety. There appear to be no convincing arguments for maintaining aneurysm repair in low volume hospitals. We have deliberately not discussed the financial implications of such centralization but these are likely to be neutral at worst with increased travel times balanced by increased quality and reduced hospital stay as units move toward national and international exemplars."[1]

Dr Forbes: "I don't doubt that a volume-outcome relationship does exist in some instances involving aneurysm care. However, case volumes don't neces-sarily equate with care quality in as simple a linear fashion as we might hope. Therefore, it is too simplistic for important health care delivery decisions, such as centralization, to depend solely on case volumes, whether it be at the surgeon or the hospital level. Patient outcomes and other quality of care indices should drive such decisions and also serve to assess their effects, and need for revision, on an ongoing basis."

B. W. Starnes, MD

Reference

1. Thompson M, Holt P, Loftus I. Part one: all major arterial interventions should now be performed in high volume centres abdominal aortic aneurysms. *Eur J Vasc Endovasc Surg.* 2011;42:411-418.

Long-term sac behavior after endovascular abdominal aortic aneurysm repair with the Excluder low-permeability endoprosthesis
Hogg ME, Morasch MD, Park T, et al (Northwestern Univ, Chicago, IL; Yonsei Univ, Seoul, Korea; et al)
J Vasc Surg 53:1178-1183, 2011

Purpose.—Sac regression is a surrogate marker for clinical success in endovascular aneurysm repair (EVAR) and has been shown to be device-specific. The low porosity Excluder endograft (Excluder low-permeability endoprosthesis [ELPE]; W. L. Gore & Associates Inc, Flagstaff, Ariz) intro-duced in 2004 was reported in early follow-up to be associated with sac regression rates similar to other endografts, unlike the original Excluder which suffered from sac growth secondary to fluid accumulation in the sac. The purpose of this study was to determine whether this behavior is durable in mid-term to long-term follow-up.

Methods.—Between July 2004 and December 2007, 301 patients under-went EVAR of an abdominal aortic aneurysm (AAA) with the ELPE at two institutions. Baseline sac size was measured by computed tomography (CT) scan at 1 month after repair. Follow-up beyond 1 year was either with a CT or ultrasound scan. Changes in sac size ≥ 5 mm from baseline were determined to be significant. Endoleak history was assessed with respect to sac behavior using χ^2 and logistic regression analysis.

Results.—Two hundred sixteen patients (mean age 73.6 years and 76% men) had at least 1-year follow-up imaging available for analysis. Mean follow-up was 2.6 years (range, 1-5 years). The average minor-axis diameter was 52 mm at baseline. The proportion of patients with sac regression was similar during the study period: 58%, 66%, 60%, 59%, and 63% at 1 to 5 years, respectively. The proportion of patients with sac growth increased over time to 14.8% at 4-year follow-up. The probability of freedom from sac growth at 4 years was 82.4%. Eighty patients (37.7%) had an endoleak detected at some time during follow-up with 29.6% (16 of 54) residual endoleak rate at 4 years; 13 of the residual 16 endoleaks were type II. All patients with sac growth had endoleaks at some time during the study compared with only 18% of patients with sac regression ($P < .0001$).

Conclusion.—A sustained sac regression after AAA exclusion with ELPE is noted up to 5-year follow-up. Sac enlargement was observed only in the setting of a current or previous endoleak, with no cases of suspected hygroma formation noted.

▶ Data from the regulatory trial for the original Gore Excluder stent graft showed aneurysm sac growth in some patients attributed to transgraft flow of serous fluid, hygroma formation, and endotension in the absence of endoleak, leading to the introduction of the Excluder low-permeability endoprosthesis (ELPE) in 2004. This study confirms earlier reports of decreased aneurysm sac enlargement with this modification, with data now extended out to long-term follow-up. In this study, sac regression was sustained out to 5 years. While the proportion of patients with sac growth did increase over the study period, all of these were attributed to endoleak, not transgraft exudate. While the clinical significance of this observation is unclear in that aneurysm sac growth from transudate is not the same as that from endoleak, the goal of stabilization or decrease in aneurysm sac size as a surrogate marker for clinical success in endovascular aneurysm repair is still a desirable marker. It is also important to remember that this problem was an outlier issue for the original Gore Excluder system, has not been seen to this extent with other US Food and Drug Administration—approved devices, and seems to have been corrected with the ELPE redesign, thereby restoring aneurysm sac growth rates to a more acceptable degree commensurate with the other stent graft systems.

M. A. Passman, MD

Effect of gender on long-term survival after abdominal aortic aneurysm repair based on results from the Medicare national database
Egorova NN, Vouyouka AG, McKinsey JF, et al (Mount Sinai School of Medicine, NY; Columbia Univ, NY; et al)
J Vasc Surg 54:1-12, 2011

Objectives.—Historically, women have higher procedurally related mortality rates than men for abdominal aortic aneurysm (AAA) repair. Although endovascular aneurysm repair (EVAR) has improved these rates for men and women, effects of gender on long-term survival with different types of AAA repair, such as EVAR vs open aneurysm repair (OAR), need further investigation. To address this issue, we analyzed survival in matched cohorts who received EVAR or OAR for both elective (eAAA) and ruptured AAA (rAAA).

Methods.—Using the Medicare Beneficiary Database (1995-2006), we compiled a cohort of patients who underwent OAR or EVAR for eAAA (n = 322,892) or rAAA (n = 48,865). Men and women were matched by propensity scores, accounting for baseline demographics, comorbid conditions, treating institution, and surgeon experience. Frailty models were used to compare long-term survival of the matched groups.

Results.—Perioperative mortality for eAAAs was significantly lower among EVAR vs OAR recipients for both men (1.84% vs 4.80%) and women (3.19% vs 6.37%, $P < .0001$). One difference, however, was that the survival benefit of EVAR was sustained for the 6 years of follow-up in women but disappeared in 2 years in men. Similarly, the survival benefit of men vs women after elective EVAR disappeared after 1.5 to 2 years. For rAAAs, 30-day mortality was significantly lower for EVAR recipients compared with OAR recipients, for both men (33.43% vs 43.70% $P < .0001$) and women (41.01% vs 48.28%, $P = .0201$). Six-year survival was significantly higher for men who received EVAR vs those who received OAR ($P = .001$). However, the survival benefit for women who received EVAR compared with OAR disappeared in 6 months. Survival was also substantially higher for men than women after emergent EVAR ($P = .0007$).

Conclusions.—Gender disparity is evident from long-term outcomes after AAA repair. In the case for rAAA, where the long-term outcome for women was significantly worse than for men, the less invasive EVAR treatment did not appear to benefit women to the same extent that it did for men. Although the long-term outcome after open repair for elective AAA was also worse for women, EVAR benefit for women was sustained longer than for men. These associations require further study to isolate specific risk factors that would be potential targets for improving AAA management (Figs 1-4, Table 2).

▶ This is a very important and interesting study that assessed the effect of gender on long-term survival following abdominal aortic aneurysm repair. Previous studies have demonstrated that women have overall worse outcomes following abdominal aortic aneurysm repair than men, especially in mortality. However, when women are treated with endovascular aortic repair, the immediate outcomes are improved over open repair. The question is whether this benefit persists in the long term. The study is a retrospective analysis with the data source for analysis derived from the Medicare Inpatient Standard Analytical and Denominator files for the years 1995 to 2006. It evaluates both women and men who underwent elective and ruptured abdominal aortic aneurysm repair. Men and women were matched by propensity scores, accounting for baseline demographics, comorbid conditions, treating institution, and surgeon experience. The major findings of this study were the following: (1) After adjusting for life expectancy and calendar

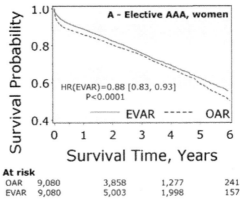

FIGURE 1.—Long-term survival of women treated with elective endovascular (*EVAR*) and open (*OAR*) repair of aortic abdominal aneurysm (*AAA*). Cases were matched by propensity score. The hazard ratio (*HR*) is the quotient of the hazard rates of the EVAR and OAR comparison groups and is expressed as a point estimate with a 95% confidence interval. (Reprinted from the Journal of Vascular Surgery, Egorova NN, Vouyouka AG, McKinsey JF, et al. Effect of gender on long-term survival after abdominal aortic aneurysm repair based on results from the Medicare national database. *J Vasc Surg*. 2011;54:1-12. Copyright 2011, with permission from The Society for Vascular Surgery.)

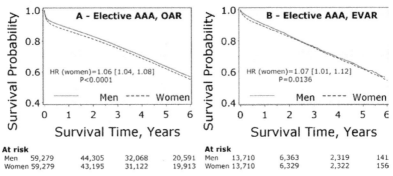

FIGURE 2.—Long-term survival after elective (**A**) open (*OAR*) and (**B**) endovascular (*EVAR*) repair of men and women with aortic abdominal aneurysms (*AAAs*). Cases were matched by propensity score. The hazard ratio (*HR*) is the quotient of the hazard rates of the two comparison groups (men and women) and is expressed as a point estimate with 95% confidence interval. (Reprinted from the Journal of Vascular Surgery, Egorova NN, Vouyouka AG, McKinsey JF, et al. Effect of gender on long-term survival after abdominal aortic aneurysm repair based on results from the Medicare national database. *J Vasc Surg*. 2011;54:1-12. Copyright 2011, with permission from The Society for Vascular Surgery.)

year, the 5-year relative survival estimates for women are decreased compared to men for both elective and ruptured abdominal aortic aneurysm repair whether the procedure was by open or endovascular repair (Table 2). (2) The 30-day mortality in women-matched groups was 6.37% after open aneurysm repair and 3.19% after endovascular repair ($P < .0001$). (3) Women undergoing elective aneurysm repair with endovascular treatment had a significant survival benefit over elective open repair that was sustained for the 6 years of observation (Fig 1a). (4) Following elective open aneurysm repair, women have a higher 30-day mortality

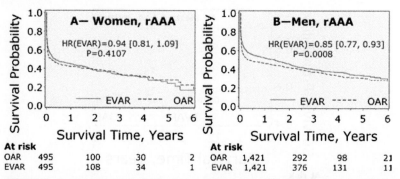

FIGURE 3.—Long-term survival of (**A**) women and (**B**) men treated with endovascular (*EVAR*) and open (*OAR*) repair of ruptured aortic abdominal aneurysm. Cases were matched by propensity score. The hazard ratio (*HR*) is the quotient of the hazard rate of the EVAR and OAR comparison groups and is expressed as a point estimate and 95% confidence interval. (Reprinted from the Journal of Vascular Surgery, Egorova NN, Vouyouka AG, McKinsey JF, et al. Effect of gender on long-term survival after abdominal aortic aneurysm repair based on results from the Medicare national database. *J Vasc Surg*. 2011;54:1-12. Copyright 2011, with permission from The Society for Vascular Surgery.)

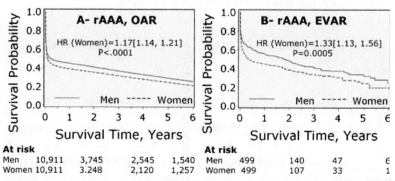

FIGURE 4.—Long-term survival after (**A**) open (*OAR*) and (**B**) endovascular (*EVAR*) repair of ruptured aortic abdominal aneurysm in men and women. Cases were matched by propensity score. The hazard ratio (*HR*) is the quotient of the hazard rates of the two comparison groups (men and women) and is expressed as a point estimate and 95% confidence interval. (Reprinted from the Journal of Vascular Surgery, Egorova NN, Vouyouka AG, McKinsey JF, et al. Effect of gender on long-term survival after abdominal aortic aneurysm repair based on results from the Medicare national database. *J Vasc Surg*. 2011;54:1-12. Copyright 2011, with permission from The Society for Vascular Surgery.)

rate in matched groups compared to men (6.43% for women and 4.98% for men, $P < .0001$) and decreased survival at 6 years (Fig 2a). (5) Following elective endovascular aneurysm repair, women have a higher 30-day mortality rate in matched groups compared to men (2.96% for women and 1.77% for men, $P < .0001$), and although overall survival was superior for men (hazard ratio [HR], 1.07; $P < .0136$), the initial survival advantage in men lessened over time, and the survival curves began to converge after 2 years (Fig 2b). (6) For ruptured abdominal aortic aneurysms, regardless of repair type (open or endovascular), the relative long-term survival for women was inferior to survival for men, with the worst survival after endovascular repair (Table 2). (7) For women, the

TABLE 2.—Five-year Relative Survival Estimates for Men and Women After Open (*OAR*) and Endovascular (*EVAR*) Repair of Abdominal Aortic Aneurysm (*AAA*)

Variable	Men % (95% CL)	Women % (95% CL)	P
Elective AAA			
OAR	86 (86, 87)	77 (76, 77)	<.0001
EVAR	87 (87, 88)	80 (78, 81)	<.0001
Excluding 90-day mortality			
OAR	93 (92, 93)	84 (84, 85)	<.0001
EVAR	91 (90, 91)	85 (83, 86)	<.0001
Ruptured AAA			
OAR	34 (33, 35)	19 (18, 21)	<.0001
EVAR	43 (39, 48)	32 (25, 39)	<.0001
Excluding 90-day mortality			
OAR	83 (82, 84)	72 (70, 74)	<.0001
EVAR	75 (67, 82)	65 (51, 78)	<.0001

CL, Confidence limit.

overall survival rate for ruptured abdominal aortic aneurysm was similar to treatment with endovascular or open repair recipients (HR, 0.94; $P = .41$), with only an advantage of survival for endovascular repair in the first 6 months (Fig 3a). (8) Unlike women, the overall survival for men after ruptured abdominal aortic aneurysms was better after endovascular than open repair, which persisted up to 6 years (Fig 3b). (9) Following open aneurysm repair for rupture, women have a higher 30-day mortality rate in matched groups compared to men (52.61% for women and 46.57% for men, $P < .0001$), and long-term survival was significantly higher for men (HR, 1.17; $P < .0001$; Fig 4a). (10) Following endovascular aneurysm repair for rupture, women have a higher 30-day mortality rate in matched groups compared to men (41.08% for women and 30.66% for men, $P < .0001$), and women had substantially lower long-term survival rates (Fig 4b). These data are compelling and clearly indicate that women have higher early and late mortality rates. Although endovascular aortic aneurysm repair offers advantages with lower complication rates and mortality initially, women clearly do not gain the same benefits as men in overall survival, regardless of whether the abdominal aortic aneurysm is repaired by open or endovascular techniques. These disparities are not entirely clear, but they certainly offer potential to maximize medical and surgical therapies. In addition, these data would suggest that the natural history for aneurysm growth and rupture is likely different for women than for men. Importantly, applying the same criteria to aneurysm interventions in women that are used in men may not be appropriate and may be responsible for some of the negative outcomes seen both short-term and long-term in women. Certainly the inferior outcomes seen in women after both elective and emergent aneurysm repair are multifactorial, including anatomical considerations, cardiovascular risk factors, age, and aggressive preoperative medical optimization. Further research in management of abdominal aortic aneurysm in women is needed to clearly define the natural history, the anatomic factors that dictate repair, medical optimization, and likely better design in endovascular grafts. Addressing these components will hopefully improve the outcomes in women with abdominal aortic aneurysm and decrease the current outcome disparity seen when compared with men.

J. D. Raffetto, MD

Impact of Aortic Grafts on Arterial Pressure: A Computational Fluid Dynamics Study

Vardoulis O, Coppens E, Martin B, et al (Ecole Polytechnique Fédérale de Lausanne, Switzerland; Katholieke Universiteit Leuven, Belgium; et al)
Eur J Vasc Endovasc Surg 42:704-710, 2011

Objective.—Vascular prostheses currently used in vascular surgery do not have the same mechanical properties as human arteries. This computational study analyses the mechanisms by which grafts, placed in the ascending aorta (proximal) and descending aorta (distal), affect arterial blood pressure.

Methods.—A one-dimensional cardiovascular model was developed and adapted to include the graft geometry with *in vitro* measured mechanical properties. Pressure at the aortic root and haemodynamic parameters were computed and compared for a control, proximal and distal graft case.

Results.—In comparison to the control case, the proximal graft increased characteristic impedance by 58% versus only 1% change for the distal graft. The proximal and distal graft increased pulse pressure by 21% and 10%, respectively.

Conclusions.—The mechanisms underlying pulse pressure increase are different for proximal and distal grafts. For the proximal graft, the primary reason for pulse pressure rise is augmentation of the forward wave, resulting from characteristic impedance increase. For the distal graft, the pulse pressure rise is associated with augmented wave reflections resulting from compliance mismatch. Overall, the proximal aortic graft resulted in greater haemodynamic alterations than the distal graft. Thus, it is likely that patients who receive ascending aorta grafts are more prone to systolic hypertension and therefore deserve closer blood pressure monitoring (Fig 3).

▶ Using computational fluid dynamics, this study evaluated the impact of proximal aortic root replacement versus thoracic aortic replacement on hemodynamic parameters. The model was based on previously reported compliance properties of the native aorta and Dacron tube grafts. Overall, aortic root replacement with Dacron grafts resulted in dramatic hemodynamic alterations (Fig 3). Most notably, the systolic blood pressure, pulse pressure, and forward pressure wave increased as a result of increasing impedance. Thoracic aortic replacement also resulted in pulse pressure increases, but relative to the aortic root replacement, there were only marginal changes in the systolic blood pressure.

The elastic properties of the aortic root have long been recognized. Replacing the dynamic aortic wall with tube grafts or endovascular stent grafts results in a rigid, noncompliant tube; the systemic effects are appreciated as an increase

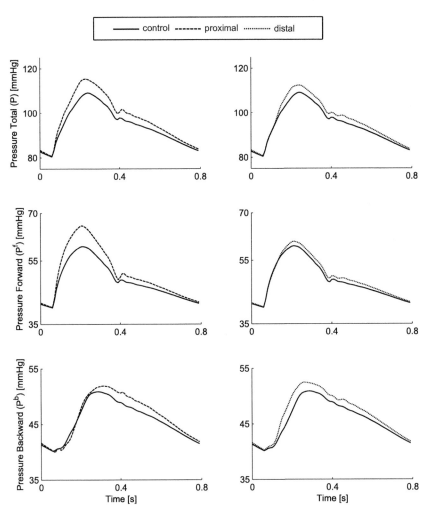

FIGURE 3.—Comparison of the pressure waves for the proximal aortic replacement (dashed lines), distal aortic replacement (dotted lines) and the control case (solid lines). The first row depicts total pressure waves. The second and third row depict forward and backward pressure waves respectively. (Reprinted from European Journal of Vascular and Endovascular Surgery, Vardoulis O, Coppens E, Martin B, et al. Impact of aortic grafts on arterial pressure: a computational fluid dynamics study. *Eur J Vasc Endovasc Surg.* 2011;42:704-710. Copyright 2011, with permission from the European Society for Vascular Surgery.)

in systolic blood pressure and pulse pressure. The long-term cardiovascular impact is unknown. Invariably, aortic root replacement results in cardiac stress secondary to increased work, which may translate into delayed cardiac morbidity.

Z. M. Arthurs, MD

A Meta-Analysis and Metaregression Analysis of Factors Influencing Mortality after Endovascular Repair of Ruptured Abdominal Aortic Aneurysms

Karkos CD, Sutton AJ, Bown MJ, et al (Aristotle Univ of Thessaloniki, Greece; Univ of Leicester, UK)

Eur J Vasc Endovasc Surg 42:775-786, 2011

Objective.—To determine factors that may influence the perioperative mortality after endovascular repair of ruptured abdominal aortic aneurysms (RAAAs) using metaregression analysis.

Methods.—A meta-analysis of all English-language literature with information on mortality rates after endovascular repair of RAAAs was conducted. A metaregression was subsequently performed to determine the impact on mortality of the following 8 factors: patient age; mid-time study point; anaesthesia; endograft configuration; haemodynamic instability; use of aortic balloon; conversion to open repair; and abdominal compartment syndrome.

Results.—The pooled perioperative mortality across the 46 studies (1397 patients) was 24.3% (95% CI: 20.7—28.3%). Of the 8 variables, only bifurcated approach was significantly associated with reduced mortality ($p = 0.005$). A moderate negative correlation was observed between bifurcated approach and haemodynamic instability (-0.35). There was still a strong association between bifurcated approach and mortality after simultaneously adjusting for haemodynamic instability, indicating that the latter was not a major factor in explaining the observed association.

Conclusions.—Endovascular repair of RAAAs is associated with acceptable mortality rates. Patients having a bifurcated endograft were less likely to die. This may be due to some surgeons opting for a bifurcated approach in patients with better haemodynamic condition. Further studies will be needed to clarify this.

▶ This review represents the most thorough analysis of contemporary results for managing ruptured abdominal aortic aneurysms with an endovascular approach. Perhaps the most striking finding of this metaregression was that a bifurcated approach was associated with a significant reduction in mortality. One possible explanation for the improved survival in the bifurcated group is that a bifurcated endograft was usually used in patients who were considered hemodynamically stable enough to tolerate the inevitable delay occurring during contralateral gate cannulation. However, there was still a strong association between a bifurcated approach and mortality after adjusting for hemodynamic instability, indicating that the latter was not a major factor in explaining this phenomenon.

Three randomized control trials are currently underway to answer this question. The French ECAR and Dutch AJAX trials have been designed to only recruit stable patients. In contrast, the UK IMPROVE trial randomizes patients immediately after diagnosis. We await the results of these important trials.

B. W. Starnes, MD

Comparative Predictors of Mortality for Endovascular and Open Repair of Ruptured Infrarenal Abdominal Aortic Aneurysms

Sarac TP, Bannazadeh M, Rowan AF, et al (Cleveland Clinic Lerner School of Medicine, OH)

Ann Vasc Surg 25:461-468, 2011

Background.—The continued success of elective endovascular aneurysm repair (EVAR) has led to an extension of this technology to ruptured aortas. The purpose of this study was to evaluate our results of ruptured infrarenal aortic aneurysm (rAAA).

Methods.—The treatment results of all patients who underwent repair of rAAAs between January 1990 and May 2008 were reviewed retrospectively. Comorbidities, intraoperative details, and postoperative complications were tabulated. EVAR and open repair were compared.

Results.—Between January 1990 and May 2008, 160 patients underwent repair of rAAA. Of these, 32 (20%) underwent EVAR for rAAA; of 160 patients, 112 were considered to have free rupture (70%) and 48 had contained rupture (30%). The average Acute Physiology and Chronic Health Evaluation II score was 13.3 ± 6.7. The Kaplan—Meier survival rates at 30 days, 6 months, 1 year, and 5 years were 69% (62,77), 57% (50,65), 50% (43,59), and 25% (19,34), respectively, with no difference seen in EVAR group as compared with open surgery ($p = 0.24$). Intraoperative mortality was 5.6%, with no patient undergoing EVAR suffering an intraoperative death ($p = 0.03$). However, 30-day mortality was 31.9% with no difference between EVAR and open surgery (31.2% vs. 32%; $p = 0.93$) results. Multivariate analysis for 30-day mortality found renal insufficiency (RI) odds ratio (OR): 2.4 (1.1, 5.3), $p = 0.04$; hypotension OR: 2.4 (1.1, 5.3), $p = 0.02$; and cardiac arrest OR: 3.8 (1.1, 11.6, $p = 0.03$), were all associated with the greatest mortality. Of all predictors analyzed, multivariate analysis found preoperative RI OR: 2.32 (1.55, 3.47), $p < 0.001$, was the only independent predictor of decreased long-term survival.

Conclusions.—Mortality rates for rAAA remain high. The use of EVAR for these procedures equals that for open repair with regard to 30-day and long-term mortality. Preoperative cardiac arrest and RI were associated with inferior results for both EVAR and open repair. Clinical judgment on when to use EVAR as a primary repair modality must be exercised (Fig 1).

▶ About half of all patients with ruptured abdominal aortic aneurysm (rAAA) die before reaching surgery.[1] When patients reach the hospital, mortality rates still range between 30% and 70% with a large meta-analysis reporting an overall 48% mortality rate.[2] Endovascular aneurysm repair (EVAR) for rAAA was first described in 1994.[3] There is clearly a trend toward increasing use of EVAR for treatment of rAAA, and most clinicians' clinical impression is that outcomes are better. This study, however, showed equal morality with open and endovascular repair of rAAA (Fig 1). The series is retrospective with different surgeons over time. We don't know the precise selection criteria for the 2 procedures, and

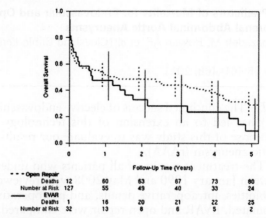

- - - Open Repair					
Deaths	12	60	63	67	73	80
Number at Risk	127	55	49	40	33	24
—— EVAR					
Deaths	1	16	20	21	22	25
Number at Risk	32	13	8	6	5	2

FIGURE 1.—Cumulative survival rates after endovascular aneurysm repair and open repair of ruptured abdominal aortic aneurysms. No significant difference was observed between two groups ($p = 0.24$). (Reprinted from the Annals of Vascular Surgery, Sarac TP, Bannazadeh M, Rowan AF, et al. Comparative predictors of mortality for endovascular and open repair of ruptured infrarenal abdominal aortic aneurysms. Ann Vasc Surg. 2011;25:461-468. Copyright 2011 with permission from Annals of Vascular Surgery, Inc.)

there may be unmeasured confounding variables. What we can really say from this article is that despite the use of EVAR for repair for rAAA, mortality remains high. EVAR is clearly a viable option for treatment of rAAA. Despite many surgeons' clinical impression, whether EVAR, when applicable, truly reduces mortality of rAAA in equal patients compared with open repair, has not been conclusively proven to everyone's satisfaction.

G. L. Moneta, MD

References

1. Acosta S, Ogren M, Bengtsson H, Bergqvist D, Lindblad B, Zdanowski Z. Increasing incidence of ruptured abdominal aortic aneurysm: a population-based study. *J Vasc Surg*. 2006;44:237-243.
2. Bown MJ, Sutton AJ, Bell PR, Sayers RD. A meta-analysis of 50 years of ruptured abdominal aortic aneurysm repair. *Br J Surg*. 2002;89:714-730.
3. Marin ML, Veith FJ, Cynamon J, et al. Initial experience with transluminally placed endovascular grafts for the treatment of complex vascular lesions. *Ann Surg*. 1995; 222:449-465.

Mid-term Outcomes following Emergency Endovascular Aortic Aneurysm Repair for Ruptured Abdominal Aortic Aneurysms

Noorani A, Page A, Walsh SR, et al (Cambridge Univ Hosps, UK)
Eur J Vasc Endovasc Surg 43:382-385, 2012

Objective.—Emergency Endovascular Aortic Aneurysm Repair (eEVAR) is a rapidly evolving approach to ruptured Abdominal Aortic Aneurysms (rAAA). Yet longer-term outcomes following eEVAR remain unclear. This study compares mid-term outcomes of eEVAR and open rAAA.

Methods.—A prospective database for all patients undergoing eEVAR and open rAAA from January 2006 to April 2010 was analysed. Patients were offered eEVAR if anatomically suitable.

Results.—52 patients (45 male, median age 78 years (62—92 years), underwent eEVAR, 50 patients (44 male, median age = 71 (62—95 years) underwent open rAAA repair. In-hospital mortalities were 12% (6/52) for eEVAR, 32% (16/50) for open repair.

There were five re-interventions (10%) in the eEVAR group. The perioperative survival benefits of eEVAR over open rAAA repair were maintained at 1 and 2 years post-operatively with open repair demonstrating a two-fold increased risk of mortality (Hazard ratio 2.2, Fisher Exact test, 95% Confidence Interval (CI) 1.108—4.62, $p = 0.0122$). Overall survival was 81% at 1 year, 73% at 2 years for eEVAR, and 62% at 1 year and 52% at 2 years for open rAAA repair.

Conclusion.—EEVAR is associated with excellent mid-term survival in this cohort. We would recommend eEVAR as the management of choice for rAAA in anatomically suitable patients where local facilities and expertise exist (Fig 1).

▶ This is yet another study that confirms my bias that emergency endovascular aneurysm repair (EVAR) should be the management of choice for patients presenting with a ruptured abdominal aortic aneurysm (rAAA). Presented is a consecutive series of patients presenting with rAAA to a tertiary center in the United Kingdom. Fifty-two patients underwent EVAR, and 50 underwent standard open repair, serving as the 2 groups for direct comparison. The in-hospital mortality rates were 12% for EVAR and 32% for open repair.

Unlike other similar studies in the literature, midterm outcomes are reported. Overall survival rates were 81% at 1 year and 73% at 2 years for EVAR compared

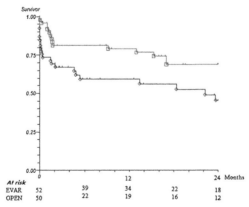

FIGURE 1.—Survival curve of open rAAA repair compared to eEVAR. eEVAR is denoted in the red, the open rAAA group in black. Log-rank $p = 0.0122$. For interpretation of the references to color in this figure legend, the reader is referred to web version of this article. (Reprinted from European Journal of Vascular and Endovascular Surgery, Noorani A, Page A, Walsh SR, et al. Mid-term outcomes following emergency endovascular aortic aneurysm repair for ruptured abdominal aortic aneurysms. *Eur J Vasc Endovasc Surg.* 2012;43:382-385. Copyright 2012, with permission from the European Society for Vascular Surgery.)

with 62% at 1 year and 52% at 2 years for open repair (Fig 1). I have a couple of criticisms on this article: (1) Nine patients were palliated during the study period, suggesting that not all patients were offered repair and, if they had been, may have increased the mortality rate in the early phase and decreased the survival rate during follow-up in either group. (2) Sixty-three percent of the EVAR patients had an aortouniiliac fem-fem construct, which, in my opinion, led to a high re-intervention rate during follow-up. The authors acknowledged this and moved toward a standard approach of bifurcated grafts toward the end of the study.

B. W. Starnes, MD

Repair of Ruptured Abdominal Aortic Aneurysm in Octogenarians

Opfermann P, von Allmen R, Diehm N, et al (Univ Hosp Berne, Switzerland)
Eur J Vasc Endovasc Surg 42:475-483, 2011

Objective.—To determine whether advanced age was independently associated with prohibitive surgical risks or impaired long-term prognosis after ruptured aortic aneurysm repair.

Design.—Post-hoc analysis of prospective cohort.

Materials.—Consecutive patients undergoing ruptured aneurysm repair between January 2001 and December 2010 at a tertiary referral centre.

Methods.—Surgical mortality (i.e., <30 days) was compared between octogenarians and younger patients using logistic regression modelling to adjust for suspected confounders and to identify prognostic factors. Long-term survival was compared with matched national populations.

Results.—Sixty of 248 involved patients were octogenarians (24%) and almost all were offered open repair ($n = 237$). Surgical mortality of octogenarians was 26.7% (adjusted odds ratio (OR) 2.1; 95% confidence interval (CI), 0.9–5.2) and confounded by cardiac disease. Hypovolaemic shock predicted perioperative death of octogenarians best (OR 5.1; 95% CI, 1.1–23.4; $P = 0.037$). After successful repair, annual mortality of octogenarians averaged 13.7% vs. 5.2% for younger patients. At 2 years, octogenarian survival was at 94% of the expected 'normal' survival in the general population (vs. 96% for younger patients).

Conclusions.—Surgical mortality of ruptured aneurysm repair was not independently related to advanced age but mainly driven by cardiac disease and manifest hypovolaemic shock. An almost normal long-term prognosis of aged patients after successful repair justifies even attempts of open repair, particularly in carefully selected patients.

▶ The fastest growing percentage of our population are those aged over 80 years. This study evaluates the repair of ruptured aortic aneurysms at a single center in octogenarians.

The most interesting data point for me in this article was the use of a "shock index," which is calculated by dividing the heart rate (beats/minute) by the systolic blood pressure (mm Hg) on admission.[1] Using this index, those octogenarians with a shock index greater than 1.0 had a fivefold increase in the risk of perioperative death, emphasizing the profound impact of hypovolemic shock in this elderly patient population ($P = .037$).

Those factors that help predict mortality with a high degree of certainty will help us choose those patients who stand to benefit most from aggressive attempts at salvage.

B. W. Starnes, MD

Reference

1. Allgöwer M, Burri C. Shock index. *Dtsch Med Wochenschr.* 1967;92:1947-1950.

Endovascular management of ascending aortic pathology
Kolvenbach RR, Karmeli R, Pinter LS, et al (Vascular Ctr Catholic Clinics Duesseldorf Augusta Hosp, Germany; Carmel Med Ctr, Haifa, Israel)
J Vasc Surg 53:1431-1438, 2011

Background.—Endovascular treatment of the ascending aorta is particularly challenging because of the anatomic features of this aortic segment. Only patients without connective tissue disorders, clinically relevant aortic regurgitation or stenosis, or concomitant coronary artery disease can be considered for an endovascular procedure. We report our results in a series of patients with aneurysms or intramural hematoma, penetrating ulcers, or floating thrombus who were scheduled for stent grafting.

Methods.—Only patients with ascending aortic pathology who were unfit for open surgery were treated with an endograft. When preoperative computed tomography imaging showed severe calcification of the aortic arch or thrombus lining, temporary clamping of the carotid arteries before wire and catheter introduction was performed. An extracorporeal bypass from the right groin to both carotid arteries with a roller pump was established and maintained during the procedure. The endograft was placed across the aortic valve into the left ventricle and deployed in a retrograde fashion. At the end of the procedure, ventriculography and, if necessary, coronary angiography was performed to rule out any damage to the left ventricle or the valve apparatus.

Result.—Eleven patients were scheduled for stent graft exclusion of ascending aortic pathology. In five cases because of discrepancies in length measurements and sizing, the thoracic endograft was cut to length intraoperatively after partial deployment on the operating table and reloaded to avoid covering of the innominate artery. The mean length of the ascending aorta covered was longer in aneurysm patients than in those with dissection. An 81-year-old patient presented with a type Ia leak. The distal landing zone in one patient was enlarged by debranching. One patient died after wire perforation of the left ventricle, and one patient sustained a cerebral stroke. Combined morbidity and mortality was 18%, and the technical success rate was 91%.

Conclusions.—Stent grafting of the ascending aorta is technically feasible but should be reserved for selected high-risk patients only, preferably in centers where vascular specialists cooperate closely with interventional cardiologists. Cardiac surgery with cardiopulmonary bypass is still the gold standard to treat ascending aortic aneurysms. Stent graft exclusion of more advanced and complex ascending aortic pathology should be performed only in centers with the necessary experience in transvalvular cardiac procedures.

▶ Studies have shown that up to a third of patients with ascending aortic pathology have such high comorbidities that they are precluded from undergoing open interposition grafting. The development of endovascular therapies of the ascending aorta and aortic arch are currently in development and may provide options for these patients. Two main strategies exist: fenestrated grafts and endovascular ascending graft conduits. The current article reports on the use of endovascular ascending aortic conduits. There are several new techniques and challenges required for the application of endovascular treatment of the ascending aorta. These include rapid ventricular pacing or cardiac arrest using adenosine, precise location of the coronary artery ostia using computer assistance, and crossing the aortic valve into the left ventricle for wire stability and purchase. Most of these techniques are used routinely in the deployment of transfemoral aortic valves (TAVI). Familiarity with the use of 3-dimensional software to analyze the aortic root dimensions and height from the aortic annulus to the coronary ostia allows vascular surgeons to be involved in acquiring the skills necessary to treat pathologies of the ascending aorta when they become available.

D. L. Gillespie, MD, FACS

7   Abdominal Aortic Endografting

Comparison of Surveillance Versus Aortic Endografting for Small Aneurysm Repair (CAESAR): Results from a Randomised Trial
Cao P, for the CAESAR Trial Group (Hosp S. Camillo — Forlanini, Rome, Italy; et al)
Eur J Vasc Endovasc Surg 41:13-25, 2011

Background.—Randomised trials have failed to demonstrate benefit from early surgical repair of small abdominal aortic aneurysm (AAA) compared with surveillance. This study aimed to compare results after endovascular aortic aneurysm repair (EVAR) or surveillance in AAA <5.5 cm.

Methods.—Patients (50—79 years) with AAA of 4.1—5.4 cm were randomly assigned, in a 1:1 ratio, to receive immediate EVAR or surveillance by ultrasound and computed tomography (CT) and repair only after a defined threshold (diameter ≥5.5 cm, enlargement >1 cm/year, symptoms) was achieved. The main end point was all-cause mortality. Recruitment is closed; results at a median follow-up of 32.4 months are here reported.

Results.—Between 2004 and 2008, 360 patients (early EVAR = 182; surveillance = 178) were enrolled. One perioperative death after EVAR and two late ruptures (both in the surveillance group) occurred. At 54 months, there was no significant difference in the main end-point rate [hazard ratio (HR) 0.76; 95% confidence interval (CI) 0.30—1.93; $p = 0.6$] with Kaplan—Meier estimates of all-cause mortality of 14.5% in the EVAR and 10.1% in the surveillance group. Aneurysm-related mortality, aneurysm rupture and major morbidity rates were similar. Kaplan—Meier estimates of aneurysms growth ≥5 mm at 36 months were 8.4% in the EVAR group and 67.5% in the surveillance group (HR 10.49; 95% CI 6.88—15.96; $p < 0.01$). For aneurysms under surveillance, the probability of delayed repair was 59.7% at 36 months (84.5% at 54 months). The probability of receiving open repair at 36 months for EVAR feasibility loss was 16.4%.

Conclusion.—Mortality and rupture rates in AAA <5.5 cm are low and no clear advantage was shown between early or delayed EVAR strategy. However, within 36 months, three out of every five small aneurysms under surveillance might grow to require repair and one out of every six might lose feasibility for EVAR. Surveillance is safe for small AAA if close supervision is applied. Long-term data are needed to confirm these results.

Clinical Trial Registration Information.—This study is registered, NCT Identifier: NCT00118573 (Figs 3 and 5).

▶ Very strong randomized controlled trials indicate that there is no advantage of surgery versus surveillance for patients with an abdominal aortic aneurysm (AAA) with a diameter between 4.1 and 5.4 cm. Some, however, have suggested that the current generation devices for endovascular aortic aneurysm repair (EVAR) decrease operative risk, are more stable, and are associated with fewer device-related complications; therefore, EVAR should be considered for early treatment of patients with small AAAs. In addition, surveillance of small AAAs may inevitably result in a small but undefined number of unpredicted ruptures, and some small aneurysms initially suitable for EVAR may become unsuitable as the aneurysm enlarges to 5.5 cm. On the other hand, early EVAR may result in overtreatment and expose patients to unnecessary risks of early procedure-related complications and unnecessary and troublesome follow-up surveillance. This study presented the midterm results of a randomized multicenter trial to compare early EVAR versus surveillance in treatment of AAAs between 4.1 and 5.4 cm in diameter. Aneurysm-related mortality in this study at 54 months was close to 0. This confirms the well-known safety of EVAR. However, the low risk of EVAR did not translate into benefit of EVAR over surveillance because of similar safety with the surveillance strategy. The risk of aneurysm-related mortality was less than 1% at 54 months in both arms of the CAESAR trial, and there was no difference in overall survival (Fig 3). The totality of available evidence indicates that there is little justification for routine repair of small AAAs with EVAR. Clearly most larger small AAAs under surveillance will eventually be repaired (Fig 5), but there is really nothing lost by waiting until the AAA reaches the generally accepted threshold

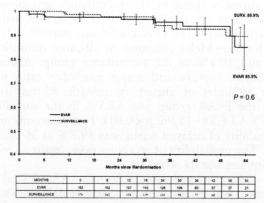

FIGURE 3.—Kaplane—Meier estimates of survival at 54 months from time of randomisation in EVAR versus Surveillance groups. *P* = 0.6. Numbers at risk are shown. (Reprinted from Cao P, for the CAESAR Trial Group. Comparison of surveillance versus aortic endografting for small aneurysm repair (CAESAR): results from a randomised trial. *Eur J Vasc Endovasc Surg.* 2011;41:13-25. Copyright 2011, with permission from European Society for Vascular Surgery.)

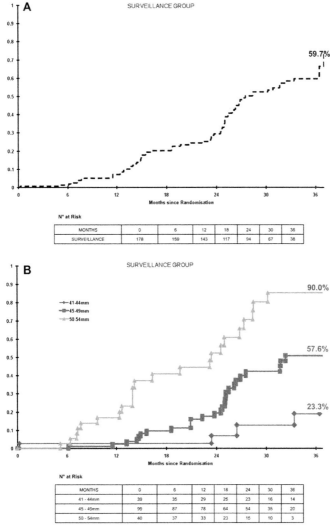

FIGURE 5.—Part A: Kaplane—Meier estimates of undergoing repair in the surveillance arm during 36 months follow-up. Part B: Kaplane—Meier estimates of undergoing repair in the surveillance arm during 36 months follow-up by baseline aneurysm diameter. (Reprinted from Cao P, for the CAESAR Trial Group. Comparison of surveillance versus aortic endografting for small aneurysm repair (CAESAR): results from a randomised trial. *Eur J Vasc Endovasc Surg.* 2011;41:13-25. Copyright 2011, with permission from European Society for Vascular Surgery.)

level of 5.5 cm for repair. It appears that health care systems will save money and patients will not be harmed by restricting EVAR to those individuals with aneurysms greater than 5.4 cm in diameter. Such a policy would seem to be a win for all involved.

G. L. Moneta, MD

Defining Perioperative Mortality after Open and Endovascular Aortic Aneurysm Repair in the US Medicare Population

Schermerhorn ML, Giles KA, Sachs T, et al (Beth Israel Deaconess Med Ctr, Boston, MA; et al)

J Am Coll Surg 212:349-355, 2011

Background.—Perioperative mortality is reported after abdominal aortic aneurysm (AAA) repair, but there is no agreed upon standard definition. Often, 30-day mortality is reported because in-hospital mortality may be biased in favor of endovascular repair given the shorter length of stay. However, the duration of increased risk of death after aneurysm repair is unknown.

Study Design.—We used propensity score modeling to create matched cohorts of US Medicare beneficiaries undergoing endovascular (n = 22,830) and open (n = 22,830) AAA repair from 2001 to 2004. We calculated perioperative mortality using several definitions including in-hospital, 30-day, and combined 30-day and in-hospital mortality. We determined the relative risk (RR) of death after open compared with endovascular repair as well as the absolute mortality difference. To define the duration of increased risk we calculated biweekly interval death rates for 12 months.

Results.—In-hospital, 30-day, and combined 30-day and in-hospital mortality for open and endovascular repair were 4.6% versus 1.1%, 4.8% versus 1.6%, and 5.3% versus 1.7%, respectively. The absolute differences in mortality were similar, at 3.5%, 3.2%, and 3.7%. The RRs of death (95% confidence interval) were 4.2 (3.6 to 4.8), 3.1 (2.7 to 3.4), and 3.2 (2.8 to 3.5). Biweekly interval death rates were highest during the first month after endovascular repair (0.6%) and during the first 2.5 months (0.5% to 2.1%) after open repair. After 2.5 months, rates were similar for both repairs (<0.5%) and stabilized after 3 months. The 90-day mortality rates for open and endovascular repair were 7.0% and 3.2%, respectively.

Conclusions.—In-hospital mortality comparisons overestimate the benefit of endovascular repair compared with 30-day or combined 30-day and in-hospital mortality. The total mortality impact of AAA repair is not realized until 3 months after repair and the duration of highest mortality risk extends longer for open repair (Figs 1 and 2).

▶ Perioperative mortality is a primary outcome report for almost any surgical procedure. However, definitions of perioperative mortality differ. Perioperative mortality may be defined as death during initial hospitalization, within 30 days of surgery, or all deaths within 30 days plus any deaths beyond 30 days that occurred before discharge from the hospital. In addition, ongoing risks due to surgery may persist beyond 30 days or beyond hospital discharge. The authors investigated the effects and implications of various methods of calculating "perioperative mortality" with respect to endovascular versus open abdominal aortic aneurysm repair. The conclusion that the use of 30-day mortality overestimates the benefit of endovascular aneurysm repair is somewhat expected. Analysis of data from the randomized trials of open versus endovascular repair suggests that the main benefit of endovascular repair is up front at the time of the

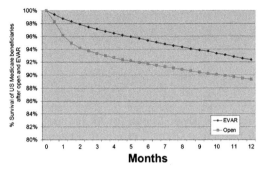

FIGURE 1.—Survival through 1 year in US Medicare beneficiaries undergoing open and endovascular abdominal aortic aneurysm repair from 2001 to 2004. EVAR, endovascular aortic aneurysm repair. (Reprinted from Journal of American College of Surgeons, Schermerhorn ML, Giles KA, Sachs T, et al, Defining perioperative mortality after open and endovascular aortic aneurysm repair in the US Medicare population. *J Am Coll Surg*. 2011;212:349-355. Copyright 2011, with permission from the American College of Surgeons.)

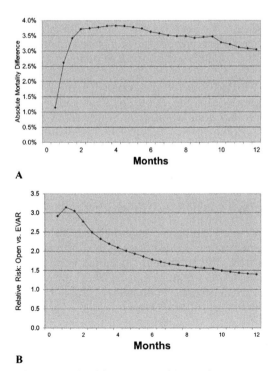

FIGURE 2.—(A) Absolute mortality differences during follow-up between open versus endovascular abdominal aortic aneurysm repair. (B) Relative risk of death after open versus endovascular abdominal aortic aneurysm repair in United States Medicare beneficiaries undergoing abdominal aortic aneurysm repair from 2001 to 2004. EVAR, endovascular aortic aneurysm repair. (Reprinted from Journal of American College of Surgeons, Schermerhorn ML, Giles KA, Sachs T, et al, Defining perioperative mortality after open and endovascular aortic aneurysm repair in the US Medicare population. *J Am Coll Surg*. 2011;212: 349-355. Copyright 2011, with permission from the American College of Surgeons.)

operation. This study helps define the length of the so-called up front period. More important, it points out that mortality impact of a major surgical procedure likely extends well beyond the traditionally reported 30-day or in-hospital time periods (Figs 1 and 2).

G. L. Moneta, MD

Elective Endovascular vs. Open Repair for Abdominal Aortic Aneurysm in Patients Aged 80 Years and Older: Systematic Review and Meta-Analysis

Biancari F, Catania A, D'Andrea V (Oulu Univ Hosp, Finland; La Sapienza Univ, Rome, Italy)
Eur J Vasc Endovasc Surg 42:571-576, 2011

Objectives.—Endovascular treatment (EVAR) of abdominal aortic aneurysm (AAA) is thought to be of benefit, particularly in patients aged ≥80 years. This issue was investigated in the present meta-analysis.

Design.—The study design involved a systematic review of the literature and meta-analysis.

Methods.—Systematic review of the literature and meta-analysis of data on elective EVAR vs. open repair of AAA in patients aged ≥80 years were performed.

Results.—Six observational studies reporting on 13 419 patients were included in the present analysis. Pooled analysis showed higher immediate postoperative mortality after open repair compared with EVAR (risk ratio 3.87, 95% confidence interval (CI) 3.19—4.68; risk difference, 6.2%, 95% CI 5.4—7.0%). The pooled immediate mortality rate after open repair was 8.6%, whereas it was 2.3% after EVAR. Open repair was associated with a significantly higher risk of postoperative cardiac, pulmonary and renal complications. Pooled analysis of three studies showed similar overall survival at 3 years after EVAR and open repair (risk ratio 1.10, 95% CI 0.77—1.57).

Conclusions.—The results of this meta-analysis suggest that elective EVAR in patients aged ≥80 years is associated with significantly lower immediate postoperative mortality and morbidity than open repair and should be considered the treatment of choice in these fragile patients. These results indicate also that, when EVAR is not feasible, open repair can be performed with acceptable immediate and late survival in patients at high risk of aneurysm rupture (Fig 4).

▶ "We are still learning how and when to place reasonable limits on our impulse to rescue all who might benefit from the dramatic technologies of contemporary surgery."[1] The decision whether to perform a major surgical procedure on the very elderly requires a sufficient burden of evidence regarding its potentially associated harms and benefits.

This is a well-conducted systematic review to evaluate open and endovascular repair of abdominal aortic aneurysms (AAA) in those patients aged 80 or older. Six studies met criteria for review, with 13 419 subjects included in the analysis. The results are remarkable and favor the bias of many endovascular

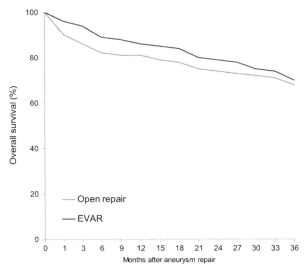

FIGURE 4.—Pooled survival after endovascular (EVAR) vs. open repair of abdominal aortic aneurysm in patients aged 80 years and older. Estimates of late survival was calculated for up to 3 years after repair as reported in three studies.[20–22] *Editor's Note*: Please refer to original journal article for full references. (Reprinted from European Journal of Vascular and Endovascular Surgery, Biancari F, Catania A, D'Andrea V. Elective endovascular vs. open repair for abdominal aortic aneurysm in patients aged 80 years and older: systematic review and meta-analysis. *Eur J Vasc Endovasc Surg*. 2011;42:571-576. Copyright 2011, with permission from the European Society for Vascular Surgery.)

specialists. Octogenarians tolerate endovascular treatment (EVAR) better than open repair, with a risk ratio of 3.87 (95% CI, 3.19-4.68). One of the unique aspects of this study is that to be included in the analysis, the publication had to have data on outcomes for at least 1 year. Fig 4 depicts the pooled survival after EVAR versus open repair for these elderly patients.

The message is sound: EVAR should be the method of first choice for repairing AAA in patients aged 80 and older.

B. W. Starnes, MD

Reference

1. McKneally MF. "We didn't expect dementia and diapers": reflections on the Nihon experience with type A aortic dissection in octogenarians. *J Thorac Cardiovasc Surg*. 2008;135:984-985.

Outcomes after Open Surgery and Endovascular Aneurysm Repair for Abdominal Aortic Aneurysm in Patients with Massive Neck Atheroma
Hoshina K, Hosaka A, Takayama T, et al (The Univ of Tokyo, Japan; Morinomiya Hosp, Osaka, Japan)
Eur J Vasc Endovasc Surg 43:257-261, 2012

Objective.—We retrospectively analysed surgically treated abdominal aortic aneurysm (AAA) in patients with massive atheroma in the aneurysmal neck and compared the outcomes of endovascular aneurysm repair (EVAR) and open surgery (OS) to determine an appropriate strategy for massive neck atheroma cases.

Methods.—A retrospective study was performed in 326 consecutive patients who underwent EVAR and in 247 patients who underwent OS. We defined massive neck atheromas if the following characteristics were observed: (1) thickness ≥ 5 mm; (2) the circumference of the infrarenal aorta $\geq 75\%$; and (3) length ≥ 5 mm. Twenty-eight patients (8.5%) in the EVAR group and 22 (8.9%) in the OS group met these criteria. We modified the previously published reporting standards on the basis of the selection of systemic and embolisation-related complications.

Results.—Patients in the EVAR group had less intra-operative blood loss, shorter operation time, and shorter hospital stays after the operation ($P < 0.01$). No perioperative deaths were observed in either group. Major complications were categorised as early (in-hospital) or late (outpatient, within 6 months). Five and three patients in the OS and EVAR groups had early complications, but the difference was not statistically significant. In contrast, 7 patients in the EVAR group had late complications, compared to no patients in the OS group ($P = 0.01$). Kaplan–Meier analysis revealed a significantly higher survival rate in the OS group ($P = 0.011$). Two of the 4 patients with suprarenal clamping developed major complications. Mild eosinophilia was observed in 10 patients in the EVAR group. Proteinuria occurred or worsened in 5 EVAR patients and 1 OS patient.

Conclusion.—Compared to OS patients, EVAR patients with massive neck atheroma tend to develop late-phase complications possibly related to cholesterol crystal embolisation. The clinical features of massive neck atheroma patients receiving EVAR should be carefully monitored even after hospital discharge (Fig 1).

▶ This article addresses early and late complications of open and endovascular treatment of aortas with so-called shaggy aorta syndrome. There are a number

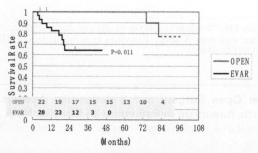

FIGURE 1.—The Kaplane–Meier curve shows superior overall survival in the OS group. The log-rank test revealed a significant difference between groups ($P = 0.011$). (Reprinted from European Journal of Vascular and Endovascular Surgery, Hoshina K, Hosaka A, Takayama T, et al. Outcomes after open surgery and endovascular aneurysm repair for abdominal aortic aneurysm in patients with massive neck atheroma. *Eur J Vasc Endovasc Surg.* 2012;43:257-261. Copyright 2012, with permission from the European Society for Vascular Surgery.)

of interesting points here. The first is that the authors offer a quantitative definition of "massive atheroma" of the infrainguinal aortic neck as detailed in the article's abstract. This definition was likely derived empirically, but nonetheless it points out that one can use a combination of length of the atheroma, thickness of the atheroma, and the percent of the circumference of the infrainguinal aorta neck involved as components of the definition. The authors examined survival and late complications related to mode of treatment of the aorta—endovascular versus open surgery. Surprisingly, they found overall survival rates of the endovascular aneurysm repair (EVAR)-treated patients with massive aortic neck atheroma were significantly less than those treated with open surgery (Fig 1). The fact the deaths were largely unrelated to the aorta suggests there may have been some selection bias in how the patients were treated. The causes of death of the EVAR patients, as detailed in the article, do not suggest that the lower survival rate in the EVAR-treated patient was a consequence of the endovascular repair. Complications related to treatment of the aorta were no different in the endovascular and open groups. Late complications, however, were higher in the EVAR group, and 9 of the 10 late complications occurred in either the kidneys or the bowel. Again, it is difficult to imagine how late complications originated above the level of the endograft could be related to earlier placement of the endograft, leading to a strong suspicion that selection bias is playing a role in the outcome of this study. It should be noted that the patients in this study were derived at 2 institutions, 1 of which primarily performs EVAR and the second of which primarily performs open procedures for infrarenal abdominal aortic aneurysm. Overall, although the authors' quantitative definition of a shaggy aorta is a useful contribution, one cannot use these data to argue one way or the other for either open or endovascular treatment of shaggy aortas.

G. L. Moneta, MD

Final Results of the Prospective European Trial of the Endurant Stent Graft for Endovascular Abdominal Aortic Aneurysm Repair
Rouwet EV, Torsello G, de Vries J-PPM, et al (Erasmus Med Ctr, Rotterdam, The Netherlands; Universitätsklinikum Münster, Germany; St Antonius Ziekenhuis, Nieuwegein, The Netherlands; et al)
Eur J Vasc Endovasc Surg 42:489-497, 2011

Objectives.—The Endurant Stent Graft System (Medtronic Vascular, Santa Rosa, CA) is specifically designed to treat patients with abdominal aortic aneurysm, including those with difficult anatomies. This is the 1-year report of a prospective, non-randomised, open-label trial at 10 European centres.

Methods.—Between November 2007 and August 2008, 80 patients were enrolled for elective endovascular aneurysm repair (EVAR) with the Endurant; 71 with moderate ($\leq 60°$) and nine with high ($60-75°$) infrarenal aortic neck angulation. Safety and stent-graft performance were assessed throughout a 1-year follow-up period.

FIGURE 1.—The Endurant Stent Graft System (with view of suprarenal anchoring pins) and the Endurant delivery system. (Reprinted from European Journal of Vascular and Endovascular Surgery, Rouwet EV, Torsello G, de Vries J-PPM, et al. Final results of the prospective European trial of the Endurant stent graft for endovascular abdominal aortic aneurysm repair. *Eur J Vasc Endovasc Surg.* 2011;42: 489-497. Copyright 2011, with permission from the European Society for Vascular Surgery.)

Results.—The device was successfully delivered and deployed in all cases. All-cause mortality was 5% (4/80), with one possibly device-related death. Serious adverse events were comparable between the high and moderate angulation groups. There were no device migrations, stent fractures, aortic ruptures or conversions to open repair. Maximal aneurysm diameter decreased >5 mm in 42.7% of cases. A total of 28 endoleaks were observed (26 type II, two undetermined). Three secondary endovascular procedures were performed for outflow vessel stenosis, graft limb occlusion and iliac extension, resulting in a secondary patency rate of 100%. No re-interventions were required in the high angulation group.

Conclusions.—The Endurant Stent Graft was successfully delivered and deployed in all cases and performed safely and effectively in all patients, including those with unfavourable proximal neck anatomy (Fig 1).

▶ The 1-year Endurant Stent Graft (Medtronic Vascular, Santa Rosa, California) results demonstrate 100% technical success, no type I or III endoleaks, and no aneurysm ruptures. Modifying the columnar strength of the graft, adding a tip-capture to the suprarenal stent, and modifying the ipsilateral limb stents were meant to treat "short necks" and "angulated necks."

The 1-year results confirm that the graft (Fig 1) can be implanted safely, but I would temper any excitement that this graft will treat shorter more angulated necks over current grafts available. Eighty patients were selected by trial coordinators; the number of patients screened is critical and not reported. Typically, for every 1 patient enrolled, 3 patients are excluded. The trial did not include all short angulated necks. In fact, only 9 patients had angulated seal zones greater than 60° with a neck length of 32 mm (range, 13−70 mm). The graft like most grafts will achieve seal in long, angulated necks. The short necks were also sparse. Of the 71 patients treated with neck angles less than 60°, the neck length was 27 mm (range, 10−73 mm).

If this is your graft of choice, the Endurant modifications offer a lower profile design with a controlled suprarenal deployment; however, the data do not support its empiric use for short angulated neck anatomy.

Z. M. Arthurs, MD

Long-term Results of Iliac Aneurysm Repair with Iliac Branched Endograft: A 5-Year Experience on 100 Consecutive Cases
Parlani G, Verzini F, De Rango P, et al (Hosp S. Maria della Misericordia, Perugia, Italy; et al)
Eur J Vasc Endovasc Surg 43:287-292, 2012

Background.—Iliac branch device (IBD) technique has been introduced as an appealing and effective solution to avoid complications occurring during repair of aorto-iliac aneurysm with extensive iliac involvement. Nevertheless, no large series with long-term follow-up of IBD are available. The aim of this study was to analyse safety and long-term efficacy of IBD in a consecutive series of patients.

Methods.—Between 2006 and 2011, 100 consecutive patients were enrolled in a prospective database on IBD. Indications included unilateral or bilateral common iliac artery aneurysms combined or not with abdominal aneurysms. Patients were routinely followed up with computed tomography. Data were reported according to the Kaplan—Meier method.

Results.—There were 96 males, mean age 74.1 years. Preoperative median common iliac aneurysm diameter was 40 mm (interquartile range (IQR): 35—44 mm). Sixty-seven patients had abdominal aortic aneurysm >35 mm (IQR: 40—57 mm) associated with iliac aneurysm. Eleven patients presented hypogastric aneurysm. Twelve patients underwent isolated iliac repair with IBD and 88 patients received associated endovascular aortic repair. Periprocedural technical success rate was 95%, with no mortality. Two patients experienced external iliac occlusion in the first month. At a median follow-up of 21 months (range 1—60) aneurysm growth >3 mm was detected in four iliac (4%) arteries. Iliac endoleak (one type III and two distal type I) developed in three patients and buttock claudication in four patients. Estimated patency rate of internal iliac branch was 91.4% at 1 and 5 years. Freedom from any reintervention rate was 90% at 1 year and 81.4% at 5 years. No late ruptures occurred.

Conclusions.—Long-term results show that IBD use can ensure persistent iliac aneurysm exclusion at 5 years, with low risk of reintervention. This technique can be considered as a first endovascular option in patients with extensive iliac aneurysm disease and favourable anatomy (Fig 1).

▶ One of the difficulties in enrolling patients into the PRESERVE trial was the requirement for specific anatomic criteria. Namely, subjects needed to have a unilateral common iliac artery aneurysm with a patent contralateral internal iliac artery. Enrollment was slow, as this clinical scenario is not a common finding.

This large consecutive series from Italy provides us with a glimpse of what we can expect from the Iliac Branch Device (IBD, COOK Inc, Bloomington, Indiana; Fig 1) once it has been formally approved by the US Food and Drug Administration.

The results are impressive. One hundred patients were treated with the IBD over a 5-year period. Twelve patients underwent isolated iliac artery aneurysm repair, and 88 had a simultaneous aortic aneurysm repair. Technical success

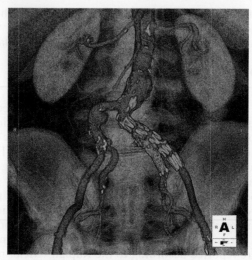

FIGURE 1.—3-Dimensional reconstruction of Computed Tomography scan with TeraRecon Aquarius Workstation in a patient with iliac side-branch repair for isolated left iliac aneurysm. (Reprinted from European Journal of Vascular and Endovascular Surgery, Parlani G, Verzini F, De Rango P, et al. Long-term results of iliac aneurysm repair with iliac branched endograft: a 5-year experience on 100 consecutive cases. *Eur J Vasc Endovasc Surg.* 2012;43:287-292. Copyright 2012, with permission from the European Society for Vascular Surgery.)

was 95% with no operative or 30-day mortality. Iliac branch device patency was 91.4% out to 60 months.

Four external iliac limbs occluded early in this series and were successfully re-intervened on in each case. This is important, as patient selection proved to be a key factor in device success. This article is important for those vascular surgeons who wish to use this device to treat aorto-iliac aneurysms in the future.

B. W. Starnes, MD

Arch and visceral/renal debranching combined with endovascular repair for thoracic and thoracoabdominal aortic aneurysms

Ham SW, Chong T, Moos J, et al (Univ of Southern California, Los Angeles)
J Vasc Surg 54:30-41, 2011

Objective.—We report a single-center experience using the hybrid procedure, consisting of open debranching, followed by endovascular aortic repair, for treatment of arch/proximal descending thoracic/thoracoabdominal aortic aneurysms (TAAA).

Methods.—From 2005 to 2010, 51 patients (33 men; mean age, 70 years) underwent a hybrid procedure for arch/proximal descending thoracic/ TAAA. The 30-day and in-hospital morbidity and mortality rates, and late endoleak, graft patency, and survival were analyzed. Graft patency was assessed by computed tomography, angiography, or duplex ultrasound imaging.

Results.—Hybrid procedures were used to treat 27 thoracic (16 arch, 11 proximal descending thoracic) and 24 TAAA (Crawford/Safi types I to III: 3; type IV: 12; type V: 9). The hybrid procedure involved debranching 47 arch vessels or 77 visceral/renal vessels using bypass grafts, followed by endovascular repair. Seventy-five percent of debranching and endovascular repair procedures were staged, with an average interval of 28 days. Major 30-day and in-hospital complications occurred in 39% of patients and included bypass graft occlusion in four, endoleak reintervention in two, and paraplegia in one. Mortality was 3.9%. During a mean follow-up of 13 months, three additional type II endoleaks required intervention, and one bypass graft occluded. No aneurysm rupture occurred during follow-up. Primary bypass graft patency was 95.3%. Actuarial survival was 86% at 1 year and 67% at 3 years.

Conclusion.—The hybrid procedure is associated with acceptable rates of mortality and paraplegia when used for treatment of arch/proximal descending thoracic/TAAA. These results support this procedure as a reasonable approach to a difficult surgical problem; however, longer follow-up is required to appraise its ultimate clinical utility.

▶ The management of patients with thoracoabdominal aortic aneurysms is undergoing a revolution. Open thoracoabdominal repair using off-loading atrial femoral bypass has been a standard for years. Specialized centers around the country have reduced the morbidity and mortality significantly. The use of fenestrated and branched endovascular aneurysm repair has the promise of reducing the morbidity and mortality even further—most notably, spinal paraplegia rates dropping from 30% to 15%. Unfortunately, these 2 operations have not allowed for the generalization of techniques outside very selective centers. The use of aortic debranching and endovascular grafting has been performed as an alternative. Although this procedure does not seem to be a great departure from the other 2, overall the outcomes have not been as optimistic. In this study, the authors report a combined morbidity of 40%, including pulmonary, renal, and graft occlusion complications. Of these the most problematic seems the postoperative assessment of bypass grafts and prevention of graft occlusion. Renal grafts may occlude asymptomatically or, if detected, require intervention immediately to avoid unsalvageable acute renal failure. To accomplish this successfully, we have adapted a policy of intraoperative arteriographic assessment with angioplasty and stenting if any defects are detected. We will have to see where the hybrid technique fits into our armamentarium after commercialization of fenestrated aortic endografts in the near future.

D. L. Gillespie, MD, FACS

EVAR Suitability is not a Predictor for Early and Midterm Mortality after Open Ruptured AAA Repair

Ten Bosch JA, Willigendael EM, van Sambeek MRHM, et al (Atrium Med Ctr Parkstad, Heerlen, The Netherlands; Catharina hosp, Eindhoven, The Netherlands; et al)
Eur J Vasc Endovasc Surg 41:647-651, 2011

Objective.—The reported mortality reduction of emergency endovascular aneurysm repair (eEVAR) compared with open repair in patients with a ruptured abdominal aortic aneurysm (rAAA), as observed in observational studies, might be flawed by selection bias based on anatomical suitability for eEVAR. In the present study, we compared mortality in EVAR suitable versus non-EVAR-suitable patients with a ruptured AAA who were all treated with conventional open repair.

Materials and Methods.—In all patients presenting with a suspected rAAA, computed tomography angiography (CTA) scanning was performed. All consecutive patients with a confirmed rAAA on preoperative CTA scan and treated with open repair between April 2002 and April 2008 were included. Anatomical suitability for eEVAR was determined by two blinded independent reviewers. Outcomes evaluated were mortality (intra-operative, 30-day, and 6-month), morbidity, complications requiring re-intervention and length of hospital stay.

Results.—A total of 107 consecutive patients presented with a rAAA and underwent preoperative CTA scanning. In 25 patients, eEVAR was performed. In the 82 patients who underwent open repair, CTA showed an EVAR-suitable rAAA in 33 patients (41.8%) and a non-EVAR-suitable rAAA in 49 patients. Thirty-day and 6-month mortality rate was 15/33 (45.5%; 95% confidence interval (CI) 28.1−63.7) and 18/33 (54.5%; 95% CI 36.4−71.9) in the EVAR-suitable group versus 24/49 (49.0%; 95% CI 34.4−63.7) (*P* = 0.75) and 29/49 (59.2%; 95% CI 44.2−73.0) (*P* = 0.68) in the non-EVAR-suitable group, respectively.

Conclusions.—The present study suggests that anatomical suitability for EVAR is not associated with lower early and midterm mortality in patients treated with open ruptured AAA repair. Therefore, the reported reduction in mortality between eEVAR and open repair is unlikely due to selection bias based on anatomical AAA configuration.

▶ Comparative series of open versus endovascular repair of ruptured abdominal aortic aneurysm (AAA) suggest a mortality benefit with endovascular aneurysm repair (EVAR) for repair of ruptured AAA.[1] However, there is no randomized study addressing this question, and selection bias with regard to treatment of more stable patients or patients with more favorable anatomic considerations with EVAR may lead to a false impression EVAR is superior to open repair for ruptured AAA. Generally, about one-half of patients with ruptured AAA are suitable for EVAR based on anatomic considerations. Unsuitable patients are treated with open repair. In this study, the authors compared mortality in EVAR-suitable versus non—EVAR-suitable patients with a ruptured AAA. All underwent preoperative computed tomography (CT) imaging, and all were treated with conventional open repair. There was no difference in the 30-day and the 60-month mortality rates in the EVAR-suitable and the EVAR-nonsuitable patients. In addition, the lower limit of the confidence interval for 30-day mortality was 28% in this series, which is higher than the morality rate of 18% to 24% reported with EVAR for ruptured AAA. The data suggest that the perceived improved mortality of ruptured AAA repair with EVAR is not due to more favorable anatomy in the EVAR patients. There are certainly a number of known (hemodynamic stability) and unknown variables that could influence morality rates in patients with ruptured AAA treated with EVAR or standard open repair. There, however, are 22 nonrandomized observational studies that, collectively taken, show reduced early mortality using EVAR for repair of ruptured AAA.[2] The overall impression is that EVAR is a positive step forward in the treatment of ruptured AAA. According to this study, the benefit is unlikely because of selection bias based on anatomic aneurysm configuration.

G. L. Moneta, MD

References

1. Ten Bosch JA, Teijink JA, Willigendael EM, Prins MH. Endovascular aneurysm repair is superior to open surgery for ruptured abdominal aortic aneurysms in EVAR-suitable patients. *J Vasc Surg*. 2010;52:13-18.
2. Hinchliffe RJ, Bruijstens L, MacSweeney ST, Braithwaite BD. A randomised trial of endovascular and open surgery for ruptured abdominal aortic aneurysm - results of a pilot study and lessons learned for future studies. *Eur J Vasc Endovasc Surg*. 2006; 32:506-513.

G. L. Moneta, MD

8 Visceral and Renal Artery Disease

Differences in anatomy and outcomes in patients treated with open mesenteric revascularization before and after the endovascular era
Ryer EJ, Oderich GS, Bower TC, et al (Mayo Clinic, Rochester, MN)
J Vasc Surg 53:1611-1618, 2011

Objective.—To compare the clinical characteristics, anatomy, and outcomes of patients treated with open mesenteric revascularization (OR) for chronic mesenteric ischemia (CMI) before and after the preferential use of endovascular revascularization (ER).

Methods.—We reviewed a prospective database of 257 patients treated for CMI with OR or ER from 1998 to 2009. Treatment trends were analyzed to identify changes in practice paradigm. Prior to 2002, OR was used in 58 of 81 patients (72%). Since 2002, ER surpassed OR as the most common treatment option; OR was indicated in 58 of 176 patients (33%) who either failed ER or had unfavorable lesions for stent placement. We analyzed differences in clinical data, anatomical characteristics, and outcomes in 116 patients treated with OR before (Pre-Endo, n = 58) and after 2002 (Post-Endo, n = 58). Anatomical characteristics were determined by a blinded investigator using conventional angiography, magnetic resonance angiography, and computed tomography angiography with centerline of flow measurements.

Results.—Both groups had similar demographics, risk factors, and clinical presentation, with the exception of higher ($P < .05$) rates of hypertension, hyperlipidemia, cardiac interventions, dysrhythmias, and higher comorbidity scores in the Post-Endo group. This group also had more extensive mesenteric artery disease, including higher incidence of three-vessel involvement (76% vs 57%; $P = .048$) and superior mesenteric artery (SMA) occlusion (67% vs 41%; $P = .005$). There were no differences ($P > .05$) in the number of vessels revascularized (1.8 ± 0.4 vs 1.7 ± 0.5) and in graft configuration (antegrade, 91% vs 78%; retrograde, 9% vs 22%; two-vessel, 69% vs 81%) in the Pre- and Post-Endo groups, respectively. There were no differences in operative mortality (1.7% vs 3.4%), morbidity (43% vs 53%), length of stay (12 ± 1 vs 12 ± 1 days), and immediate symptom improvement (88% vs 86%) in the Pre- and Post-Endo groups, respectively. Mean follow-up was 57 ± 6 months for patients treated before 2002 and 29 ± 6 months for those treated after 2002 ($P = .0001$). At 5 years, primary and secondary patency rates and recurrence-free survival were 82%, 86%, and 84% in the Pre-Endo and 81%, 82%, and 76% in the Post-Endo groups (*P* > .05).

Conclusion.—OR has been used in approximately one-third of patients treated for CMI since 2002. Despite more comorbidities and more extensive mesenteric artery disease in patients now treated with OR, outcomes have not changed compared with those operated prior to the preferential use of mesenteric stents before 2002 (Fig 2).

▶ Endovascular revascularization is a common practice and in many instances is a primary treatment modality for many patients with lower extremity and visceral arterial disease. Treatment for patients with chronic mesenteric ischemia can be either open or endovascular; however, the latter can have up to 50% failures in the first year, requiring reintervention, and this must be taken into account in the decision-making process. Endovascular treatment for chronic mesenteric ischemia is favorable in lesions that have short-length stenoses with minimal calcifications. Unfavorable lesions in visceral vessels are those that are long or occluded or lesions

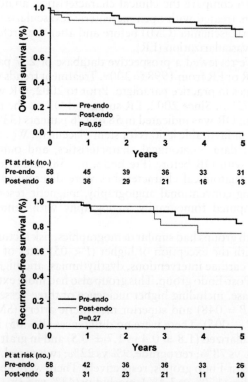

FIGURE 2.—Kaplan-Meier estimates of overall patient survival and recurrence-free survival in 116 patients treated with open mesenteric revascularizations for chronic mesenteric ischemia before (*Pre-endo*) and after (*Post-endo*) the preferential use of mesenteric stents. (Reprinted from the Journal of Vascular Surgery, Ryer EJ, Oderich GS, Bower TC, et al. Differences in anatomy and outcomes in patients treated with open mesenteric revascularization before and after the endovascular era. *J Vasc Surg.* 2011;53:1611-1618. Copyright 2011, with permission from The Society for Vascular Surgery.)

with extensive calcification or thrombus. Despite these shortcomings, endovascular treatment of chronic mesenteric ischemia has several advantages, including decreased in-hospital mortality and length of hospital stay when compared to open surgery. In this study, the authors performed a retrospective review of 257 patients with chronic mesenteric ischemia from 1998 to 2009. The authors noted that from 1998 to 2002, 73% of revascularization for patients with chronic mesenteric ischemia were treated by open revascularization, but after 2002 only 33% of the procedures were performed by open surgery because endovascular revascularization was not possible, failed, or the anatomy was considered unfavorable due to occlusion, severe calcification, or long-segment stenosis. The study then evaluated all patients treated with open revascularization in the preendovascular (group A, 58 patients) versus their postendovascular (group B, 58 patients) era, with an arbitrary cutoff point after 2002 because of the change in treatment paradigm shifting in favor of endovascular interventions after 2002. Clinical presentation was similar in both groups except for greater frequency of food fear, postprandial abdominal pain, and need for preoperative total parenteral nutrition in group B. Significant findings were that group B had more extensive mesenteric artery disease, including higher incidence of 3-vessel involvement (76% vs 57%; $P = .048$) and superior mesenteric artery occlusion (67% vs 41%; $P = .005$). There were no differences in the number of vessels revascularized (1.8 ± 0.4 vs 1.7 ± 0.5) and graft configuration (antegrade, 91% vs 78%; retrograde, 9% vs 22%; two-vessel, 69% vs 81%) in group A and group B, respectively. The most common graft configuration in both groups was a supraceliac aorta to celiac and superior mesenteric artery bypass, which was used in 76% of patients. There were no differences in operative mortality (1.7% vs 3.4%), morbidity (43% vs 53%), length of stay (13.1 ± 1 vs 12 ± 3 days), and immediate symptom improvement (88% vs 86%) in group A and group B, respectively. Five-year survival and freedom from recurrence were similar in both groups (Fig 2). Five-year primary and secondary patency rates for celiac artery reconstructions were 87% and 92% in group A, and 84% and 84% in group B, respectively. For superior mesenteric artery reconstructions, 5-year primary and secondary patency rates were 79% and 82% and 80% and 82%, respectively. Between the groups, the patency rates were not different. Of importance, this study demonstrated that for patients with significant risk factors (age > 80 years, forced expiratory volume in the first second of expiration < 800 mL, diffusion capacity for carbon monoxide < 50%, resting pCO_2 > 50 mm Hg, resting O_2 < 60 mm Hg, home oxygen therapy, ejection fraction < 25%, New York Heart Association [NYHA] class III or class IV angina, positive cardiac stress testing, myocardial infarction < 90 days, or Cr > 3.0), the mortality increased significantly (7.4%). Despite the increased use of endovascular treatment of chronic mesenteric ischemia, patients who are offered open surgical reconstructions in an era of endovascular therapies have similar outcomes to those who were treated by open surgery in an era with less endovascular options. Although endovascular therapy for chronic mesenteric ischemia offers many advantages over open surgical revascularization, it is critical that we offer these newer therapies to properly selected patients or those with significant risk factors so that the best possible outcomes may be achieved.

J. D. Raffetto, MD

Contemporary Management of Splanchnic and Renal Artery Aneurysms: Results of Endovascular Compared with Open Surgery from Two European Vascular Centers

Cochennec F, Riga CV, Allaire E, et al (Hosp Henri Mondor, Créteil, France; St Mary's Hosp, London, UK; et al)
Eur J Vasc Endovasc Surg 42:340-346, 2011

Introduction.—Splanchnic and renal artery aneurysms (SRAAs) are uncommon but potentially life-threatening in case of rupture. Whether these aneurysms are best treated by open repair or endovascular intervention is unknown. The aim of this retrospective study is to report the results of open and endovascular repairs in two European institutions over a fifteen-year period. We have reviewed the available literature published over the 10 last years.

Methods.—All patients with SRAAs diagnosed from 1995 to 2010 in St Marys Hospital (London, UK) and Henri Mondor Hospital (Créteil, France) were reviewed. Preoperative clinical and anatomical data, operative management and outcomes were recorded from the charts and analyzed.

Results.—40 patients with 51 SRAAs were identified. There were 21 males and 19 females with a mean age of 57 ± 14.9 years. The aneurysms locations were: 14 (27%) renal, 11 (22%) splenic, 7 (14%) celiac trunk, 7 (14%) superior mesenteric artery, 4 (8%) hepatic, 4 (8%) pancreaticoduodenal arcades, 3 (6%) left gastric and 1 (2%) gastroduodenal. 4 patients presented with a ruptured SRAA. 17 SRAAs in 16 patients were treated by open repair, 15 in 15 patients were treated endoluminally and 17 (mean diameter: 18 mm, range: 8—75 mm) were managed conservatively. One patient with metastatic pulmonary cancer with two mycotic aneurysms of the superior mesenteric artery (75 mm) and celiac trunk (15 mm) was palliated. After endovascular treatment, the immediate technical success rate was 100%.

There was no significant difference between open repair and endovascular patients in terms of 30-day post-operative mortality rate and perioperative complications. No in-hospital death occurred in patients treated electively. Postoperatively, four patients (1 ruptured and 3 elective) suffered non-lethal mild to severe complication in the open repair group, as compared with one in the endovascular group (*p* = .34). The mean length of stay was significantly higher after open repair as compared with endovascular repair (17 days, range: 8—56 days vs. 4 days, range: 2—6; *p* < .001).

The mean follow-up time was 17.8 months (range: 0—143 months) after open repair, 15.8 months (range: 0—121 months) after endovascular treatment, and 24.8 (range: 3—64 months) for patient being managed conservatively. No late death related to the VAA occurred. In each group, 2 successful reoperations were deemed necessary. In the endovascular group, two patients presented a reperfusion of the aneurysmal sac at 6 and 24 months respectively.

Conclusion.—No significant difference in term of 30-day mortality and post-operative complication rates could be identified between open repair and endovascular treatment in the present series. Endovascular treatment is a safe alternative to open repair but patients are exposed to the risk of aneurysmal reperfusion. This mandates careful long-term imaging follow up in patients treated endoluminally.

▶ Splanchnic and renal artery aneurysms occur infrequently, such that most reports are relegated to small heterogenous populations. This report accumulates patients over 15 years from 2 separate hospital systems in 2 countries, attempting to overcome the limitations of an infrequent disorder. Unfortunately, only 40 patients were identified with aneurysms primarily in the renal arteries, and the remainder displaced across the mesenteric circulation. This paper describes 40 patients but does not add to our current understanding of their treatment.

The authors highlight a 100% technical success rate for both endovascular and open repair, yet no definition of technical success was provided. In the case of renal artery aneurysms, the decision to treat using an endovascular approach as opposed to open aneurysmorrhaphy is often related to the ability to preserve renal branch vessels and renal function. In the case of pancreaticoduodenal aneurysms, embolization of all feeding branch vessels is necessary but can also be extremely challenging. Technical endpoints for both open and endovascular repair would have supported their conclusions that both treatment modalities offer similar results. In practice, a strong selection bias exists given that most of these aneurysms anatomically favor either an endovascular or open approach.

Z. M. Arthurs, MD

9 Thoracic Aorta

A microRNA profile comparison between thoracic aortic dissection and normal thoracic aorta indicates the potential role of microRNAs in contributing to thoracic aortic dissection pathogenesis
Liao M, Zou S, Weng J, et al (Second Military Med Univ, Shanghai, China)
J Vasc Surg 53:1341-1349, 2011

Objectives.—Our aim was to identify important microRNAs (miRNAs) that might play an important role in contributing to aortic dissection by conducting a miRNA profile comparison between thoracic aortic dissection (TAD) and normal thoracic aorta.

Methods.—The differentially expressed miRNA profiles of the aortic tissue between TAD patients (n = 6) and age-matched donors without aortic diseases (NA; n = 6) were analyzed by miRNA microarray. Quantitative reverse transcription polymerase chain reaction (qRT-PCR) was further performed to verify the expression of 12 selected miRNAs with an increased number of samples (TAD n = 12; NA n = 8). The potential targets of the differentially expressed miRNAs were predicted using computational searches. Bioinformatic analyses of the predicted target genes (gene ontology, pathway and network analysis) were done for further research. Additionally, Western blotting was performed to confirm the bioinformatics findings.

Results.—The miRNA microarray revealed differentially expressed miRNAs between the TAD and NA groups. In the TAD group, 18 miRNAs were upregulated and 56 were down regulated (fold change >2, $P < .01$). qRT-PCR verified statistically consistent expression of seven selected miRNAs with microarray analysis. Combined with our previous proteomics study, target gene prediction revealed that some miRNAs reciprocally expressed with their targeted proteins. Target gene-related pathway analysis showed a significant change in five pathways in the TAD group compared with the NA group, especially the focal adhesion and the mitogen-activated protein kinase (MAPK) signaling pathways. By further conducting miRNA gene network analysis, we found that the mir-29 and mir-30 families are likely to play a role in the regulation of these two pathways, respectively.

Conclusions.—Our results indicate that miRNAs expression profiles in aortic media from TAD were significantly changed. These results may provide important insights into TAD disease mechanisms. This study also suggests that the focal adhesion and MAPK signaling pathways might play important roles in the pathogenesis of TAD.

▶ Aortic dissection can lead to devastating life-threatening consequences, especially when malperfusion syndrome occurs. A clear understanding of the biochemical changes taking place in patients with aortic dissections would provide further information in the pathogenesis of the disease, and possibly new avenues for therapy. In this well-designed study, the authors evaluate the role of microRNA (miRNA), which is a group of highly conserved, small noncoding RNAs of 21 to 25 nucleotides that usually negatively modulate gene expression at the posttranscriptional level by incomplete or complete complementary binding to target sequences within the 3' untranslated region (3' UTR) of mRNA. Therefore, miRNAs have an important role in regulating gene expression. miRNAs are involved in many important biological processes, some of which are related to regulation of cell proliferation, differentiation, apoptosis, and tumorigenesis, and aberrant and/or absent expression of miRNA is often associated with pathophysiologic disorders. In this study, the authors obtain tissue from patients with aortic dissections from the ascending aorta during surgical repair (n = 12) and from control ascending aorta of age- and sex-matched organ donors (n = 8). Nine of the 12 patients with aortic dissection were taking antihypertensive medications, but none were taking statins. The study found that compared with normal controls, in the aortic dissection group, there were 18 miRNAs upregulated, and 56 were downregulated (fold change > 2, P < .01). Target gene—related pathway analysis showed a significant change in 5 pathways in the aortic dissection group compared with the control group, especially the focal adhesion and the mitogen-activated protein kinase signaling pathways. Further miRNA gene network analysis found that the mir-29 and mir-30 families are likely regulating the focal adhesion and mitogen-activated protein kinase pathways, respectively. The differentially expressed miRNA found in the aortic dissection group regulate important biologic functions that include cell communication, signal transduction, RNA metabolic process, transcription, and cell differentiation. The authors speculate that the underexpression of the specific miRNA hsa-miR-29a and hsa-miR-29c may lead to the increased collagen deposition in the aortic wall and contribute to the pathogenesis of aortic dissection. In addition, the miRNA mir143/145 are underexpressed in aortic dissection tissue, which may help explain why vascular smooth muscle cells are underdifferentiated, leading to dysfunction and aortic wall remodeling in aortic dissection. A limitation of this study is that it only included male subjects. Whether the same changes in miRNA are also present in the dissected aorta of women is not known, and further research in this area is required. In addition, it would be interesting to know whether statins, which have a many pleiotropic effects, have an effect on the expression of miRNA in aortic dissection tissue. This area of investigating miRNA is exciting in vascular diseases and will provide further insight in gene regulation and the potential for advanced therapy, hopefully before the events of aortic dissection and its catastrophic complications.

J. D. Raffetto, MD

Pravastatin Reduces Marfan Aortic Dilation
McLoughlin D, McGuinness J, Byrne J, et al (Royal College of Surgeons in Ireland, Dublin; et al)
Circulation 124:S168-S173, 2011

Background.—The sequelae of aortic root dilation are the lethal consequences of Marfan syndrome. The root dilation is attributable to an imbalance between deposition of matrix elements and metalloproteinases in the aortic medial layer as a result of excessive transforming growth factor-beta signaling. This study examined the efficacy and mechanism of statins in attenuating aortic root dilation in Marfan syndrome and compared effects to the other main proposed preventative agent, losartan.

Methods and Results.—Marfan mice heterozygous for a mutant allele encoding a cysteine substitution in fibrillin-1 (C1039G) were treated daily from 6 weeks old with pravastatin 0.5 g/L or losartan 0.6 g/L. The end points of aortic root diameter (n=25), aortic thickness, and architecture (n=10), elastin volume (n=5), dp/dtmax (maximal rate of change of pressure) (cardiac catheter; n=20), and ultrastructural analysis with stereology (electron microscopy; n=5) were examined. The aortic root diameters of untreated Marfan mice were significantly increased in comparison to normal mice (0.161 ± 0.001 cm vs 0.252 ± 0.004 cm; $P<0.01$). Pravastatin (0.22 ± 0.003 cm; $P<0.01$) and losartan (0.221 ± 0.004 cm; $P<0.01$) produced a significant reduction in aortic root dilation. Both drugs also preserved elastin volume within the medial layer (pravastatin 0.23 ± 0.02 and losartan 0.29 ± 0.03 vs untreated Marfan 0.19 ± 0.02; $P=0.01$; normal mice 0.27 ± 0.02). Ultrastructural analysis showed a reduction of rough endoplasmic reticulum in smooth muscle cells with pravastatin (0.022 ± 0.004) and losartan (0.013 ± 0.001) compared to untreated Marfan mice (0.035 ± 0.004; $P<0.01$).

Conclusions.—Statins are similar to losartan in attenuating aortic root dilation in a mouse model of Marfan syndrome. They appear to act through reducing the excessive protein manufacture by vascular smooth muscle cells, which occurs in the Marfan aorta. As a drug that is relatively well-tolerated for long-term use, it may be useful clinically.

▶ Marfan syndrome is a connective tissue disorder that affects multiple systems. Life-threatening complications are mostly cardiovascular, particularly dilation of the aortic root and development of thoracic aorta aneurysm and dissection. Marfan syndrome derives from a relative lack of, or abnormal, fibrillin-1. This results in vascular smooth muscle cells loosing ability to sense aortic wall strain. This in turn leads to excessive transforming growth factor beta (TGF-β) release from the connective tissue matrix resulting in excessive activation of smooth muscle cells and an inappropriate and haphazard remodeling process. The result is progressive dilation and weakening of aorta and aortic root. Pravastatin, an HMG-CoA reductase inhibitor statin medication, has pleiotropic anti-inflammatory effects. It has been shown to reduce cardiac expression of transforming growth factor beta.[1] Because TGF-β dysregulation can be attributed to fibrillin-1 deficiency, pravastatin is a theoretic potential therapeutic agent to prevent aortic complications of Marfan syndrome. The authors therefore examined the efficacy and mechanisms of action of statins in attenuating aortic root dilation in Marfan syndrome and compared these effects with those of losartan, a medication already found to have favorable effects in the mouse model of Marfan syndrome. Pravastatin had a beneficial effect in attenuating aortic root dilation and preserving aortic elastin in a mouse model of Marfan syndrome. Losartan also reduced aortic root dilation to the same degree but seemed to have a greater effect of preserving elastin within the aortic wall and in reducing aortic wall thickening. Both likely work through some modulation of TGF-β. Theoretically, losartan with its antihypertensive effect and reduction in pulse pressure and hemodynamic strain on the aortic root should have more favorable long-term effects. Statins, however, are well tolerated in the long term and now need to be investigated as both monotherapy and as combination therapy with losartan in animal models of Marfan syndrome and eventually in humans with Marfan syndrome.

G. L. Moneta, MD

Reference

1. Yu Y, Ohmori K, Chen Y, et al. Effects of pravastatin on progression of glucose intolerance and cardiovascular remodeling in a type II diabetes model. *J Am Coll Cardiol.* 2004;44:904-913.

Meta-Analysis of Usefulness of D-Dimer to Diagnose Acute Aortic Dissection
Shimony A, Filion KB, Mottillo S, et al (Jewish General Hosp/McGill Univ, Montreal, Quebec, Canada; Univ of Minnesota, Minneapolis)
Am J Cardiol 107:1227-1234, 2011

Numerous studies have examined whether plasma D-dimer (DD) can be used to identify patients with acute aortic dissection (AAD). These studies have been inconclusive because of their limited sample sizes and the different cut-off values employed. We aimed to conduct a systematic review and meta-analysis to examine the utility of plasma DD as a screening tool for AAD. We systematically searched EMBASE and MEDLINE and hand-searched relevant articles to identify studies investigating plasma DD as a screening tool for AAD. A value of 500 ng/ml was defined as the threshold for a positive plasma DD finding because it is widely used for ruling out pulmonary emboli. Using DerSimonian—Laird random-effects models we pooled data across studies to estimate sensitivity, specificity, positive and negative predictive values, and positive and negative likelihood ratios (LRs). We identified 7 studies involving 298 subjects with AAD and 436 without. When data were pooled across studies, sensitivity (0.97, 95% confidence interval [CI] 0.94 to 0.99) and negative predictive value (0.96, 95% CI 0.93 to 0.98) were high. Specificity (0.56, 95% CI 0.51 to 0.60) and positive predictive value (0.60, 95% CI 0.55 to 0.66) were low. Negative LR showed an excellent discriminative ability (0.06, 95% CI 0.03 to 0.12), whereas positive LR did not (2.43, 95% CI 1.89 to 3.12).

In conclusion, our meta-analysis suggests that plasma DD <500 ng/ml is a useful screening tool to identify patients who do not have AAD. Plasma DD may thus be used to identify subjects who are unlikely to benefit from further aortic imaging.

▶ It has been suggested that analysis of plasma D-dimer levels can be useful to rule out acute aortic dissection (AAD).[1,2] The idea is that if D-dimer levels are normal, AAD is effectively ruled out, and further imaging studies are not needed. Previous studies, however, have had relatively limited sample sizes and have used different D-dimer cutoff values as indicative of normal versus abnormal (100-900 ng/mL). Some studies have also not had control groups, precluding calculations of specificity, positive and negative predictive values, and positive and negative likelihood ratios. The authors' goal was to perform a systematic review and meta-analysis to examine the use of plasma D-dimer as a screening tool for AAD. The high sensitivity and high negative predictive value reported here indicate plasma D-dimer level is a potential useful screening tool to identify patients who do not have AAD and therefore may not need additional imaging studies to rule out AAD. Thus, in patients being considered for a diagnosis of AAD, plasma D-dimer levels can help to identify subjects unlikely to benefit from further aortic imaging. It is, however, important to remember that untreated AAD has a high mortality rate. Excluding patients from definitive imaging studies based on a negative plasma D-dimer level may be unwise, particularly in patients with a higher risk profile, such as those with Marfan syndrome or uncontrolled hypertension. D-dimer to rule out AAD is most likely to be useful in subjects with low to moderate risk to actually have to AAD. Additional evaluation of D-dimer under specific clinical circumstances is needed before the test can be advocated as a "stand-alone" test to exclude AAD.

G. L. Moneta, MD

References

1. Sodeck G, Domanovits H, Schillinger M, et al. D-dimer in ruling out acute aortic dissection: a systematic review and prospective cohort study. *Eur Heart J*. 2007; 28:3067-3075.
2. Marill KA. Serum D-dimer is a sensitive test for the detection of acute aortic dissection: a pooled meta-analysis. *J Emerg Med*. 2008;34:367-376.

Long-term follow-up of acute type B aortic dissection: Ulcer-like projections in thrombosed false lumen play a role in late aortic events
Miyahara S, Mukohara N, Fukuzumi M, et al (Hyogo Brain and Heart Ctr at Himeji, Japan)
J Thorac Cardiovasc Surg 142:e25-e31, 2011

Objective.—Patients with Stanford type B dissection treated medically during the acute phase have a risk of surgery and aortic rupture during the chronic phase. We investigated the predictors for late aortic events by focusing on the false lumen status with computed tomography.

Methods.—A total of 160 patients were enrolled in the study, with a mean follow-up interval of 44.6 ± 25.4 months. Patients were divided into 3 groups according to the false lumen status at the time of onset: group T, thrombosed in 49 patients (30.6%); group U, thrombosed with ulcer-like projections in 52 patients (32.5%); and group P, patent in 59 patients (36.9%).

Results.—The mean aortic enlargement rate of groups U and P was greater than that of group T (0.40 ± 0.91 mm/month in group U, 0.44 ± 0.49 mm/month in group P, and −0.016 ± 0.23 mm/month in group T). The event-free rate in groups U and P was lower than in group T: 5-year event-free rates of 67.4% ± 8.2% in group U and 57.7% ± 10.9% in group P versus 95.0% ± 4.9% in group T (group T vs group U: *P* = .0011, group U vs group

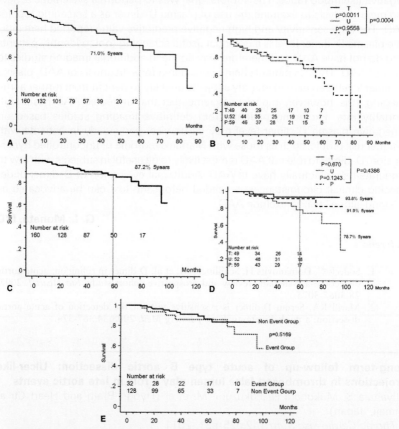

FIGURE 2.—A, Freedom from aortic events in entire study group. B, Freedom from aortic events in each group; *P* values were calculated by the log-rank test. C, Cumulative survival of entire study group. D, Cumulative survival of each group; *P* values were calculated by the log-rank test. E, Cumulative survival of event group (N = 32) and non-event group (N = 128); *P* values were calculated by the log-rank test. (Reprinted from the Journal of Thoracic and Cardiovascular Surgery, Miyahara S, Mukohara N, Fukuzumi M, et al. Long-term follow-up of acute type B aortic dissection: ulcer-like projections in thrombosed false lumen play a role in late aortic events. *J Thorac Cardiovasc Surg.* 2011;142:e25-e31. Copyright 2011, with permission from The American Association for Thoracic Surgery.)

P: $P = .96$, group P vs group T: $P = .0004$). Cox regression analysis revealed that the false lumen status (patent or ulcer-like projections) ($P = .029$), maximum aortic diameter at onset ($P < .0001$), and patient age ($P = .0069$) were predictors of the late aortic events.

Conclusions.—In type B aortic dissection, a thrombosed false lumen with ulcer-like projections and a patent false lumen had an influence on late aortic dilation and late aortic events (Figs 2 and 3).

▶ Patients with acute type B aortic dissection who present without complications of rupture, malperfusion, or persistent pain are usually treated medically. However, a significant proportion of these patient will go on to have late aortic rupture or serial aortic dilation, requiring intervention. It is known that patients with type B aortic dissection and a patent false lumen at presentation have poorer outcomes than those with a thrombosed false lumen (ie, intramural hematoma). At least 2 types of intramural hematoma are recognized: those with and those without ulcerlike projections (ULPs) (Fig 3). There is controversy over the appropriate management of thrombosed false lumens with ULPs. Widespread availability of thoracic endografts has added to the controversy as to the best

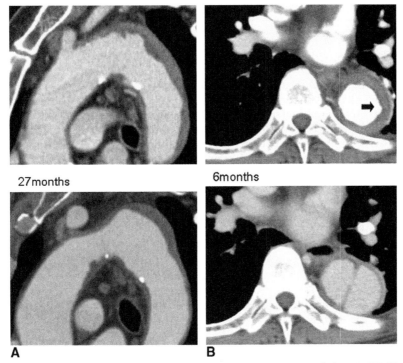

27 months

6 months

A   **B**

FIGURE 3.—A, ULP in distal arch progressed to a saccular aneurysm 27 months later. B, ULP (*black arrow*) in descending aorta recanalized into false lumen 6 months later. (Reprinted from the Journal of Thoracic and Cardiovascular Surgery, Miyahara S, Mukohara N, Fukuzumi M, et al. Long-term follow-up of acute type B aortic dissection: ulcer-like projections in thrombosed false lumen play a role in late aortic events. *J Thorac Cardiovasc Surg.* 2011;142:e25-e31. Copyright 2011, with permission from The American Association for Thoracic Surgery.)

way to treat patients with acute aortic dissection. At one end of the extreme is to use medical management for all patients except those with obvious complications of rupture or malperfusion. At the other end of the extreme is placement of an endograft in anyone who presents with acute type B aortic dissection, regardless of the presence of complications at the time of presentation. A bit of a middle ground is to determine which patients with acute type B aortic dissection are at greatest risk for late aortic events such as late rupture or progressive dilation. Data such as these (Fig 2) are helpful in determining whether a middle ground for acute treatment of patients with acute aortic dissection is reasonable. Natural history data are vitally important in helping determine how best to target interventional therapy in patients with acute aortic dissection.

G. L. Moneta, MD

Type-Selective Benefits of Medications in Treatment of Acute Aortic Dissection (from the International Registry of Acute Aortic Dissection [IRAD])
Suzuki T, Isselbacher EM, Nienaber CA, et al (Univ of Tokyo, Japan; Massachusetts General Hosp, Boston; Univ Hosp, Rostock, Germany; et al)
Am J Cardiol 109:122-127, 2012

The effects of medications on the outcome of aortic dissection remain poorly understood. We sought to address this by analyzing the International Registry of Acute Aortic Dissection (IRAD) global registry database. A total of 1,301 patients with acute aortic dissection (722 with type A and 579 with type B) with information on their medications at discharge and followed for ≤5 years were analyzed for the effects of the medications on mortality. The initial univariate analysis showed that use of β blockers was associated with improved survival in all patients ($p = 0.03$), in patients with type A overall ($p = 0.02$), and in patients with type A who received surgery ($p = 0.006$). The analysis also showed that use of calcium channel blockers was associated with improved survival in patients with type B overall ($p = 0.02$) and in patients with type B receiving medical management ($p = 0.03$). Multivariate models also showed that the use of β blockers was associated with improved survival in those with type A undergoing surgery (odds ratio 0.47, 95% confidence interval 0.25 to 0.90, $p = 0.02$) and the use of calcium channel blockers was associated with improved survival in patients with type B medically treated patients (odds ratio 0.55, 95% confidence interval 0.35 to 0.88, $p = 0.01$). In conclusion, the present study showed that use of β blockers was associated with improved outcome in all patients and in type A patients (overall as well as in those managed surgically). In contrast, use of calcium channel blockers was associated with improved survival selectively in those with type B (overall and in those treated medically). The use of angiotensin-converting enzyme inhibitors did not show association with mortality (Figs 1 and 2).

▶ There is no evidence-based consensus on medical management of aortic dissection. Medical management of aortic dissection depends primarily on opinion

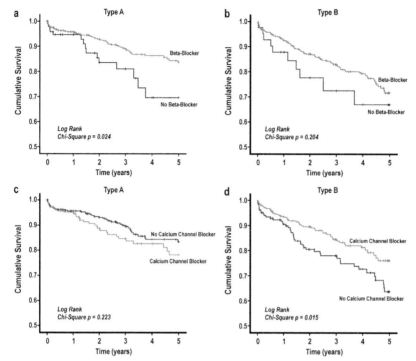

FIGURE 1.—Kaplan-Meier survival curves for effects of medications on mortality. β Blockers in patients with (*A*) type A dissection and (*B*) type B dissection; and calcium channel blockers in those with (*C*) type A and (*D*) type B. (Reprinted from the American Journal of Cardiology, Suzuki T, Isselbacher EM, Nienaber CA, et al. Type-selective benefits of medications in treatment of acute aortic dissection (from the International Registry of Acute Aortic Dissection [IRAD]). *Am J Cardiol.* 2012;109:122-127. Copyright 2012, with permission from Elsevier.)

and historic observational studies.[1] β-blockers are generally regarded as first-line medications, and calcium channel blockers are also frequently used. Recent studies have also suggested benefit with inhibitors of the renin angiotensin system.[2] The lack of solid evidence as to which drugs to use for medical management of aortic dissection has let to disparate guidelines from the European Society for Cardiology, Japanese Circulation Society, and the American Heart Association. The bottom line here, within the limitations of the article, is that β-blockers are beneficial in patients with type A dissection, the largest majority of whom are managed surgically, and in patients with type B dissection, whether they are managed surgically or medically. However, calcium channel blockers appear to be only beneficial in the medical management of type B dissection (Figs 1 and 2). No benefit could be found for the use of angiotensin-converting enzyme (ACE) inhibitors. There have, however, been recent studies, primarily in patients with Marfan syndrome, suggesting a benefit in using ACE inhibitors. A separate analysis of patients with Marfan syndrome in the International Registry of Acute Aortic Dissection (IRAD) was not performed in this study. In addition, the IRAD database predates the current increased use of angiotensin receptor

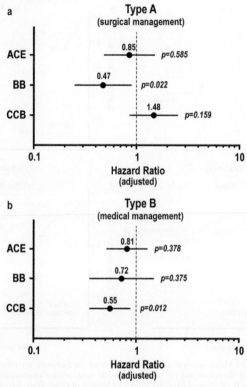

a

Type A
(surgical management)

ACE 0.85 p=0.585

BB 0.47 p=0.022

CCB 1.48 p=0.159

0.1   1   10

Hazard Ratio
(adjusted)

b

Type B
(medical management)

ACE 0.81 p=0.378

BB 0.72 p=0.375

CCB 0.55 p=0.012

0.1   1   10

Hazard Ratio
(adjusted)

FIGURE 2.—Effects of medications on outcomes. *(A)* Patients with type A who underwent surgery; and *(B)* those with type B treated medically. ACE = angiotensin-converting enzyme; BB = β blocker; CCB = calcium channel blocker. (Reprinted from the American Journal of Cardiology, Suzuki T, Isselbacher EM, Nienaber CA, et al. Type-selective benefits of medications in treatment of acute aortic dissection (from the International Registry of Acute Aortic Dissection [IRAD]). *Am J Cardiol.* 2012;109:122-127. Copyright 2012, with permission from Elsevier.)

blockers. The data also did not allow authors to test the combination of drugs and different dosages on mortality. The strongest conclusions from the data are that β-blockers appear useful in all patients with aortic dissection, and calcium channel blockers, as single agents, may only be useful in the medical management of type B dissection.

G. L. Moneta, MD

References

1. Hiratzka LF, Bakris GL, Beckman JA, et al. 2010 ACCF/AHA/AATS/ACR/ASA/SCA/SCAI/SIR/STS/SVM guidelines for the diagnosis and management of patients with Thoracic Aortic Disease: a report of the American College of Cardiology Foundation/American Heart Association Task Force on Practice Guidelines, American Association for Thoracic Surgery, American College of Radiology, American Stroke Association, Society of Cardiovascular Anesthesiologists, Society for Cardiovascular Angiography and Interventions, Society of Interventional Radiology, Society of Thoracic Surgeons, and Society for Vascular Medicine. *Circulation.* 2010;121:e266-e369.

2. Sawada T, Yamada H, Dahlöf B, Matsubara H; KYOTO HEART Study Group. Effects of valsartan on morbidity and mortality in uncontrolled hypertensive patients with high cardiovascular risks: KYOTO HEART Study. *Eur Heart J.* 2009;30:2461-2469.

Endovascular Stent-graft Treatment for Stanford Type A Aortic Dissection

Ye C, Chang G, Li S, et al (Sun Yat-Sen Univ, Guangzhou, People's Republic of China)
Eur J Vasc Endovasc Surg 42:787-794, 2011

Objective.—The aim of the study is to summarise our experience of endovascular stent grafting for Stanford type A aortic dissection.

Design.—Retrospective analysis at single centre.

Methods.—From January 2001 to January 2009, we treated 45 cases of Stanford type A aortic dissection with endovascular stent grafting. The entry tear was located at the ascending aorta in 10 cases (DeBakey type I), the aortic arch in 14 cases and the distal aortic arch or proximal

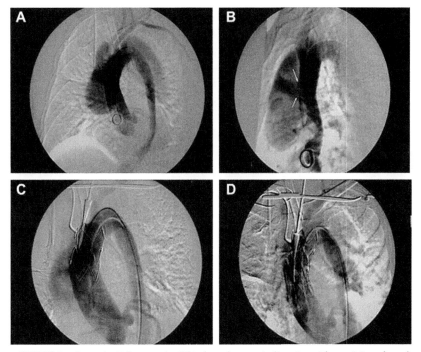

FIGURE 1.—Group A. A) Preoperative DSA showed an aortic dissection with tear 1.5 cm from the right innominate artery, 5 cm from the ostium of coronary artery, and B) 2.0 cm in diameter. C) Endoleak remained after the first stent was implanted through LCCA. D) A second stent was implanted to close the tear and the leakage stopped. (Reprinted from European Journal of Vascular and Endovascular Surgery, Ye C, Chang G, Li S, et al. Endovascular stent-graft treatment for Stanford type A aortic dissection. *Eur J Vasc Endovasc Surg.* 2011;42:787-794. Copyright 2011, with permission from the European Society for Vascular Surgery.)

descending aorta in 21 cases in which the ascending aorta was also involved by the dissection.

Results.—The surgical success rate was 97.8% (44/45) and 30-day mortality rate was 6.7% (3/45). Type I endoleaks occurred in 10 cases: one patient died intra-operatively, four were successfully treated with ballooning, four were sealed with aortic cuffs and one case caused by left subclavian artery (LSA) reflux was sealed with an occluder. Average follow-up time was 35.5 ± 5.4 months. Up to the most recent review or death, 32 patients had complete thrombosis and 10 had partial thrombosis inside the false lumen. Two deaths occurred after 30-days postoperatively.

Conclusion.—Endovascular stent-graft treatment is a minimally invasive and effective method to treat Stanford type A aortic dissection (Figs 1-3).

▶ For anyone who manages aortic dissection, this article is a must-read! This impressive 8-year experience of managing type A aortic dissections with endografts warrants a thorough review.

Patients were placed in three groups based on the location of the entry tear. Group A included 10 subjects who had an entry tear between the coronary ostia and the innominate artery, group B included 14 subjects with an entry tear in

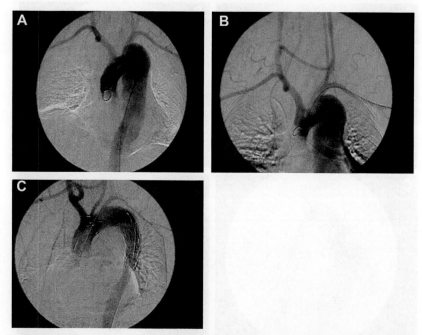

FIGURE 2.—Group B. A) Tear on aortic arch between LCCA and LSA. Another tear was located below the level of the renal artery. B) Postoperative DSA showed good circulation in the carotid artery bypass. C) The right femoral artery was exposed, the aortic stent delivery system was inserted into brachiocephalic artery, the bare stent frame was placed to the left of the brachiocephalic artery, and the stent was released. (Reprinted from European Journal of Vascular and Endovascular Surgery, Ye C, Chang G, Li S, et al. Endovascular stent-graft treatment for Stanford type A aortic dissection. *Eur J Vasc Endovasc Surg.* 2011;42:787-794. Copyright 2011, with permission from the European Society for Vascular Surgery.)

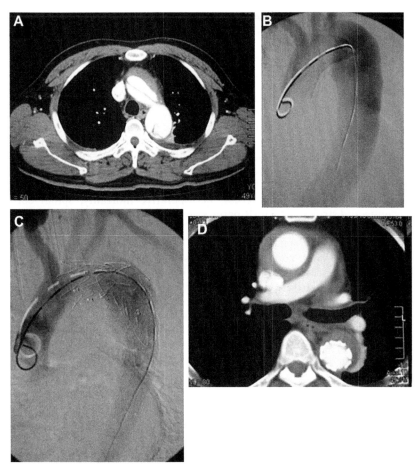

FIGURE 3.—Group C. A) CTA revealed Stanford type A dissection. B) DSA showed tear at the distal LSA. C) Stent graft implanted. D) CTA 3 months postoperatively indicated the dissection is no longer present and thrombus formation inside the dissection cavity. (Reprinted from European Journal of Vascular and Endovascular Surgery, Ye C, Chang G, Li S, et al. Endovascular stent-graft treatment for Stanford type A aortic dissection. *Eur J Vasc Endovasc Surg.* 2011;42:787-794. Copyright 2011, with permission from the European Society for Vascular Surgery.)

the aortic arch, and group C had 21 subjects with an entry tear distal to the left subclavian artery with retrograde extension of the dissection. The main strategy here was to seal the entry tear (Figs 1, 2, and 3).

The results were incredible. The technical success rate was 97.8% (44/45) and the 30-day mortality rate and stroke rate were both only 6.7% (3/45).

Since two-thirds of all aortic dissection cases in the United States are of the Stanford type A variety, an "endovascular first" strategy warrants intensive review.

B. W. Starnes, MD

Analysis of Stroke after TEVAR Involving the Aortic Arch

Melissano G, Tshomba Y, Bertoglio L, et al (Università Vita-Salute, Milano, Italy)
Eur J Vasc Endovasc Surg 43:269-275, 2012

Objective.—To analyse the incidence of stroke after thoracic endovascular aortic repair (TEVAR) for aortic arch disease.

Methods.—In the last decade, 393 patients received TEVAR at our Institution; in 143 cases the aortic arch was involved (32 zones '0', 35 zones '1' and 76 zone '2'). The left subclavian artery (LSA) was revascularised selectively in 75 cases; the proximal LSA was ligated or occluded with a plug in 55 cases before endograft (EG) deployment.

Results.—Initial clinical success, perioperative mortality, spinal cord ischaemia and stroke in TEVAR patients with or without arch involvement were, respectively, 86.7% vs. 94.4%, 4.2% vs. 2.4%, 2.1% vs. 3.6% and 2.8% vs. 1.2%. The stroke rate was 9.4% ($P < 0.02$) in 'zone 0', 0% in 'zone 1' and 1.3% in 'zone 2' with scans showing severe atheroma and/or thrombus in all cases. Stroke was observed in patients with 2.6% or without 2.9% LSA revascularisation; however, it was never observed in patients in whom the LSA was occluded before EG deployment and in 4.5% of patients in whom it was patent at the time of EG deployment.

Conclusions.—Stroke after TEVAR is not infrequent especially when the arch is involved. Careful patient selection together with a strategy to

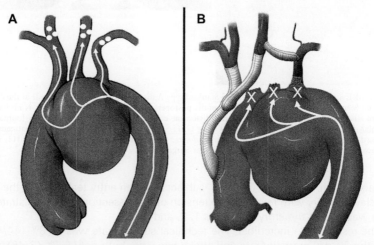

FIGURE 2.—(A) Guidewire manipulation of the aortic arch prior to surgical debranching may cause cerebral embolisation of atherothrombotic material through the patent supraaortic vessels. (B) Surgical by-passing of all the supra-aortic trunks, associated with ligation of the origin of the innominate artery and left common carotid, and endovascular occlusion of the LSA are performed prior to guidewire engagement of the aortic arch in order to reduce the risk of cerebral embolisation. (Reprinted from European Journal of Vascular and Endovascular Surgery, Melissano G, Tshomba Y, Bertoglio L, et al. Analysis of stroke after TEVAR involving the aortic arch. *Eur J Vasc Endovasc Surg.* 2012;43:269-275. Copyright 2012, with permission from the European Society for Vascular Surgery.)

TABLE 5.—Table Showing the Incidence of Stroke in Two Different Groups in the Series of Patients who Underwent Hybrid or Endovascular Repair of the Aortic Arch at Our Centre Between 1999 and 2011 (*n* = 143). *Group A*: Patients who Underwent LSA Revascularization; *Group B*: Patients who did not Undergo LSA revascularization. The Difference of Stroke Rate in the Two Groups was not Statistically Significant (*P* = 0.6 at Fisher Exact Test)

Overall 143 Patients	A. LSA Revascularization	B. NO LSA Revascularization
No stroke	73	66
Stroke	2	2

Data are reported as number of patients.
Abbreviations: LSA: left subclavian artery.

TABLE 6.—Table Showing the Incidence of Stroke in Two Different Groups in the Series of Patients who Underwent Hybrid or Endovascular Repair of the Aortic Arch at Our Centre Between 1999 and 2011 (*n* = 143). *Group A*: Patients who Underwent Endograft Deployment in the Aortic Arch After Occlusion of LSA; *Group B*: Patients who Underwent Endograft Deployment in the Aortic Arch Before LSA Occlusion. The Difference of Stroke Rate in the Two Groups was not Statistically Significant (*P* = 0.13 at Fisher Exact Test)

Overall 143 Patients	A. LSA Occluded During TEVAR	B. LSA Patent During TEVAR
No stroke	55	84
Stroke	0	4

Data are reported as number of patients.
Abbreviations: LSA: left subclavian artery; TEVAR: thoracic endovascular aortic repair.

reduce embolisation such as occlusion of supra-aortic trunks before EG deployment may play a beneficial role (Fig 2, Tables 5-7).

▶ This highly experienced group of surgeons led by Germano Melissano has given us some very valuable information regarding their experience with thoracic endovascular aortic repair (TEVAR) over the last 12 years. Specifically, these authors sought to evaluate the incidence of stroke after TEVAR for aortic arch disease. Using the classification put forth by Ishimaru,[1] the authors divided patients by zones of aortic arch coverage and into groups based on whether a debranching procedure was done before TEVAR or concurrent with TEVAR. Not surprisingly, hybrid arch procedures and those in which the stent graft was deployed in zone 0 had a higher incidence of stroke. Overall, TEVAR in patients with arch involvement had twice the mortality and stroke rate as TEVAR in patients without arch involvement. Unlike other large series, there was no difference in stroke rate in 143 arch TEVAR patients regardless of whether they underwent left subclavian artery revascularization or no revascularization (Table 5). The most interesting aspect of this article is that the authors were able to show that if they performed left subclavian artery plug occlusion prior to TEVAR, they were able to reduce their rate of stroke to zero (Tables 6 and 7). In the context

TABLE 7.—Table Showing the Incidence of Stroke in Two Different Groups in the Sub-Group of "Zone 0 Patients" who Underwent Hybrid or Endovascular Repair of the Aortic Arch at Our Centre Between 1999 and 2011 ($n = 32$). *Group A*: Patients who Underwent Endograft Deployment in Aortic Arch After Occlusion of LSA; *Group B*: Patients who Underwent Endograft Deployment in the Aortic Arch Before LSA Occlusion. The Difference of Stroke Rate in the Two Groups was Statistically Significant ($P = 0.04$ at Fisher Exact Test)

32 "Zone 0 Patients"	A. LSA Occluded During TEVAR	B. LSA Patent During TEVAR
No stroke	20	9
Stroke	0	3

Data are reported as number of patients.
Abbreviations: LSA: left subclavian artery; TEVAR: thoracic endovascular aortic repair.

of ongoing efforts to reduce stroke rate, the authors highlighted the following recommendations:

- Exclusion from TEVAR of patients with aortic arches at higher risk of embolism (shaggy aorta, heavily calcified aortic wall, floating thrombus);
- The use of endovascular materials specifically designed for aortic arch, such as precurved stiff guide wires, introducers and EG shafts;
- Utmost attention in any endomanipulation of the aortic arch, limiting maneuvers to those strictly necessary;
- A procedural plan favoring the endovascular manipulation in the aortic arch after arch debranching and left subclavian artery occlusion (Fig 2).

B. W. Starnes, MD

Reference

1. Ishimaru S. Endografting of the aortic arch. *J Endovasc Ther.* 2004;11:II62-II71.

A Systematic Review of Mid-term Outcomes of Thoracic Endovascular Repair (TEVAR) of Chronic Type B Aortic Dissection

Thrumurthy SG, Karthikesalingam A, Patterson BO, et al (St George's Vascular Inst, London, UK)
Eur J Vasc Endovasc Surg 42:632-647, 2011

Objective and Design.—The role of Thoracic Endovascular Repair (TEVAR) in chronic type B aortic dissection remains controversial and its mid-term success as an alternative to open repair or best medical therapy remains unknown. The aim of the present study was to provide a systematic review of mid-term outcomes of TEVAR for chronic type B aortic dissection.

Materials and Methods.—Medline, trial registries, conference proceedings and article reference lists from 1950 to January 2011 were searched to identify case series reporting mid-term outcomes of TEVAR in chronic type B dissection. Data were extracted for review.

Results.—17 studies of 567 patients were reviewed. The technical success rate was 89.9% (range 77.6−100). Mid-term mortality was 9.2% (46/499) and survival ranged from 59.1 to 100% in studies with a median follow-up of 24 months. 8.1% of patients (25/309) developed endoleak, predominantly type I. Re-intervention rates ranged from 0 to 60% in studies with a median follow-up of 31 months. 7.8% of patients (26/332) developed aneurysms of the distal aorta or continued false lumen perfusion with aneurysmal dilatation. Rare complications included delayed retrograde type A dissection (0.67%), aorto-oesophageal fistula (0.22%) and neurological complications (paraplegia 2/447, 0.45%; stroke 7/475, 1.5%).

Conclusion.—The absolute benefit of TEVAR over alternative treatments for chronic B-AD remains uncertain. The lack of natural history data for medically treated cases, significant heterogeneity in case selection and absence of consensus reporting standards for intervention are significant obstructions to interpreting the mid-term data. High-quality data from registries and clinical trials are required to address these challenges (Fig 5).

▶ This is a must read for anyone who treats chronic aortic dissection (CAD) with endovascular methods. It remains controversial whether thoracic endovascular repair (TEVAR) is indicated in patients with CAD. This is the first focused, systematic review of midterm outcomes of TEVAR for patients presenting with Stanford Type B aortic dissections of more than 14 days from time of presentation. Seventeen articles made the cut, which encompassed the endovascular management of 567 patients. Neurologic complications were rare, with stroke occurring in 0.82% (4/489) and paraplegia or paraparesis in 0.43% (2/462). The most common delayed complication (7.8%) was the development of aneurysms of the distal aorta or continued false lumen perfusion with aneurysmal dilation (26/332).

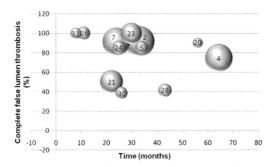

FIGURE 5.—Scatterplot to illustrate mid-term incidence of complete false-lumen thrombosis after TEVAR for chronic BAD. Each of the 12 studies is represented by a single datapoint. The sample size of each study (range 14−84) is reflected by the size of its respective datapoint. The reference number of each study is also displayed within the respective datapoint. (Reprinted from European Journal of Vascular and Endovascular Surgery, Thrumurthy SG, Karthikesalingam A, Patterson BO, et al. A systematic review of mid-term outcomes of thoracic endovascular repair (TEVAR) of chronic type B aortic dissection. *Eur J Vasc Endovasc Surg.* 2011;42:632-647. Copyright 2011, with permission from the European Society for Vascular Surgery.)

Of the studies that reported on subtype of endoleak, only 1 type 1B endoleak was reported (1/232). Rates of complete false lumen thrombosis ranged from 38.5% to 100%. It should be noted that no mid- or long-term data currently exist for the open surgical treatment of CAD. With midterm outcomes being ill defined, such data are required for meaningful and direct comparison of outcomes with TEVAR. The authors correctly point out that consistent reporting standards are urgently required.

B. W. Starnes, MD

Endovascular Repair of Complicated Acute Type-B Aortic Dissection with Stentgraft: Early and Mid-term Results

Shu C, He H, Li Q-M, et al (The Second Xiangya Hosp of Central South Univ, Changsha, Hunan, China)
Eur J Vasc Endovasc Surg 42:448-453, 2011

Objectives.—To analyse the experience of a single centre and evaluate the early and mid-term results of endovascular repair of complicated acute type B aortic dissection with stentgrafts.

Method.—From July 2002 to January 2009, 45 patients (12 women, 33 men) with complicated acute type B aortic dissection (mean age, 42.6 years; range, 31−47 years) were treated with Thoracic Endovascular Aortic Repair (TEVAR). Indications for treatment included rupture in 6(13%), hemathorax with impending rupture in 27(60%), malperfusion syndrome in 11 (22%), and transient paraplegia in one patient (2.2%). Five kinds of commercially available thoracic stentgrafts were used. Follow up was 100% during a period of 13 months (range, 1−36 months).

Results.—Technical success (coverage of the primary tear site) was achieved in all 45 patients (100%) including deliberate partial or total coverage of the LSA in 7 patients (15.6%). The 30-day and in-hospital mortality was 4.4% including one late rupture case. Overall survival was 95.6% at 1 and 3-years' follow-up. None of the patients with malperfusion required adjunct distal stents. All hemothoces resolved within 3 months including 5 patient required thoracentesis and one had tube thoracostomy. And 7 patients required temporary dialysis. In-hospital complications occurred in 26.7% of patients and re-intervention was required in one patient and no patient had postoperative paraplegia. Postoperative CT angiography showed 25 patients (58.1%) with complete thrombosis of the false lumen and re-expansion of the true lumen.

Conclusions.—Endovascular repair of complicated acute type B aortic dissection with stentgraft is proven to be a technically feasible and effective in this relatively difficult patient cohort. The short and mid-term efficacy are persuasive, however, the long-term efficacy needs to be evaluated further.

▶ I recently returned from my first visit to China. There, I made an independent observation of what seemed to be an unusually high percentage of people on the street in wheelchairs with what appeared to be the obvious results of a stroke. I later learned from one of my colleagues that in fact the number one cause of death in China is stroke. This is thought to be due to the high-salt diet and the high rate of uncontrolled and untreated hypertension. Given these facts, it is not surprising that the rate of aortic dissection is also high.

These authors from a single institution in Changsha, China, report their 7-year experience of managing complicated type B aortic dissection (rupture, impending rupture, and malperfusion) with thoracic endovascular aortic repair (TEVAR). The results are remarkable. The 30-day and in-hospital mortality was only 4.4%.

One of the glaring weaknesses of this study is the lack of follow-up. The longest follow-up was only 36 months (range, 1-36 months) even though the study period was 7 years.

I think we are going to see a large amount of experience in treating type B aortic dissection with TEVAR emerging from China.

B. W. Starnes, MD

Predictors of Outcome after Endovascular Repair for Chronic Type B Dissection
Mani K, Clough RE, Lyons OTA, et al (Guy's and St Thomas NHS Foundation Trust, London, UK)
Eur J Vasc Endovasc Surg 43:386-391, 2012

Objectives.—To assess the durability of endovascular repair (TEVAR) in chronic type B dissection (CD) and identify factors predictive of outcome.

Design.—Retrospective analysis of a prospective database.

Materials.—Patients undergoing TEVAR for CD at a tertiary referral centre 2000—2010.

Methods.—Analysis of pre-operative characteristics, operative outcome, false lumen thrombosis, aortic diameter and survival.

Results.—58 consecutive patients were included (49 elective, 9 urgent, mean age 66 years). Mean aortic diameter was 6.4 cm (Standard deviation SD 1.3 cm). Three patients died perioperatively (5%, 1 urgent, 2 elective). Complications included retrograde type A dissection ($n = 3$), paraplegia (1), and transient ischaemic attack (1). Estimated survival (Kaplan—Meier) was 89% (1-year) and 64% (3-years). Forty-seven patients had mid-term imaging follow-up at mean 38 months. Reintervention rate was 15% at 1-year and 29% at 3-years. Aortic diameter decreased in 24, was stable in 15 and increased in 8. Mid-term survival was higher in patients with aortic remodelling (reduction of aortic diameter >0.5 cm; 3-year 89%) than without (54%; Log Rank $p = 0.005$). Remodelling occurred with extensive false lumen thrombosis.

Conclusion.—Satisfactory mid-term outcome after TEVAR for CD remains a challenge. Survival is associated with aortic remodelling, which is related to persistence of flow in the false lumen.

▶ Endovascular treatment of chronic aortic dissection is controversial. This series is one of the largest to date to assess the performance of endovascular stent grafts in managing these difficult situations. Remember, the goal of this strategy is to treat the aneurysm that results from the dissection and thus prevent death due to rupture. The goal is *not* to treat the aortic dissection.

These authors have shown that favorable aortic remodeling occurs in 50% of patients and is related to false lumen thrombosis. Therefore, future strategies should include methods to obliterate persistent flow in the false lumen. We have had similar results managing patients with chronic aortic dissections using this approach.

B. W. Starnes, MD

Combined Proximal Endografting With Distal Bare-Metal Stenting for Management of Aortic Dissection

Hofferberth SC, Foley PT, Newcomb AE, et al (The Univ of Melbourne, Fitzroy, Victoria, Australia; St Vincent's Hosp Melbourne, Fitzroy, Victoria, Australia)
Ann Thorac Surg 93:95-102, 2012

Background.—Established endovascular treatments for aortic dissection often result in incomplete aortic repair, potentially leading to late complications involving the distal aorta. To address the problems of incomplete true lumen reconstitution and late aneurysmal change, we report the midterm results of combined proximal endografting with distal true lumen bare-metal stenting (STABLE: Staged Total Aortic and Branch vesseL Endovascular reconstruction) in Stanford type A and B aortic dissection.

Methods.—Between January 2003 and January 2010, 31 patients underwent staged total aortic and branch vessel endovascular reconstruction for management of acute (type A, 13; type B, 11) and chronic (type B, 7) aortic dissection. Proximal endografting was combined with bare-metal Z stent implantation in the distal true lumen. Patients with type A dissection underwent adjunctive treatment at operation. Computed tomography angiography was performed at baseline, 1 year, and annually thereafter to assess aortic remodelling.

Results.—Primary technical success was 97%. Thirty-day rates of death, stroke, and permanent paraplegia/paresis were 3% (n = 1), 0%, and 0%, respectively. Mean follow-up was 57.3 months (range, 5 to 100 months). Overall survival was 60% at 100 months. Aortic-specific survival was 93%. Four patients (13%) underwent device-related reintervention. One (3%) late aortic-related death occurred. Thoracic ($p = 0.64$) and abdominal ($p = 0.14$) aortic dimensions were stable. The true lumen index increased significantly at follow-up.

Conclusions.—Staged total aortic and branch vessel endovascular reconstruction is a feasible ancillary endovascular technique to address the problems of distal true lumen collapse, incomplete aortic remodelling, and late aneurysm formation in aortic dissection (Fig 4).

▶ Stent graft repair of acute aortic dissection was initially reported in 1999.[1] The idea is to decompress the false lumen to encourage false lumen thrombosis

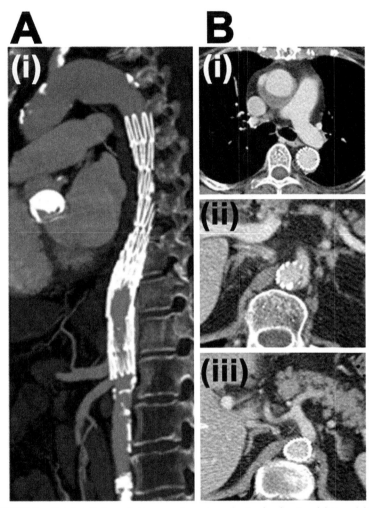

FIGURE 4.—(A, i; B, i, ii) Computed tomography angiography 4 years after staged thoracoabdominal and branch vessel endoluminal repair demonstrates complete remodelling of the descending thoracic aorta. There was residual false lumen perfusion, but improved true lumen index without dilatation. (B, iii) Celiac axis perfusion was not compromised. (This article was published in The Annals of Thoracic Surgery, Hofferberth SC, Foley PT, Newcomb AE, et al. Combined proximal endografting with distal bare-metal stenting for management of aortic dissection. *Ann Thorac Surg.* 2012;93:95-102. © The Society of Thoracic Surgeons.)

and aortic remodeling, thereby providing stabilization of the dissection and aortic dimensions. However, endograft closure can result in incomplete repair, and the aorta can fail to remodel in 50% to 80% of patients.[2] To potentially avoid late complications of aneurysm change, repeat dissections, and rupture, the authors have augmented proximal endografting with distal deployment of bare-metal Z stents, a concept termed Staged Total Aortic and Branch vesseL Endovascular (STABLE) reconstruction. In this article the authors describe use of the STABLE technique in treatment of 31 patients with either Stanford type A or Stanford type B aortic dissection (Fig 4). At the end of the article, the authors call for a controlled trial and longer follow-up prior to introduction of the STABLE technique into broad clinical practice. Nevertheless, there is a decidedly positive spin placed by the authors on this technique. In an invited commentary printed in the original article, Leonard Girardi from Cornell Medical College in New York presents a somewhat different interpretation of the data. Girardi contends "the data presented by Hofferberth and colleagues did not advance the case of endovascular intervention of uncomplicated aortic dissections." He points out that while the STABLE technique improved true lumen perfusion and diameter, it did not suppress false lumen patency, with the false lumen remaining patent in 74% of the cases. In addition, the goal of minimizing additional procedures was not met as adjunctive procedures were required in 40% of patients prior to discharge. An additional 15% required branch vessel intervention, and 17% required a late aortic procedure for stent-related complications, including rupture. Girardi notes that a patent false lumen was present in all of the patients who needed aortic reintervention and in the 1 patient who had an aortic-related death. He appropriately argues that prior to introducing techniques such as STABLE into general clinical practice, results must be rigorously analyzed in the context of what can be achieved with standard techniques.

G. L. Moneta, MD

References

1. Dake MD, Kato N, Mitchell RS, et al. Endovascular stent-graft placement for the treatment of acute aortic dissection. *N Engl J Med.* 1999;340:1546-1552.
2. Eggebrecht H, Nienaber CA, Neuhäuser M, et al. Endovascular stent-graft placement in aortic dissection: a meta-analysis. *Eur Heart J.* 2006;27:489-498.

Computational Study of Haemodynamic Effects of Entry- and Exit-Tear Coverage in a DeBakey Type III Aortic Dissection: Technical Report
Karmonik C, Bismuth J, Shah DJ, et al (The Methodist Hosp, Houston, TX; et al)
Eur J Vasc Endovasc Surg 42:172-177, 2011

Objectives.—Outcome prediction in DeBakey Type III aortic dissections (ADs) remains challenging. Large variations in AD morphology, physiology and treatment exist. Here, we investigate if computational fluid dynamics (CFD) can provide an initial understanding of pressure changes in an AD computational model when covering entry and exit tears and removing the intra-arterial septum (IS).

Design.—A computational mesh was constructed from magnetic resonance images from one patient (one entrance and one exit tear) and CFD simulations performed (scenario #1). Additional meshes were derived by virtually (1) covering the exit tear (false lumen (FL) thrombus progression) (scenario #2), (2) covering the entrance tear (thoracic endovascular treatment, TEVAR) (scenario #3) and (3) completely removing the IS (fenestration) (scenario #4). Changes in flow patterns and pressures were quantified relative to the initial mesh.

Results.—Systolic pressures increased for #2 (300 Pa increase) with largest inter-luminal differences distally (2500 Pa). In #3, false lumen pressure decreased essentially to zero. In #4, systolic pressure in combined lumen reduced from 2400 to 800 Pa.

Conclusions.—CFD results from computational models of a DeBakey type III AD representing separate coverage of entrance and exit tears correlated with clinical experience. The reported results present a preliminary look at a complex clinical problem (Fig 3).

▶ This is a very interesting preliminary look at a complex clinical problem. These authors used computational fluid dynamics (CFD) assessing true and false lumen pressure changes in 4 simulated scenarios for a patient presenting with a type B aortic dissection. They used a sagittal 3-dimensional contrast-enhanced magnetic resonance angiographic (3D ceMRA) image data set. The 4 scenarios correlated with the clinical presentation of (1) baseline pressure measurement, (2) coverage of the exit tear simulating false lumen thrombosis, (3) coverage of the entry tear

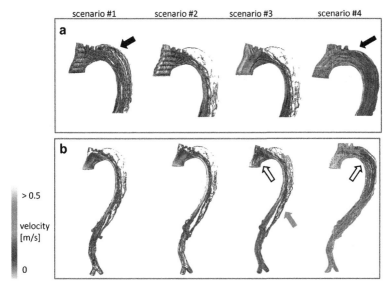

FIGURE 3.—a: Flow Patterns in proximal aorta during systole. Ordered laminar flow can be appreciated in TL and FL for scenario #1 and in the combined lumen for scenario #4 (filled arrow). Inflow into FL diminished in scenario #2 and was absent in scenario #3. b: Flow Patterns during retrograde flow. Compared to systolic flow, recirculation patterns were visible immediately proximal to the origin of the innominate artery (open arrow); in addition, retrograde flow occurred in the FL in scenario #3 (red arrow) and smaller deviations from laminar flow appeared in the combined lumen in scenario #4 (open arrow). For interpretation of the references to color in this figure legend, the reader is referred to web version of this article. (Reprinted from European Journal of Vascular and Endovascular Surgery, Karmonik C, Bismuth J, Shah DJ, et al. Computational study of haemodynamic effects of entry- and exit-tear coverage in a DeBakey type III aortic dissection: technical report. *Eur J Vasc Endovasc Surg.* 2011;42:172-177. Copyright 2011, with permission from the European Society for Vascular Surgery.)

simulating thoracic endovascular treatment, and (4) removal of the septum mimicking fenestration (Fig 3). As is observed clinically, for scenarios 1 and 2, false lumen pressure exceeded true lumen pressure. For scenario 3, maximum true lumen pressure was cut in half while essentially depressurizing the entire false lumen. For scenario 4, maximum pressures in the combined lumens decreased 75%. Obviously, CFD is still considered to be theoretical and in need of verification and validation. It is a shame that these authors did not obtain consent to directly measure at least the pressures in each lumen at baseline to help validate these methods. Nonetheless, this does represent proof of concept and is exciting. Think about it. If one possessed a validated tool to assess the outcome of any given patient with aortic dissection based on the initial pretreatment MRA, one would then be able to best select the method of repair, tailored to that individual patient. A lot of work remains to be done in this area, but the potential is enormous.

B. W. Starnes, MD

Paraplegia prevention branches: A new adjunct for preventing or treating spinal cord injury after endovascular repair of thoracoabdominal aneurysms
Lioupis C, Corriveau MM, MacKenzie KS, et al (McGill Univ, Montreal, Quebec, Canada; Royal Victoria Hosp, Montreal, Quebec, Canada; et al)
J Vasc Surg 54:252-257, 2011

In this report, we describe a technique that could potentially be used for both prevention and treatment of spinal cord ischemia (SCI) in endovascular repair of thoracoabdominal aneurysms. This technique involves using a specially designed endograft with side branches (paraplegia prevention branches [PPBs]), which are left patent to perfuse the aneurysmal sac and any associated lumbar or intercostal arteries in the early postoperative period. The use of PPBs with this technique is feasible and allows for a temporary controlled endoleak that may be useful for preventing or reversing spinal cord injury. This technique may be considered as an adjunct to the more standard perioperative physiological manipulations such as permissive hypertension and spinal fluid drainage.

▶ Spinal cord ischemia and consequent paraplegia is reported to occur in 0% to 17% of patients undergoing open or endovascular repair of thoracoabdominal aortic aneurysms (TAAAa). In this case report, the authors detail their experience using a new novel method of maintaining spinal cord perfusion for a period after endovascular repair of a type II thoracoabdominal aortic aneurysm. Conceived by Krassi Ivancev, the device uses 2 paraplegia prevention branches built into the EVAR portion of their endograft components. The concept creates a planned type Ib endoleak using these side branches, which are later closed using an Amplatzer plug technique. The concept is similar to an emergent postoperative fenestration technique reported last year by Reilly and Chuter.[1] Such measures may be most useful in patients with type II TAAAs, previous aortic surgery, impaired vertebrobasilar blood flow, or advanced age. Clearly, continued improvement in our approach to this problem is necessary if we are to generalize the 2.5% paraplegia rate reported at specialized centers. This technique, while successful in case reports, carries numerous risks such as delayed aneurysm rupture while "staging" complete aneurysm exclusion, which will need to be explored more in larger series.

D. L. Gillespie, MD, FACS

Reference

1. Reilly LM, Chuter TA. Reversal of fortune: induced endoleak to resolve neurological deficit after endovascular repair of thoracoabdominal aortic aneurysm. *J Endovasc Ther.* 2010;17:21-29.

A propensity score—matched comparison of deep versus mild hypothermia during thoracoabdominal aortic surgery
Weiss AJ, Lin H-M, Bischoff MS, et al (Mount Sinai School of Medicine, NY)
J Thorac Cardiovasc Surg 143:186-193, 2012

Objective.—By using deep hypothermic circulatory arrest and non—deep hypothermic circulatory arrest approaches, we examined the impact of distal ischemia time and temperature on intra-abdominal reversible adverse outcomes and permanent adverse outcomes during descending thoracic aortic and thoracoabdominal aortic aneurysm operations.

Methods.—A retrospective review of all patients who underwent descending thoracic aortic and thoracoabdominal aortic aneurysm repair between January 2002 and December 2008 was undertaken, including relevant preoperative, intraoperative, and postoperative data, and followed by a propensity score—matched analysis. Of the total of 262 patients, 240 had data complete enough to permit analysis, and 90 were suitable for the propensity-matched study. Reversible adverse outcomes included renal failure, liver failure, and temporary hemodialysis. Permanent adverse outcomes included paraplegia, permanent hemodialysis, and 30-day mortality.

Results.—Thirty-day mortality was 7.1% (17/240). Overall, reversible adverse outcomes developed in 40.8% of patients and permanent adverse outcomes developed in 10% of patients. The propensity score analysis identified statistically significant decreased odds of developing reversible adverse outcomes in patients undergoing deep hypothermic circulatory arrest (odds ratio, 0.32; confidence interval, 0.12—0.85). Specifically, significantly lower rates of acute renal failure (22% vs 46.4%, $P = .03$) and liver failure (17.8% vs 34.3%, $P = .04$) were observed in the deep hypothermic circulatory arrest group compared with the non—deep hypothermic circulatory arrest group. In addition, there were decreased odds of reversible adverse outcomes (odds ratio, 0.22; confidence interval, 0.06—0.79) developing in patients with a stage II elephant trunk procedure.

Conclusions.—During descending thoracic aortic and thoracoabdominal aortic aneurysm repairs, the use of deep hypothermic circulatory arrest results in improved postoperative adverse outcome rates compared with non–deep hypothermic circulatory arrest techniques. The development of reversible adverse outcomes is strongly associated with the development of permanent adverse outcomes.

▶ Many patients with descending thoracic aneurysms (DTA) and thoracoabdominal aneurysms (TAAA) are treated with open surgical techniques. For open surgeries, there are many perfusion techniques possible. These include clamp and sew, mild hyperthermia with atriofemoral or femoral-femoral bypass, and deep hypothermic circulatory arrest (DHCA). Although some surgeons routinely used DHCA in DTA and TAAA repairs, the technique is largely restricted to high-volume aortic centers and used selectively. Potential advantages of deep hypothermic circulatory arrest include a bloodless field and minimalization of aortic dissection, with no need for proximal and sequential aortic clamping. In addition, profound hypothermia theoretically offers protection to visceral organs by decreasing metabolic rate and oxygen debt of the organ. Potential disadvantages of deep hypothermic circulatory arrest are the increased time of cardiopulmonary bypass for cooling, increased coagulopathy, and increased blood-product usage. In addition, experienced surgeons appear to be able to obtain similar results with a combination of mild hypothermia, cerebrospinal fluid drainage, rapid renal cooling, and selective intercostal implantation.[1] One must weigh the increased complexity of deep hypothermic circulatory arrest with potential but not necessarily proven improvement in ischemic complications following thoracic aneurysm and thoracoabdominal aneurysm repair.

G. L. Moneta, MD

Reference

1. Acher C, Wynn M. Outcomes in open repair of the thoracic and thoracoabdominal aorta. *J Vasc Surg.* 2010;52:3S-9S.

10 Leg Ischemia and Aortoiliac Disease

Supervised Exercise Versus Primary Stenting for Claudication Resulting From Aortoiliac Peripheral Artery Disease: Six-Month Outcomes From the Claudication: Exercise Versus Endoluminal Revascularization (CLEVER) Study

Murphy TP, for the CLEVER Study Investigators (Rhode Island Hosp, Providence; et al)

Circulation 125:130-139, 2012

Background.—Claudication is a common and disabling symptom of peripheral artery disease that can be treated with medication, supervised exercise (SE), or stent revascularization (ST).

Methods and Results.—We randomly assigned 111 patients with aortoiliac peripheral artery disease to receive 1 of 3 treatments: optimal medical care (OMC), OMC plus SE, or OMC plus ST. The primary end point was the change in peak walking time on a graded treadmill test at 6 months compared with baseline. Secondary end points included free-living step activity, quality of life with the Walking Impairment Questionnaire, Peripheral Artery Questionnaire, Medical Outcomes Study 12-Item Short Form, and cardiovascular risk factors. At the 6-month follow-up, change in peak walking time (the primary end point) was greatest for SE, intermediate for ST, and least with OMC (mean change versus baseline, 5.8 ± 4.6, 3.7 ± 4.9, and 1.2 ± 2.6 minutes, respectively; $P<0.001$ for the comparison of SE versus OMC, $P=0.02$ for ST versus OMC, and $P=0.04$ for SE versus ST). Although disease-specific quality of life as assessed by the Walking Impairment Questionnaire and Peripheral Artery Questionnaire also improved with both SE and ST compared with OMC, for most scales, the extent of improvement was greater with ST than SE. Free-living step activity increased more with ST than with either SE or OMC alone (114 ± 274 versus 73 ± 139 versus -6 ± 109 steps per hour), but these differences were not statistically significant.

Conclusions.—SE results in superior treadmill walking performance than ST, even for those with aortoiliac peripheral artery disease. The contrast between better walking performance for SE and better patient-reported quality of life for ST warrants further study.

Clinical Trial Registration.—URL: http://clinicaltrials.gov/ct/show/ NCT00132743?order=1. Unique identifier: NCT00132743.

▶ Intermittent claudication is a significant health problem, limiting physical function, quality of life, and self-perceived ambulatory function and resulting in a more sedentary lifestyle. Clinical trials have demonstrated the efficacy of cilostazol, supervised exercise, and endovascular revascularization in improving quality of life and objective measures of walking performance in patients with intermittent claudication. Although drug therapy, revascularization, and supervised exercise are all documented effective therapies for intermittent claudication, the relative effectiveness of these measures is unknown. There have been no multicenter clinical trials directly comparing strategies of pharmacology alone or supervised exercise versus endovascular intervention. The CLEVER study is a randomized clinical trial comparing the benefits of optimal medical care, supervised exercise, and stent revascularization on walking outcomes and measures of quality of life in patients with intermittent claudication secondary to aortoiliac disease. CLEVER was a well-conducted clinical trial, but it was hampered by low enrollment, a common problem with comparative effectiveness trials. It is, however, difficult to know what to do with the data. The primary endpoint of the trial, walking on a treadmill, is perhaps not all that relevant to real life. In addition, the primary endpoint was measured at the time patients completed supervised exercise, and whether the effects of supervised exercise will hold up in the long term compared with stenting is unknown. One wonders whether the improvement of patients' perceived quality of life with stent therapy reflects the placebo effect of having undergone intervention or whether the improved performance on the treadmill with exercise therapy reflects a training effect.

G. L. Moneta, MD

Walking Performance and Health-related Quality of Life after Surgical or Endovascular Invasive versus Non-invasive Treatment for Intermittent Claudication – A Prospective Randomised Trial

Nordanstig J, Gelin J, Hensäter M, et al (Sahlgrenska Univ Hosp, Sweden; et al)
Eur J Vasc Endovasc Surg 42:220-227, 2011

Objectives.—Despite limited scientific evidence for the effectiveness of invasive treatment for intermittent claudication (IC), revascularisation procedures for IC are increasingly often performed in Sweden. This randomised controlled trial compares the outcome after 2 years of primary invasive (INV) versus primary non-invasive (NON) treatment strategies in unselected IC patients.

Materials/Methods.—Based on arterial duplex and clinical examination, IC patients were randomised to INV (endovascular and/or surgical, $n = 100$) or NON ($n = 101$). NON patients could request invasive treatment if they deteriorated during follow-up. Primary outcome was maximal walking performance (MWP) on graded treadmill test at 2 years and secondary outcomes included health-related quality of life (HRQL), assessed with Short Form (36) Health Survey (SF-36).

Results.—MWP was not significantly ($p = 0.104$) improved in the INV versus the NON group. Two SF-36 physical subscales, Bodily Pain ($p < 0.01$) and Role Physical ($p < 0.05$) improved significantly more in the INV versus the NON group. There were 7% crossovers against the study protocol in the INV group.

Conclusions.—Although invasive treatment did not show any significant advantage regarding MWP, the HRQL improvements associated with invasive treatment tentatively suggest secondary benefits of this regimen. On the other hand, a primary non-invasive treatment strategy seems to be accepted by most IC patients.

▶ This randomized prospective study attempts to identify the best strategy in treating patients with intermittent claudication. Outcomes over 2 years were evaluated in 2 groups of patients randomized to invasive treatment (INV) versus noninvasive treatment (NON). The noninvasive group underwent best medical therapy and nonsupervised exercise training, while the invasive groups underwent open and endovascular revascularization. Maximal walking performance (MWP) and health-related quality of life (HRQL) were assessed in each group. In the INV group, baseline MWP was 66 ± 25 W, and at 24 months, the MWP had increased by 10 W, which was significant within this group. In the NON group, the baseline MWP was 67 ± 24 W and increased by approximately 5 W, which was not statistically significant within this group, and comparison between the NON and INV groups did not reveal a statistically significant difference. Most patients in the INV group stopped their posttreatment treadmill test because of generalized fatigue, whereas the NON group stopped the treadmill test because of intolerable claudication. Regarding HRQL, RP (role physical, limitations in social functioning caused by physical condition) and BP (bodily pain or discomfort) improved significantly in the INV group in comparison with the NON group.

Claudication continues to be the most commonly encountered symptom of the peripheral arterial system, and although the course is benign in regard to limb loss, surgical and endovascular intervention is commonly performed in the hope of regaining improved ambulatory function. The study did not use a supervised exercise program and still did not reveal any significant difference in MWP between the 2 groups. It has been shown that intervention alone does not improve walking distance versus supervised exercise alone, but when both modalities (intervention + supervised exercise program) are combined, it is better than the single-modality therapy.[1] This disease process is a marker for atherosclerotic burden elsewhere (4% mortality over 2 years), and as was seen in this study, an invasive pathway did not lead to statistically improved MWP, but the patient's perception in the HRQL did show a positive effect, and it is potentially this result that may allow for behavior modification and increased compliance with an exercise program after an intervention.

N. Singh, MD

Reference

1. Ahimastos AA, Pappas EP, Buttner PG, Walker PJ, Kingwell BA, Golledge J. A meta-analysis of the outcome of endovascular and noninvasive therapies in the treatment of intermittent claudication. *J Vasc Surg.* 2011;54:1511-1521.

Systematic review of exercise training or percutaneous transluminal angioplasty for intermittent claudication

Frans FA, Bipat S, Reekers JA, et al (Academic Med Centre, Amsterdam, The Netherlands)
Br J Surg 99:16-28, 2012

Background.—The aim was to summarize the results of all randomized clinical trials (RCTs) comparing percutaneous transluminal angioplasty (PTA) with (supervised) exercise therapy ((S)ET) in patients with intermittent claudication (IC) to obtain the best estimates of their relative effectiveness.

Methods.—A systematic review was performed of relevant RCTs identified from the MEDLINE, Embase and Cochrane Library databases. Eligible RCTs compared PTA with (S)ET, included patients with IC due to suspected or known aortoiliac and/or femoropopliteal artery disease, and compared their effectiveness in terms of functional outcome and/or quality of life (QoL).

Results.—Eleven of 258 articles identified (reporting data on eight randomized clinical trials) met the inclusion criteria. One trial included patients with isolated aortoiliac artery obstruction, three trials studied those with femoropopliteal artery obstruction and five included those with combined lesions. Two trials compared PTA with advice on ET, four PTA with SET, two PTA plus SET with SET and two PTA plus SET with PTA. Although the endpoints in most trials comprised walking distances and QoL, pooling of data was impossible owing to heterogeneity. Generally, the effectiveness of PTA and (S)ET was equivalent, although PTA plus (S)ET improved walking distance and some domains of QoL scales compared with (S)ET or PTA alone.

Conclusion.—As IC is a common healthcare problem, defining the optimal treatment strategy is important. A combination of PTA and exercise (SET or ET advice) may be superior to exercise or PTA alone, but this needs to be confirmed.

▶ One goal in patients with intermittent claudication is to improve their walking distance with the thought that this will subsequently improve their quality of life. Percutaneous transluminal angioplasty (PTA), surgery, drugs, and exercise therapy (ET) all can improve symptoms in patients with intermittent claudication. Systematic reviews have found superiority of supervised exercise therapy (SET) over unsupervised ET for both increasing pain-free and maximum walking distance.[1,2] A Cochran review[3] indicted that there was greater short-term benefit with PTA than exercise in patients with intermittent claudication but that the effect was not sustained after 1 to 2 years. A second review found medical treatment (home or SET plus risk factor modification) resulted in longer walking distances than PTA at 1 to 2 years.[4] The authors noted that since this review, there have been 6 additional randomized clinical trials comparing PTA and ET over the last 5 years. They therefore decided to perform a systematic review to summarize the results of all randomized clinical trials comparing PTA with ET therapy. Their goal was to obtain the best estimate of the relative effectiveness of these 2 approaches. The article does indeed provide a good summary of the most up-to-date information currently available on the effectiveness of ET and PTA in patients treated for intermittent claudication. The data suggest that both SET and PTA can be effective in improving walking distance in patients with claudication. Neither therapy is perfect. ET is noninvasive, seemingly relatively inexpensive with less risk compared with PTA. However, PTA may be more universally applicable and more quickly effective than ET. Eventual failure rates are high with PTA treatment of femoral popliteal disease, but angioplasty of infrainguinal arteries is a moving target with improvements of percutaneous techniques such as drug-eluted balloons and stents potentially shortly down the road. Two important questions not addressed in this study include the cost effectiveness of each treatment strategy and the potential for each treatment strategy to convert patients from claudicates to critical limb ischemia with therapy failure.

G. L. Moneta, MD

References

1. Bendermacher BL, Willigendael EM, Teijink JA, Prins MH. Supervised exercise therapy versus non-supervised exercise therapy for intermittent claudication. *Cochrane Database Syst Rev.* 2006;(2):CD005263.
2. Wind J, Koelemay MJ. Exercise therapy and the additional effect of supervision on exercise therapy in patients with intermittent claudication. Systematic review of randomised controlled trials. *Eur J Vasc Endovasc Surg.* 2007;34:1-9.
3. Fowkes FG, Gillespie IN. Angioplasty (versus non surgical management) for intermittent claudication. *Cochrane Database Syst Rev.* 2000;(2):CD000017.
4. Wilson SE. Trials of endovascular treatment for superficial femoral artery occlusive lesions: a call for medically managed control patients. *Ann Vasc Surg.* 2010;24:498-502.

Comparison of the effect of upper body-ergometry aerobic training vs treadmill training on central cardiorespiratory improvement and walking distance in patients with claudication

Bronas UG, Treat-Jacobson D, Leon AS (Univ of Minnesota, Minneapolis)

J Vasc Surg 53:1557-1564, 2011

Background.—Supervised treadmill-walking exercise programs have been proven to be a highly effective in improving walking distance in peripheral arterial disease (PAD) patients with lifestyle-limiting claudication. Limited information is available on the contributions of central cardiorespiratory functions for improving these patients' walking capacity with exercise training.

Methods.—This study randomized 28 participants (21 men; age, 65.6 years; 92.7% smoking history, 36.6% with diabetes) with lifestyle-limiting PAD-related claudication to 3 hours/week of supervised exercise training for 12 weeks, using arm-ergometry (n = 10) or treadmill-walking (n = 10) vs a usual-care control group (n = 8). Cardiorespiratory function measurements were assessed before and after training at a submaximal workload and at the onset of claudication (pain-free walking distance [PFWD]) and at maximal walking distance (MWD). Changes in these functions from baseline were analyzed among the groups with analysis of covariance. Associations between variables were determined by Pearson's partial correlations.

Results.—The mean baseline demographic, medical, and exercise variables were similar among the groups. There were similar significant differences in the submaximal double product (heart rate × systolic blood pressure) and at MWD, ventilatory threshold, ventilatory oxygen uptake (VO_2) at onset of claudication, and VO_2 peak in response to training in both exercise groups vs the control group. Statistically significant, moderate correlations ($r = 0.60$-0.68) were found between changes in all cardiorespiratory variables and changes in PFWD or MWD.

Conclusion.—Improvements in cardiorespiratory function after arm-ergometry or treadmill-training were significantly associated with improvements in both PFWD and MWD, providing supporting evidence of systemic contributions to exercise training-related improvements in walking capacity seen in patients with claudication.

▶ Claudication is a common problem in the aging population, especially when cardiovascular risks factors are present. An important aspect of treatment is risk factor modification and exercise. Multiple studies have demonstrated that structured exercise is an important aspect in the overall treatment of claudication. The recent CLEVER trial demonstrated that supervised exercise resulted in superior treadmill walking performance at 6 months in patients with claudication than endovascular stent revascularization in patients with aortoiliac occlusive disease. What is less known is whether upper extremity ergometric aerobic training helps with cardiovascular function and walking distances in patients with claudication. In this interesting study, the authors randomized 3 groups of patients to the following exercise programs: 3 hours per week of supervised exercise training for 12 weeks, using (1) arm-ergometry aerobic exercise (n = 10) or (2) treadmill walking (n = 10) versus (3) a usual-care control group (n = 8). The study found that cardiorespiratory function as measured by ventilator threshold, minute ventilation, heart rate × systolic blood pressure (double product), a surrogate measure of myocardial oxygen demands and coronary blood flow, ventilatory oxygen consumption (VO_2) at onset of claudication, VO_2 peak, and peak metabolic equivalents dramatically improved in both the arm-ergometry aerobic exercise and treadmill-walking exercise groups compared with control; these improvements were associated with concomitant improvements in both pain-free walking distance and maximal walking distance. Interestingly, there was no improvement from baseline in ankle-brachial index after 12 weeks in any of the study groups. These data support the hypothesis that arm-exercise training improves the cardiopulmonary system, an adaptation that is systemic and not localized to the ischemia-induced local muscle vascular and metabolic changes. Both arm aerobic exercise and treadmill exercise improved walking ability and physical fitness, which is associated with central cardiorespiratory function and improved oxygen delivery in patients with claudication. An important finding from this study is that patients with claudication and significant limitations in walking distance could potentially improve their overall cardiorespiratory function with arm aerobic exercise, and then likely improve their walking ability and ultimately their quality of life. Some limitations of this study are that the majority of participants were male and Caucasian; therefore, future studies need to assess whether female patients and other races with claudication also demonstrate similar improvement in cardiopulmonary function and walking distances following arm-ergometry aerobic exercise.

J. D. Raffetto, MD

Influence of peripheral arterial disease and supervised walking on heart rate variability
Leicht AS, Crowther RG, Golledge J (James Cook Univ, Townsville, Queensland, Australia)
J Vasc Surg 54:1352-1359, 2011

Objective.—To examine the influence of peripheral arterial disease (PAD) on heart rate variability (HRV) in patients, and to examine the influence of an intense long-term (12 months) exercise program on HRV in PAD patients.

Methods.—This study involved ambulatory patients attending a local hospital and university center. Participants were twenty-five patients with diagnosed PAD and intermittent claudication and 24 healthy, age-matched adults. Interventions involved random allocation of PAD patients to 12 months of conservative medical treatment (Conservative) or medical treatment with supervised treadmill walking (Exercise). The main outcome measures were time- and frequency-domain, nonlinear HRV measures during supine rest, and maximal walking capacity prior to and following the intervention.

Results.—Despite significantly worse walking capacity (285 ± 190 m vs 941 ± 336 m; $P < .05$), PAD patients exhibited similar resting HRV to healthy adults. At the 12-month follow-up, Exercise patients exhibited a significantly greater improvement in walking capacity ($183\% \pm 185\%$ vs $57\% \pm 135\%$; $P = .03$) with similar small nonsignificant changes in HRV compared with Conservative patients.

Conclusions.—The current study demonstrated that PAD patients exhibited similar resting HRV to healthy adults with 12 months of intense supervised walking producing similar HRV changes to that of conservative medical treatment. The greater walking capacity of healthy adults and

PAD patients following supervised exercise does not appear to be associated with enhanced HRV.

▶ The authors present a well-structured but underpowered study on heart rate variability (HRV) and its association with peripheral arterial disease (PAD), specifically, intermittent claudication. While the numbers of patients at final analysis were low, their finding of increase in walking distance with supervised exercise program does support the current evidence. Their lack of a relationship with HRV makes one question the utility of this complex measurement. While we know from epidemiology data that PAD patients are at high risk for cardiac morbidity, their supposition that PAD and coronary artery disease patients are different based on a lack of HRV is hard to understand. Overall, the emphasis on vascular medicine and a further understanding of the pathophysiology of PAD is important but likely needs a much larger patient population to draw general conclusions. Most importantly, they do provide some evidence that the beneficial effects of exercise on intermittent claudication are not mediated through a heart rate/cardiac pathway.

A. Chandra, MD

Additional Supervised Exercise Therapy After a Percutaneous Vascular Intervention for Peripheral Arterial Disease: A Randomized Clinical Trial
Kruidenier LM, Nicolaï SP, Rouwet EV, et al (Orbis Med Centre, Sittard, the Netherlands; Maxima Med Centre, Eindhoven, the Netherlands; Erasmus Med Centre, Rotterdam, the Netherlands; et al)
J Vasc Interv Radiol 22:961-968, 2011

Purpose.—To determine whether a percutaneous vascular intervention (PVI) combined with supplemental supervised exercise therapy (SET) is more effective than a PVI alone in improving walking ability in patients with symptomatic peripheral arterial disease (PAD).

Materials and Methods.—In this prospective randomized trial, patients with PAD treated with a PVI were eligible. Exclusion criteria were major amputation or tissue loss, comorbidity preventing physical activity, insufficient knowledge of the Dutch language, no insurance for SET, and prior participation in a SET program. All patients received a PVI and subsequently were randomly assigned to either the PVI alone group (n = 35) or the PVI + SET group (n = 35). The primary outcome parameter was the absolute claudication distance (ACD). This trial was registered at Clinicaltrials.gov, NCT00497445.

Results.—The study included 70 patients, most of whom were treated for an aortoiliac lesion. The mean difference in ACD at 6 months of follow-up was 271.3 m (95% confidence interval [CI] 64.0–478.6, $P = .011$) in favor of additional SET. In the PVI alone group, 1 (3.7%) patient finished the complete treadmill test compared with 11 (32.4%) patients in the PVI + SET group ($P = .005$). Physical health—related quality-of-life score was 44.1 ± 7.8

in the PVI alone group compared with 41.9 ± 9.5 in the PVI + SET group, which was a nonsignificant difference (*P* = .34).

Conclusions.—SET following a PVI is more effective in increasing walking distance compared with a PVI alone. These data indicate that SET is a useful adjunct to a PVI for the treatment of PAD.

▶ Inter-Society Consensus for the Management of Peripheral Arterial Disease (TASC II) guidelines suggest supervised exercise therapy (SET) is the first choice of therapy for treatment of peripheral arterial disease (PAD). However, despite TASC guidelines, percutaneous interventions are increasingly used for initial treatment of PAD. Immediate technical success in most cases exceeds 90%. Many patients, however, after a peripheral vascular intervention (PVI), and despite patency of the treated arterial segment, have persistent or recurrent symptoms. It has been suggested that SET combined with a PVI may provide better therapy than PVI alone for patients with stable intermittent claudication secondary to infrainguinal PAD.[1] The current study is a randomized, prospective clinical trial evaluating the combination of a PVI of either aortoiliac disease or infrainguinal disease in combination with supplemental SET. The study raises interesting questions about the role of PVIs for treatment of claudication. One may ask what is it that matters, an increase in walking distance or an increase in patient quality of life (QOL)? In this study, an increase in walking distance did not translate directly into QOL improvement for the patients. This suggests better selection methods for treatment of patients with PVIs for claudication may be needed or that perhaps the generic QOL instruments utilized here lacked sensitivity to detect meaningful QOL changes in patients likely afflicted by numerous additional comorbidities. Different results may have been obtained with a disease-specific QOL instrument, such as the walking impairment questionnaire.

G. L. Moneta, MD

Reference

1. Mazari FA, Gulati S, Rahman MN, et al. Early outcomes from a randomized, controlled trial of supervised exercise, angioplasty, and combined therapy in inter-mittent claudication. *Ann Vasc Surg.* 2010;24:69-79.

A meta-analysis of the outcome of endovascular and noninvasive therapies in the treatment of intermittent claudication
Ahimastos AA, Pappas EP, Buttner PG, et al (Baker IDI Heart and Diabetes Inst, Melbourne, Australia; James Cook Univ, Brisbane, Australia; et al)
J Vasc Surg 54:1511-1521, 2011

Purpose.—Intermittent claudication is a common symptom of peripheral arterial disease. Currently, there is a lack of consensus on the most effective therapies for this problem. We conducted a meta-analysis of randomized trials assessing the efficacy of endovascular therapy (EVT) compared with noninvasive therapies for the treatment of intermittent claudication.

Methods.—Randomized trials comparing the efficacy of EVT and noninvasive therapies, such as medical therapy (MT) and supervised exercise (SVE) in patients with intermittent claudication were identified by a systematic search. Data were pooled, and combined overall effect sizes (standardized differences of mean values) were calculated for a random effect model in terms of ankle-brachial index (ABI) and treadmill walking for initial claudication distance (ICD) and maximum walking distance (MWD). Nine eligible trials (873 participants) were included: two compared EVT and MT alone, four compared EVT and SVE, and three trials compared EVT plus SVE vs SVE alone.

Results.—Heterogeneity between studies was marked. Quantitative data analysis suggested that EVT improved outcomes over MT alone at early follow-up evaluations. Outcomes of EVT plus SVE were better than those of SVE alone in terms of both ABI and treadmill walking at immediate, early, and intermediate follow-up. No substantial differences in outcomes of EVT alone compared with SVE alone were found.

Conclusion.—In patients with intermittent claudication, current evidence supports improved ABI and treadmill walking when EVT is added to MT or SVE during early and intermediate follow-up. There is no evidence that EVT alone provides improved outcome over SVE alone. There is low confidence in these findings for a number of reasons, including the small number of trials, the small size of these studies, the heterogeneity in study design, and the limited use of quality of life tools in assessing outcomes. More consistent data from larger, more homogenous studies, including longer follow-up, are required.

▶ Peripheral arterial disease is a significant problem with a prevalence that reaches 29% in individuals 70 years or older and of these, up to 33% have symptoms of intermittent claudication. Endovascular treatment of peripheral arterial disease is common practice. There is a paucity of data to suggest that endovascular treatment alone is of benefit or that combined with medical treatment and exercise outcomes are improved. In this excellent meta-analysis, the authors investigate the question by assessing randomized trials to determine the efficacy of endovascular therapy compared with noninvasive therapies for the treatment of intermittent claudication. The main findings of this study were the following: (1) Nine trials met the study primary endpoints (contained ankle-brachial index, initial claudication distance, maximum claudication distance), and quality-of-life data as a secondary endpoint were not available from the studies reviewed meeting the primary endpoint. (2) Detailed information of the extent of the lesion in the lower extremity was only available in 3 of the 9 trials. (3) In 1 study, only 17 of 61 patients underwent angioplasty, whereas 44 underwent surgical intervention. Thus, this group was not very representative of endovascular treatment alone, but represented patients actually having surgery. (4) Treatment failures after endovascular therapy ranged between 0% and 25%. (5) Major complications ranged between 0% and 5%. (6) No related deaths due to angioplasty were reported. (7) Ankle-brachial index values at baseline were comparable between studies, but significant heterogeneity was observed for baseline initial claudication distance and maximum walking distance values among the individual studies. (8) Compared with medical treatment, endovascular treatment offered improved hemodynamic and treadmill-walking outcomes at early (up to 12 months) and intermediate (up to 24 months) time points. (9) Compared with supervised exercise, endovascular treatment had no advantage in treadmill-walking distances (immediate and maximum claudication distances). (10) Compared with supervised exercise alone, endovascular treatment in addition to supervised exercise offered improved hemodynamic and treadmill-walking outcomes at early (up to 12 months) and intermediate (up to 24 months) time points. Some of the limiting factors when assessing various studies for meta-analysis are that the randomized trials qualifying for analysis have significant heterogeneity and lack standardization in methodology, have small and variable sample sizes, have intermediate follow-up, and lack important patient-related outcomes with relation to quality of life. In the future, to understand which thera-pies for intermittent claudication are the most effective will require large random-ized, controlled trials or comparative analysis. More importantly, using outcomes that include ankle-brachial index, initial claudication distance, and maximum walking distance is at best a surrogate measured outcome. Trials should focus on adding health value to the overall condition of the patient, taking into account patient-perceived improvements that can be assessed with proper quality-of-life tools both general and disease specific, in addition to having an assessment of the total costs for providing care for the entire duration of the specific disease condition.

J. D. Raffetto, MD

Effect of Hypoxia-Inducible Factor-1α Gene Therapy on Walking Performance in Patients With Intermittent Claudication

Creager MA, Olin JW, Belch JJF, et al (Brigham and Women's Hosp and Harvard Med School, Boston, MA; Mount Sinai Med Ctr, NY; Univ of Dundee, Scotland, UK; et al)
Circulation 124:1765-1773, 2011

Background.—Hypoxia-inducible factor-1α (HIF-1α) is a transcrip-tional regulatory factor that orchestrates cellular responses to hypoxia. It increases collateral vessel growth and blood flow in models of hind-limb ischemia. This study tested whether intramuscular administration of Ad2/HIF-1α/VP16, an engineered recombinant type 2 adenovirus vector encoding constitutively active HIF-1α, improves walking time in patients with peripheral artery disease and intermittent claudication.

Methods and Results.—Two hundred eighty-nine patients with claudi-cation were randomized in a double-blind manner to 1 of 3 doses of Ad2/HIF-1α/VP16 (2×10^9, 2×10^{10}, or 2×10^{11} viral particles) or placebo, administered by 20 intramuscular injections to each leg. Graded treadmill tests were performed at baseline and then 3, 6, and 12 months after treat-ment. The primary end point was the change in peak walking time from baseline to 6 months. The secondary end point was change in claudication onset time, and tertiary end points included changes in ankle-brachial index and quality-of-life assessments. Median peak walking time increased by 0.82 minutes (interquartile range, $-0.05-1.93$ minutes) in the placebo group and by 0.82 minutes (interquartile range, $-0.07-2.12$ minutes), 0.28 minutes (interquartile range, $-0.37-1.70$ minutes), and 0.78 minutes (interquartile range, $-0.02-2.10$ minutes) in the HIF-1α 2×10^9, 2×10^{10}, and 2×10^{11} viral particle groups, respectively (P=NS between placebo and each HIF-1α treatment group). There were no significant differences in claudication onset time, ankle-brachial index, or quality-of-life measurements between the placebo and each HIF-1α group.

Conclusions.—Gene therapy with intramuscular administration of Ad2/HIF-1α/VP16 is not an effective treatment for patients with intermittent claudication.

Clinical Trial Registration.—URL: http://www.clinicaltrials.gov. Unique identifier: NCT00117650.

▶ Interventional treatment for patients with peripheral arterial disease (PAD) is generally reserved for those with limb-threatening ischemia or disabling symptoms of intermittent claudication. Induction of angiogenesis of lower extremity arteries via protein, gene-based, or cellular therapy may result in new blood vessel formation, thereby improving blood flow in affected limbs of patients with PAD and improving symptoms of claudication. Hypoxia-inducible factor 1α (HIF-1α) is a transcriptional regulatory factor with important roles in cellular response to changes in oxygen tension.[1] HIF-1α exerts control on multiple genes, providing adaptive responses to hypoxia at the cellular level. HIF-1α/VP16 is hybrid transcription factor comprised of a truncated HIF-1α sequence fused to herpes simplex virus (VP16) transactivator. A previous phase 1 trial of patients with critical limb ischemia indicated that Ad2/HIF-1α/VP16 and engineered recombinant type 2 adenovirus vector encoding active HIF-1α provided resolution of rest pain and ulcer healing.[2] The authors postulated that intramuscular administration of Ad2/HIF-1α/VP16 could improve peak walking time in patients with intermittent claudication secondary to PAD. This was a negative study. Other than the possibility HIF-1α is ineffective in inducing angiogenesis, there are other possible reasons the study failed to prove the hypothesis that HIF-1α could improve walking time in patients with intermittent claudication. In the discussion portion of the article, the authors speculate that there may be differences in biologic activity of HIF-1α in patients with claudication compared with those with critical limb ischemia. Adenovirus transfection is perhaps not efficient in skeletal muscle, and duration of gene expression may be too short for development and subsequent maintenance of collateral vessels. It is also possible the distance between injection sites was too great to enable efficient collateral development. There may be compounding effects of mechanisms other than blood supply that limit walking distance in the intermittent claudication patient population. Finally, despite attempts to mitigate the placebo response, patients randomly assigned to placebo increased peak walking distance by approximately 30%. This study should be regarded only as negative under the conditions used in the study. Cellular- and gene-based therapies remain intriguing possibilities in the treatment of PAD. Unfortunately, it is going to be both time consuming and expensive to prove they are not just intriguing but also effective.

G. L. Moneta, MD

References

1. Semenza GL. Life with oxygen. *Science*. 2007;318:62-64.
2. Rajagopalan S, Olin J, Deitcher S, et al. Use of a constitutively active hypoxia-inducible factor-1alpha transgene as a therapeutic strategy in no-option critical limb ischemia patients: phase I dose-escalation experience. *Circulation*. 2007; 115:1234-1243.

Autologous bone marrow mononuclear cell therapy is safe and promotes amputation-free survival in patients with critical limb ischemia
Murphy MP, Lawson JH, Rapp BM, et al (Indiana Univ School of Medicine, Indianapolis; Duke Univ Med Ctr, Durham, NC)
J Vasc Surg 53:1565-1574, 2011

Objective.—The purpose of this Phase I open label nonrandomized trial was to assess the safety and efficacy of autologous bone marrow mononuclear cell (ABMNC) therapy in promoting amputation-free survival (AFS) in patients with critical limb ischemia (CLI).

Methods.—Between September 2005 and March 2009, 29 patients (30 limbs), with a median age of 66 years (range, 23–84 years; 14 male, 15 female) with CLI were enrolled. Twenty-one limbs presented with rest pain (RP), six with RP and ulceration, and three with ulcer only. All patients were not candidates for surgical bypass due to absence of a patent artery below the knee and/or endovascular approaches to improving perfusion was not possible as determined by an independent vascular surgeon. Patients were treated with an average dose of $1.7 \pm 0.7 \times 10^9$ ABMNC injected intramuscularly in the index limb distal to the anterior tibial tuberosity. The primary safety end point was accumulation of serious adverse events, and the primary efficacy end point was AFS at 1 year. Secondary end points at 12 weeks posttreatment were changes in first toe pressure (FTP), toe-brachial index (TBI), ankle-brachial index (ABI), and transcutaneous oxygen measurements (TcPO2). Perfusion of the index limb was measured with positron emission tomography-computed tomography (PET-CT) with intra-arterial infusion of H_2O^{15}. RP, using a 10-cm visual analogue scale, quality of life using the VascuQuol questionnaire, and ulcer healing were assessed at each follow-up interval. Subpopulations of endothelial progenitor cells were quantified prior to ABMNC administration using immunocytochemistry and fluorescent-activated cell sorting.

Results.—There were two serious adverse events; however, there were no procedure-related deaths. Amputation-free survival at 1 year was 86.3%. There was a significant increase in FTP (10.2 ± 6.2 mm Hg; $P = .02$) and TBI (0.10 ± 0.05; $P = .02$) and a trend in improvement in

ABI (0.08 ± 0.04; $P = .73$). Perfusion index by PET-CT H_2O^{15} increased by 19.3 ± 3.1, and RP decreased significantly by 2.2 ± 0.6 cm ($P = .02$). The VascuQol questionnaire demonstrated significant improvement in quality of life, and three of nine ulcers (33%) healed completely. KDR^+ but not $CD34^+$ or $CD133^+$ subpopulations of ABMNC were associated with improvement in limb perfusion.

Conclusion.—This Phase I study has demonstrated safety, and the AFS rates suggest efficacy of ABMNC in promoting limb salvage in "no option" CLI. Based on these results, we plan to test the concept that ABMNCs improve AFS at 1 year in a Phase III randomized, double-blinded, multicenter trial.

▶ Over the past decade, there have been evolving observations of effective cell-mediated angiogenesis from putative stem cells, both circulating and bone marrow derived, and their role in blood vessel development. More recently, there has been increasing attention on bone marrow—derived endothelial progenitor cells in patients with critical limb ischemia (CLI), as highlighted in both this study and the study by Powell et al.[1] The study by Murphy et al, sponsored by Biomet Biologics (Warsaw, IN), is a phase I study evaluating patients with CLI and no revascularization options treated with autologous bone marrow mononuclear cells derived from proprietary techniques for cell processing performed onsite followed by intramuscular delivery into the ischemic limb within a short timeframe. As a phase I study, primary endpoints of safety and amputation-free survival were achieved. In the study by Powell et al, the RESTORE-CLI trial sponsored by Aastrom Biosciences (Ann Arbor, MI), the sample population is relatively similar with CLI patients and no revascularization options, but bone marrow mononuclear cells are targeted using a different proprietary cell-processing technique in a closed automated cell manufacturing system offsite for 12 days, with cells returned to the original location for subsequent intramuscular injections into the index limb. As a phase II, multicenter, randomized, double-blinded, placebo-controlled study, endpoints of safety and decreased clinical endpoints associated with atherosclerotic disease progression are also realized. Although both of these studies on bone marrow—derived endothelial progenitor cells for treatment of CLI show safety, efficacy, and potential promise, pivotal proof of concept is still lacking and awaiting phase III extended randomized, double-blinded, multicenter investigation.

M. A. Passman, MD

Reference

1. Powell RJ, Comerota AJ, Berceli SA, et al. Interim analysis results from the RESTORE-CLI, a randomized, double-blind multicenter phase II trial comparing expanded autologous bone marrow-derived tissue repair cells and placebo in patients with critical limb ischemia. *J Vasc Surg.* 2011;54:1032-1041.

Interim analysis results from the RESTORE-CLI, a randomized, double-blind multicenter phase II trial comparing expanded autologous bone marrow-derived tissue repair cells and placebo in patients with critical limb ischemia
Powell RJ, Comerota AJ, Berceli SA, et al (Dartmouth-Hitchcock Med Ctr, Lebanon, NH; Jobst Vascular Ctr, Toledo, OH; Malcolm Randall VAMC and Univ of Florida, Gainesville; et al)
J Vasc Surg 54:1032-1041, 2011

Objectives.—Cell therapy is a novel experimental treatment modality for patients with critical limb ischemia (CLI) of the lower extremities and no other established treatment options. This study was conducted to assess the safety and clinical efficacy of intramuscular injection of autologous tissue repair cells (TRCs).

Methods.—A prospective, randomized double-blinded, placebo controlled, multicenter study (RESTORE-CLI) was conducted at 18 centers in the United States in patients with CLI and no option for revascularization. Enrollment of 86 patients began in April 2007 and ended in February 2010. For the prospectively planned interim analysis, conducted in February 2010, 33 patients had the opportunity to complete the trial (12 months of follow-up), and 46 patients had completed at least 6 months of follow-up. The interim analysis included analysis of both patient populations. An independent physician performed the bone marrow or sham control aspiration. The aspirate was processed in a closed, automated cell manufacturing system for approximately 12 days to generate the TRC population of stem and progenitor cells. An average of $136 \pm 41 \times 10^6$ total viable cells or electrolyte (control) solution were injected into 20 sites in the ischemic lower extremity. The primary end point was safety as evaluated by adverse events, and serious adverse events as assessed at multiple follow-up time points. Clinical efficacy end points included major amputation-free survival and time to first occurrence of treatment failure (defined as any of the following: major amputation, death, de novo gangrene, or doubling of wound size), as well as major amputation rate and measures of wound healing.

Results.—There was no difference in adverse or serious adverse events between the two groups. Statistical analysis revealed a significant increase in time to treatment failure (log-rank test, $P = .0053$) and amputation-free survival in patients receiving TRC treatment, (log-rank test, $P = .038$). Major amputation occurred in 19% of TRC-treated patients compared to 43% of controls ($P = .14$, Fisher exact test). There was evidence of improved wound healing in the TRC-treated patients when compared with controls at 12 months.

Conclusions.—Intramuscular injection of autologous bone marrow-derived TRCs is safe and decreases the occurrence of clinical events associated with disease progression when compared to placebo in patients with lower extremity CLI and no revascularization options.

▶ Over the past decade, there have been evolving observations of effective cell-mediated angiogenesis from putative stem cells, both circulating and bone marrow derived, and their role in blood vessel development. More recently, there has been increasing attention on bone marrow—derived endothelial progenitor cells in patients with critical limb ischemia (CLI), as highlighted in both this study and the study by Murphy et al.[1] The study by Murphy et al, sponsored by Biomet Biologics (Warsaw, IN), is a phase I study evaluating patients with CLI and no revascularization options treated with autologous bone marrow mononuclear cells derived from proprietary techniques for cell processing performed onsite followed by intramuscular delivery into the ischemic limb within a short timeframe. As a phase I study, primary endpoints of safety and amputation-free survival were achieved. In this study by Powell et al, the RESTORE-CLI trial sponsored by Aastrom Biosciences (Ann Arbor, MI), the sample population is relatively similar with CLI patients and no revascularization options, but bone marrow mononuclear cells are targeted using a different proprietary cell-processing technique in a closed, automated cell-manufacturing system offsite for 12 days, with cells returned to the original location for subsequent intramuscular injections into the index limb. As a phase II, multicenter, randomized, double-blinded, placebo-controlled study, endpoints of safety and decreased clinical endpoints associated with atherosclerotic disease progression are also realized. Although both of these studies on bone marrow—derived endothelial progenitor cells for treatment of CLI show safety, efficacy, and potential promise, pivotal proof of concept is still lacking and awaiting phase III extended randomized, double-blinded, multicenter investigation.

M. A. Passman, MD

Reference

1. Murphy MP, Lawson JH, Rapp BM, et al. Autologous bone marrow mononuclear cell therapy is safe and promotes amputation-free survival in patients with critical limb ischemia. *J Vasc Surg.* 2011;53:1565-1574.

Endovascular treatment as first line approach for infrarenal aortic occlusive disease
Schwindt AG, Panuccio G, Donas KP, et al (St Franziskus Hosp, Münster, Germany; et al)
J Vasc Surg 53:1550-1556.e1, 2011

Introduction.—The purpose of this study was to report the early and late results of primary stenting for focal atherosclerotic lesions of the infrarenal aorta.

Methods.—A retrospective analysis of 52 consecutive patients treated for infrarenal occlusive aortic disease with primary stenting between January 2002 and November 2009 was performed. Original angiographic imaging, medical records, and noninvasive testing were reviewed. Primary stenting was the first line of treatment. Perioperative technical success and Kaplan-Meier estimates for patency and survival were calculated.

Results.—The majority of the patients (43) were treated for severe claudication (Rutherford III; 82.7%), 5 for ischemic rest pain (Rutherford IV; 9.6%), and 4 for minor tissue loss (Rutherford V; 7.7%). Aortic stenosis was found in 40 cases (76.9%) and occlusion in 12 (23%). Perioperative hemodynamic success was 100%. All patients had an improvement of ankle brachial index (ABI) >0.10. Clinical improvement was found in 96%. Early surgical revision was necessary for aortic rupture in 1 patient. One death occurred for pneumonia. The mean follow-up time was 39.4 ± 27.2 months. Ten reinterventions (19%) were needed for symptom recurrence. The estimated assisted primary patency at 9 years was 96% and the mean survival time was 86.6 months.

Conclusion.—Primary stenting offers safe and durable results and should be considered as the first line of treatment for focal aortic lesions.

▶ The operative approach is considered standard treatment for infrarenal aortic occlusive disease, but with expansion of endovascular techniques, primary stenting of infrarenal aortic occlusive pathology has become more feasible and may be an alternative to primary operative options. The sample population in this study focused on patients with occlusive disease of infrarenal aortic segment with or without iliac artery involvement, whereas those with isolated iliac occlusive disease were excluded. Of the 52 patients, 39 (75%) underwent isolated infrarenal aortic stenting and 13 (25%) had combined aortoiliac stenting, which included 10 patients who required additional concomitant procedures such as femoral endarterectomy or femorofemoral crossover bypass. Overall complication rates were low, and although primary patency was worse for TransAtlantic Inter-Society Consensus D class disease, cumulative assisted primary patency (11 patients requiring reintervention) was 96% at 9 years. As a retrospective study over an extended time period, these results are qualified by selection bias, changes in stent technology and the use of many types of stents and endovascular techniques during the study period, and lack of a control group comparing primary operative approaches. Although the authors' conclusion that primary stenting did offer safe and durable results is supported by the data set, their statement that primary stenting should be considered first-line treatment for focal aortic lesions is not supported. When deciding best options for patients with occlusive disease of the infrarenal aorta with or without iliac involvement, reported results from this study should be factored into clinical decision making along with other patient-related factors to determine whether an endovascular or operative approach is most optimal.

M. A. Passman, M.D

Effect of Physician and Hospital Experience on Patient Outcomes for Endovascular Treatment of Aortoiliac Occlusive Disease
Indes JE, Tuggle CT, Mandawat A, et al (Yale Univ School of Medicine, New Haven, CT)
Arch Surg 146:966-971, 2011

Objective.—To evaluate the effect of physician volume and specialty and hospital volume on population-level outcomes after endovascular repair of aortoiliac occlusive disease (AIOD).

Design.—A retrospective cross-sectional analysis of all inpatients undergoing endovascular repair of AIOD. Physician volume was classified as low (<17 procedures per year [<50th percentile]) or high (≥17 procedures per year). Physicians were defined as surgeons if they performed at least 1 carotid, aortic, or iliac endarterectomy; open aortic repair; above- or below-knee amputation; or aortoiliac-femoral bypass. Hospital volume was low (<116 procedures per year [<50th percentile]) or high (≥116 procedures per year).

Patients.—Eight hundred eighteen inpatients who underwent endovascular repair of AIOD in the Healthcare Cost and Utilization Project Nationwide Inpatient Sample from January 2003 through December 2007.

Setting.—National hospital database.

Main Outcome Measures.—In-hospital complications and mortality, length of stay, and cost.

Results.—Of the 818 procedures, 59.0% of high-volume physicians were surgeons and 65.0% practiced at high-volume hospitals. Unadjusted complication rates were significantly higher for low-volume compared with high-volume physicians (18.7% vs 12.6%; $P = .02$); rates were not significantly different by physician specialty ($P = .88$) or hospital volume ($P = .16$). Shorter length of stay was associated with high-volume physicians ($P = .001$), high-volume hospitals ($P = .001$), and surgeon providers ($P = .03$), whereas decreased cost was associated with physician specialty ($P = .004$). On multivariate analysis, high physician volume was associated with significantly lower complications ($P = .04$); high hospital volume, with shorter length of stay ($P = .002$); and nonsurgeons, with higher costs ($P = .05$).

Conclusions.—Overall, volume at the physician and hospital levels appears to be a robust predictor of patient outcomes after endovascular interventions for AIOD. Surgeons performing endovascular procedures for AIOD have a decreased associated hospital cost compared with nonsurgeons.

▶ It has been shown that patients undergoing some vascular and cancer procedures have a decreased risk of operative death when the procedures are performed in high-volume hospitals. For many procedures, associations between operative mortality and hospital volume are mediated through surgeon volume.[1] Whereas the relationship between open vascular procedures and surgeon and hospital volume has been frequently studied, there is little information available on the relationship between physician volume, hospital volume, and the outcomes of endovascular procedures for arterial disease. In a recent study, physician specialty was not associated with outcomes or complications for lower extremity percutaneous angioplasty.[2] In this study, the authors evaluated the effects of physician volume, especially in-hospital volume, on outcomes of endovascular repair in patients with aortoiliac occlusive disease (AIOD), and they conclude that volume matters. In this comment, Dr Karl Illig suggests that the article adds aortoiliac endovascular intervention to the list of procedures best performed by high-volume physicians and high-volume institutions. He may be correct, but there are too many problems with this article to justify the conclusion. First, the study only looked at in patients, and most patients undergoing endovascular interventions for AIOD are treated as outpatients. In addition, this study does not look at the appropriateness of interventions. In some cases it has been shown that high-volume specialists are sometimes associated with a higher volume of marginal or inappropriate procedures as well. This study represents a clearly skewed sample of the patients undergoing endovascular treatment for AIOD for indications that may or may not be appropriate. It is not possible to do a drill down with these data as to why shorter lengths of stay may be associated with higher-volume physicians or why surgeons were associated with lower hospital costs. It is certainly possible that patients may not have been stratified equally among the providers and the hospitals. Overall, this article really provides no insight as to the relationship between physician and hospital volume for endovascular treatment of patients with AIOD.

G. L. Moneta, MD

References

1. Birkmeyer JD, Siewers AE, Finlayson EV, et al. Hospital volume and surgical mortality in the United States. *N Engl J Med.* 2002;346:1128-1137.
2. Vogel TR, Dombrovskiy VY, Carson JL, Haser PB, Graham AM. Lower extremity angioplasty: impact of practitioner specialty and volume on practice patterns and healthcare resource utilization. *J Vasc Surg.* 2009;50:1320-1324.

Stent-assisted Remote Iliac Artery Endarterectomy: An Alternative Approach to Treating Combined External Iliac and Common Femoral Artery Disease
Simó G, Banga P, Darabos G, et al (Szent Imre Hosp, Budapest, Hungary)
Eur J Vasc Endovasc Surg 42:648-655, 2011

Objective.—Stent-assisted remote iliac endarterectomy (SA-RIEA) is a hybrid minimally invasive technique for treating patients with combined external iliac and common femoral disease, when the only alternative would be conventional open revascularisation.

Design.—This was a retrospective, single-centre study.

Materials and Methods.—From January 2004 to April 2010, 155 SA-RIEA procedures were performed. The patients' mean age was 62 (range, 43–86) years. Indications for surgery were: severe claudication in 79 (51%), rest pain in 43 (28%) and gangrene in 33 (21%) cases. The mean length of follow-up was 21 months.

Result.—Initial technical success was achieved in 145 (93.5%) procedures. Ten patients required conversion to a conventional iliofemoral reconstructive procedure. The 1-, 3- and 5-year primary, primary-assisted and secondary patency rates were 80.2%, 74.7% and 69.3%; 84.8%, 82.4% and 78.2%; and 86.8%, 84.2% and 79.6%, respectively. Within the first 30 days, there were no early reocclusions, one (0.6%) perioperative death due to myocardial infarction, five (3.4%) minor wound complications and two (1.3%) limb losses. During follow-up, seven patients underwent open reconstruction due to symptomatic reocclusion, and four were re-operated on due to symptomatic restenosis (three percutaneous transluminal angioplasties (PTAs), one reendarterectomy).

Conclusion.—In patients with combined common femoral and external iliac disease, SA-RIEA appears to offer a safe and effective alternative to conventional open surgery.

▶ The authors report their 6-year experience performing combined common femoral endarterectomy and retrograde iliac remote endarterectomy with angioplasty and stenting. The common femoral artery has become the common access point for the treatment of aneurysms and peripheral artery disease. In the case of peripheral arterial disease, it is technically feasible to perform a common femoral endarterectomy, profundaplasty, retrograde iliac recanalization with angioplasty and stenting, and antegrade superficial artery recanalization with angioplasty and stenting—all performed through a 5- to 7-cm groin incision. How does endovascular surgical bypass compare with open surgical bypass?

Their report is limited by the constraints of a retrospective report. Their selection bias is clear; they do not provide the true denominator in the report. What was the outcome of surgical bypasses at their hospital? It is clear that some cases are favorable for endovascular attempts and others for open repair. They report their learning curve but provide no insight into the patients who were excluded. In addition, they report revascularization outcomes on 2 distinct populations that should rarely be reported in the same article: claudicants and critical limb ischemia patients.

This is a technical report and should be regarded as such. Their success rate of 94% is excellent, but how and when to use this procedure is still relegated to the surgeon's clinical judgment, not objective data.

Z. M. Arthurs, MD

Impact of renal insufficiency on clinical outcomes in patients with critical limb ischemia undergoing endovascular revascularization
Willenberg T, Baumann F, Eisenberger U, et al (Swiss Cardiovascular Ctr, Bern, Switzerland)
J Vasc Surg 53:1589-1597, 2011

Background.—Patients with renal insufficiency (RI) are frequently excluded from trials assessing various endovascular revascularization concepts in critical limb ischemia (CLI) although information on clinical outcomes is scarce.

Methods.—Consecutive patients with CLI undergoing endovascular lower limb revascularization during a 4.5-year time interval at a tertiary referral center were prospectively followed over a 12-month period. Patients were grouped according to renal function defined as normal (estimated glomerular filtration rate [eGFR] $\geq$60 mL/min/1.73 m^2; n = 108, 49.5%), moderate RI (eGFR $\geq$30-59 mL/min/1.73 m^2; n = 86, 39.5%) and severe RI, including dialysis (eGFR <30 mL/min/1.73 m^2; n = 24,

11%). Clinical endpoints assessed were sustained clinical success, peri- and postprocedural mortality and major, above-the-ankle amputation. Sustained clinical improvement was defined as an upward shift of at least one category on the Rutherford classification compared with baseline to a level of claudication without repeated revascularization or unplanned amputation in surviving patients. Survival analysis was performed using the Kaplan–Meier method. Multivariate regression analysis was conducted in separate models for all above-mentioned clinical endpoints.

Results.—A total of 208 patients (218 limbs, mean age 77.1 ± 9.5, 131 men) underwent endovascular revascularization. Technical success rate was 95.2%, 92.5%, and 100% in patients without, moderate or severe RI. Sustained clinical success was 81.7%, 74.1%, and 51.5% in patients with normal renal function, 87.8%, 67.0%, and 63.3% with moderate, and 81.0%, 64.6%, and 50.2% with severe RI ($P = .87$ by log-rank) at 2, 6, and 12 months. Accordingly, major amputation rates were 9.9%, 18.2%, and 20.8% vs 9.9%, 22.6%, and 24% vs 12.5%, 16.7%, and 21.1% ($P = .83$, by log-rank). Mortality rates were 8.4%, 17.6%, and 26.5% in patients with normal renal function, 9.6%, 17.6%, and 30.1% with moderate and 17.5%, 26.6%, and 31.9% in patients with severe RI ($P = .77$, by log-rank) at corresponding intervals. Multivariate analysis revealed eGFR (hazard ratio [HR], 1.016; 95% confidence interval [CI],

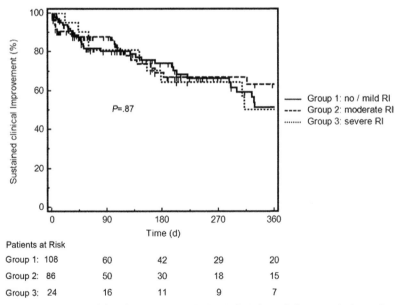

FIGURE 1.—Sustained clinical improvement in 218 critically ischemic limbs, categorized according to renal function. *RI*, Renal insufficiency. (Reprinted from the Journal of Vascular Surgery, Willenberg T, Baumann F, Eisenberger U, et al. Impact of renal insufficiency on clinical outcomes in patients with critical limb ischemia undergoing endovascular revascularization. *J Vasc Surg*. 2011;53:1589-1597. Copyright 2011, with permission from The Society for Vascular Surgery.)

1.001-1.031; $P = .036$), age (HR, 1.12; 95% CI, 1.061-1.189; $P < .0001$) and cigarette smoking (HR, 3.14; 95% CI, 1.153-8.55; $P = .026$) to be predictors for increased mortality within 1 year of follow-up.

Conclusion.—While functional lower limb outcomes were not influenced by renal function in this study, presence of RI was an independent predictor for higher mortality in CLI patients undergoing endovascular revascularization (Figs 1, 3, and 4).

▶ Endovascular treatment for critical limb ischemia has become a primary mode of treatment, especially in patients with significant risk factors. A concern when offering this form of therapy to patients with limb ischemia is the status of their renal function. There are data to support that patients with significant renal dysfunction or who are on dialysis have worse limb outcomes following endovascular interventions, higher limb loss rates, increased restenosis rates, and higher mortality rates. For these reasons, many patients with renal insufficiency are not entered into trial to assess the efficacy of novel therapies. In this study, the authors evaluate limb outcomes and mortality in patients with normal renal function (estimated glomerular filtration rate [eGFR] > 60 mL/min, n = 108 limbs), moderate renal insufficiency (eGFR 30–59 mL/min, n = 86 limbs), and severe renal insufficiency, including those patients on dialysis (eGFR < 30 mL/min, n = 24 limbs) who present with critical limb ischemia (rest pain and tissue loss) and undergo

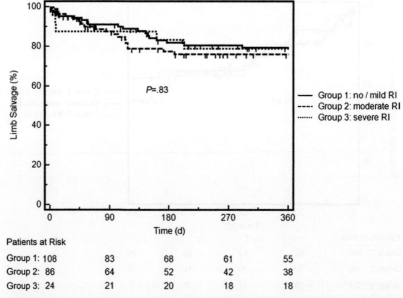

FIGURE 3.—Limb salvage rates in 218 critically ischemic limbs, categorized according to renal function. *RI*, Renal insufficiency. (Reprinted from the Journal of Vascular Surgery, Willenberg T, Baumann F, Eisenberger U, et al. Impact of renal insufficiency on clinical outcomes in patients with critical limb ischemia undergoing endovascular revascularization. *J Vasc Surg.* 2011;53:1589-1597. Copyright 2011, with permission from The Society for Vascular Surgery.)

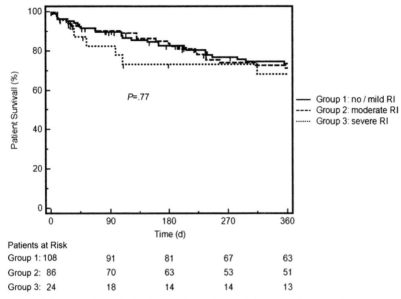

Patients at Risk

Group 1:	108	91	81	67	63
Group 2:	86	70	63	53	51
Group 3:	24	18	14	14	13

FIGURE 4.—Survival of 208 critical limb ischemia (CLI) patients, categorized according to renal function. *RI*, Renal insufficiency. (Reprinted from the Journal of Vascular Surgery, Willenberg T, Baumann F, Eisenberger U, et al. Impact of renal insufficiency on clinical outcomes in patients with critical limb ischemia undergoing endovascular revascularization. *J Vasc Surg.* 2011;53:1589-1597. Copyright 2011, with permission from The Society for Vascular Surgery.)

endovascular revascularizations. The anatomic levels of angioplasty were similar among the 3 groups, as was the use of stents. Surprisingly, the authors find that the initial technical success, sustained clinical success at 2, 6, and 12 months (Fig 1), cumulative rates of repeat endovascular revascularizations at 2, 6, and 12 months, limb salvage outcomes at 2, 6, and 12 months (Fig 3), and mortality rates at 2, 6, and 12 months (Fig 4) were all similar among the 3 groups. Not surprisingly, in their regression model, creatinine clearance at baseline was an independent predictor of mortality, along with age and cigarette smoking. The lesson learned from this study is that we should carefully select our patients for revascularization in the setting of critical limb ischemia, and the presence of renal insufficiency should not preclude from performing endovascular interventions for limb salvage and improvement in quality of life. Some shortcomings of this study are that it is nonrandomized, the group with severe renal insufficiency is small, it is a single center, and the follow-up is short. In addition, it is unclear if the patients' symptoms or tissue loss improved during the study period, as these data are not available or, more importantly, whether the patients' quality-of-life improved. Further study is required before we know whether the best value of care delivered is both outcome- and cost-effective in patients with critical limb ischemia and renal insufficiency.

J. D. Raffetto, MD

Impact of cilostazol after endovascular treatment for infrainguinal disease in patients with critical limb ischemia

Soga Y, Iida O, Hirano K, et al (Kokura Memorial Hosp, Kitakyushu, Japan; Kansai Rosai Hosp, Amagasaki, Japan; Saiseikai Yokohama-city Eastern Hosp, Japan; et al)
J Vasc Surg 54:1659-1667, 2011

Background.—Cilostazol reduces restenosis and repeat revascularization after endovascular therapy (EVT) in claudicant patients with femoropopliteal lesions. However, the efficacy of cilostazol in patients with critical limb ischemia (CLI) is unclear. Therefore, we investigated the effect of cilostazol on outcomes in patients with CLI.

Methods.—From January 2004 to December 2009, 618 patients (30.8% women, 356 treated with cilostazol, 72.4 ± 7.3 years old) with CLI underwent EVT for de novo infrainguinal lesions. Their data were retrospectively analyzed. The primary outcome measure was amputation-free survival (AFS), The secondary outcome measures were overall survival, limb salvage, freedom from repeat revascularization, and freedom from surgical conversion. Mean follow-up was 21 ± 14 months.

Results.—AFS and the limb salvage rate at 5 years were significantly higher in the cilostazol-treated group (47.7% vs 32.7%, $P < .01$; 86.6% vs 75.3%, $P < .01$; respectively). However, overall survival and freedom from repeat revascularization at 5 years did not differ significantly between the two groups (43.9% vs 46.0%, $P = .24$; 39.9% vs 31.8%, $P = .21$, respectively). Freedom from surgical conversion at 5 years was significantly higher in the cilostazol-treated group (91.0% vs 81.2%, $P < .01$). After correcting all end points with baseline variables, cilostazol was effective for prevention of AFS (hazard ratio [HR], 0.67; 95% confidential interval [CI], 0.49-0.91; adjusted $P = .01$) and improvement of limb salvage rate (HR, 0.42; 95% CI, 0.25-0.69; adjusted $P < .01$). There was no significant difference in overall survival, repeat revascularization, and surgical conversion between the groups.

Conclusions.—Cilostazol may improve AFS and limb salvage rate after EVT for infrainguinal disease in patients with CLI.

▶ The authors present the effects of cilostazol on a retrospective series of patients who underwent endovascular therapy for critical limb ischemia. Much of the data in this article are valuable to continue building the overall data set for percutaneous revascularization for this patient population and agree with much of the existing literature regarding overall limb salvage, amputation-free survival, and overall survival. The most glaring issue with the authors' data set is the significantly higher number of renal failure patients in the cilostazol group, which they (and the reviewers) show in Table 1 but do not state in the results. The subsequent "adjustment" analysis and univariate analysis show that there is no effect of cilostazol for renal failure patients. Overall, the retrospective nature of the study and the

TABLE 1.—Patients' Characteristics

Variable[a]	Cilostazol Therapy Yes (n = 356)	No (n = 262)	P
Age, years	72.0 ± 11.3	71.3 ± 9.5	.44
Male (%)	242 (68.0)	165 (63.0)	.20
BMI, kg/m²	21.4 ± 3.4	21.9 ± 2.9	.09
Hypertension	291 (81.7)	213 (81.3)	.89
Dyslipidemia	252 (70.8)	189 (72.1)	.71
Diabetes (%)	258 (72.5)	205 (78.2)	.10
Hemodialysis	170 (47.8)	151 (57.6)	.02
Current smoker	107 (30.1)	61 (23.3)	.06
COPD	22 (6.2)	13 (5.0)	.52
CVD	131 (36.8)	92 (35.1)	.67
CAD	179 (50.3)	150 (57.3)	.09
LV dysfunction[b]	31 (8.7)	18 (6.9)	.40
Rutherford class			.65
4	96	62	
5	197	151	
6	63	49	
CLI in other leg	58 (16.3)	43 (16.4)	.97
Poor runoff	258 (72.3)	183 (69.8)	.48
Ambulatory	160 (44.9)	115 (43.9)	.80
ABI			
Preprocedure	0.67 ± 0.30	0.69 ± 0.31	.57
Postprocedure	0.84 ± 0.27	0.84 ± 0.25	.88
SPP, mm Hg			
Preprocedure	30.6 ± 19.2	29.1 ± 19.1	.35
Postprocedure	49.8 ± 19.9	44.2 ± 22.0	.002
CRP, mg/dL	2.3 ± 3.6	2.7 ± 4.7	.25
Procedure success	332 (93.3)	236 (90.1)	.15
Lesion location			
FP	122 (34.3)	92 (35.1)	.44
BTK	221 (62.1)	165 (63.0)	
FP + BTK	13 (3.7)	5 (1.9)	
Medication			
Aspirin	310 (87.8)	216 (82.4)	.06
Thienopyridine	96 (27.2)	134 (51.3)	<.0001
ACEI/ARB	106 (29.8)	94 (35.9)	.11
Calcium antagonist	218 (61.2)	153 (58.4)	.48
β-Blockade	23 (6.5)	14 (5.3)	.56
Statins	78 (22.1)	56 (21.5)	.85
Warfarin	63 (17.8)	47 (18.0)	.95

ABI, Ankle-brachial index; *ACEI*, angiotensin converting enzyme inhibitors; *ARB*, angiotensin receptor blockers; *BTK*, below-the-knee; *CLI*, critical limb ischemia; *COPD*, chronic obstructive pulmonary disease; *CRP*, C-reactive protein; *CVD*, cardiovascular death; *FP*, femoropopliteal; *LV*, left ventricular; *SPP*, skin perfusion pressure.
[a]Continuous data are presented as mean ± standard deviation; categoric data as number (%).
[b]LV dysfunction was defined as a left ventricular ejection fraction <40%.

physician's choice as to cilostazol treatment make changing clinical practice based on these results.

A. Chandra, MD

Femoropopliteal Balloon Angioplasty vs. Bypass Surgery for CLI: A Propensity Score Analysis

Korhonen M, Biancari F, Söderström M, et al (Helsinki Univ Central Hosp, Finland; Oulu Univ Hosp, Finland)
Eur J Vasc Endovasc Surg 41:378-384, 2011

Objectives.—To compare the outcomes of femoropopliteal percutaneous transluminal angioplasty (PTA) and bypass surgery for critical limb ischaemia (CLI).

Design.—The study is retrospective in nature.

Materials and Methods.—This study included 858 consecutive patients, who underwent femoropopliteal revascularisation for CLI at Helsinki University Central Hospital during 2000—2007. As many as 517 patients

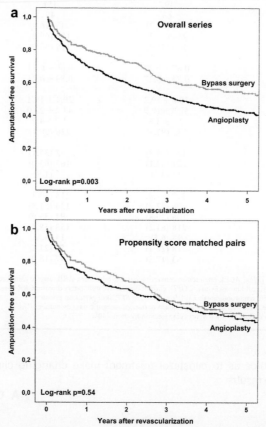

FIGURE 2.—Amputation-free survival after femoropopliteal percutaneous transluminal angioplasty and bypass surgery for critical limb ischaemia a) in the overall series and b) in 241 propensity score-matched pairs. (Reprinted from Korhonen M, Biancari F, Söderström M, et al. Femoropopliteal balloon angioplasty vs. bypass surgery for CLI: a propensity score analysis. *Eur J Vasc Endovasc Surg.* 2011;41:378-384. Copyright 2011, with permission from European Society for Vascular Surgery.)

(60%) underwent PTA and 341 (40%) bypass surgery. Propensity score analysis was used for risk adjustment in multivariable analysis and for one-to-one matching.

Results.—In the overall series, PTA had poorer long-term results than bypass (5-year leg salvage, 78.2% vs. 91.8%, $p < 0.0001$; survival 49.2% vs. 57.1%, $p = 0.048$; amputation-free survival, 42.0% vs. 53.7%, $p = 0.003$; freedom from surgical re-intervention 86.2% vs. 94.3%, $p < 0.0001$).

When treatment method was adjusted for propensity score as well as in the propensity score-matched pairs, leg salvage and freedom from surgical re-intervention were worse after PTA than after bypass (among the 241 propensity score-matched pairs, 74.3% vs. 88.2%, $p = 0.031$, and 86.1% vs. 89.8%, $p = 0.025$, respectively). Differences in survival, amputation-free survival and freedom from any re-intervention were not observed.

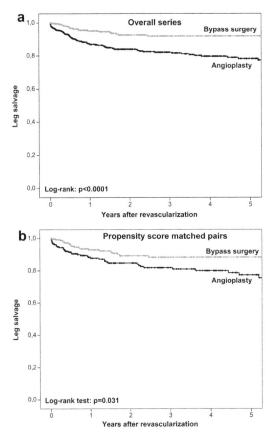

FIGURE 3.—Leg salvage after femoropopliteal percutaneous transluminal angioplasty and bypass surgery for critical limb ischaemia a) in the overall series and b) in 241 propensity score-matched pairs. (Reprinted from Korhonen M, Biancari F, Söderström M, et al. Femoropopliteal balloon angioplasty vs. bypass surgery for CLI: a propensity score analysis. *Eur J Vasc Endovasc Surg.* 2011;41:378-384. Copyright 2011, with permission from European Society for Vascular Surgery.)

Conclusions.—In CLI patients, femoropopliteal PTA seems to be associated with poorer long-term leg salvage and freedom from surgical reintervention than bypass surgery. However, the treatment method did not affect long-term amputation-free survival (Figs 2 and 3).

▶ Endovascular procedures in patients with critical limb ischemia (CLI) have rapidly increased over the past decade, but evidence supporting this approach is largely anecdotal. The BASIL trial, with all its flaws, remains the only large randomized trial comparing the 2 treatment methods.[1] It is indeed commonly observed that comparisons of surgical and endovascular therapy with randomized trials is troublesome because it is difficult to form comparable groups. Propensity score analysis potentially allows for a more accurate comparison between treatment arms by adjusting for differences between treatment groups. Propensity score analysis is a measure of the likelihood that a patient would have been treated similarly using covariant scores. Theoretically, propensity scores reduce bias and increase precision by adjusting for risk factors and calculating for the effective treatment.[2] The authors in this study adjusted for treatment method with the most relevant covariants in their 1:1 propensity-matched pairs. They found no significant difference in amputation-free survival between open and endovascular treatment of CLI but did note that bypass surgery was associated with better long-term limb salvage. They postulate that the overall high mortality of patients with CLI overwhelm the effect of better long-term leg salvage using the combined endpoint of amputation-free survival (Figs 2 and 3). There is beginning to be a slow accumulation of non-anecdotal data that support long-term benefits of bypass surgery over percutaneous transluminal angioplasty in treatment of CLI in patients with longevity expected to be at least 2 years.

G. L. Moneta, MD

References

1. Adam DJ, Beard JD, Cleveland T, et al. Basil trial participants. Bypass versus angioplasty in severe ischaemia of the leg (BASIL): multicentre, randomised controlled trial. *Lancet.* 2005;366:1925-1934.
2. D'Agostino RB Jr. Propensity score methods for bias reduction in the comparison of a treatment to a non-randomized control group. *Stat Med.* 1998;17:2265-2281.

Functional Ability in Patients with Critical Limb Ischaemia is Unaffected by Successful Revascularisation
Cieri E, Lenti M, De Rango P, et al (Univ of Perugia, Italy; et al)
Eur J Vasc Endovasc Surg 41:256-263, 2011

Objective.—Patient- and society-oriented measures of outcome have a critical role in determining the effectiveness of any treatment in patients with critical limb ischaemia (CLI). In particular, the impact of an intervention on patient's dependency and functional performance is relevant but is largely unknown.

The aim of the study was to investigate whether the limitations encountered in the activities of daily living (ADLs) measured with the Katz Index (KI) in patients with CLI were changed by the treatment.

Methods.—During the period 2006–2008, 248 consecutive patients undergoing repair for CLI were investigated with an ADL questionnaire for assessing KI before and after a mean of 16.19 months from treatment. Changes in KI were stratified by type of treatment and outcome.

Results.—There were 165 males and 83 females, mean age 73.3 ± 8.3 years; 125 patients showed tissue loss and 123 rest pain alone, 98 received surgical bypass and 150 endovascular repair. Pre-operative KI mean was 10.42. At the post-operative assessment, there was significant worsening in patients' functional outcome (mean KI decreased to 9.78) despite relief of pain (81.5%), tissue healing (72%), good vessel patency (83.8%) and low amputation rate (9.7%). Deterioration of KI was not significantly higher in patients undergoing endovascular repair. Patients receiving major amputation started with worse pre-operative functional score (KI mean 9.42) and did further deteriorate (KI mean 7.71) after demolition surgery. However, patients who received successful revascularisation showed deterioration in the dependence index.

Conclusions.—Successful vascular treatment is not associated with improved functional ability in patients with CLI, especially when already highly dependent in their activities. Large nationwide preventive and educational programmes should be implemented to prevent irreversible and severe health deterioration in populations with CLI (Fig 1).

▶ In many patients with critical limb ischemia (CLI), it can be difficult to decide whether to treat by revascularization, amputation, or medical therapy alone. Limb

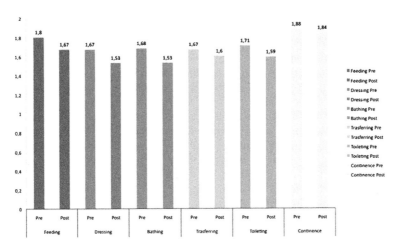

FIGURE 1.—Katz index pre and post revascularisation by specific function. (Reprinted from European Journal of Vascular and Endovascular Surgery, Cieri E, Lenti M, De Rango P, et al. Functional ability in patients with critical limb ischaemia is unaffected by successful revascularisation. *Eur J Vasc Endovasc Surg.* 2011;41:256-263. Copyright 2011, with permission from the European Society for Vascular Surgery.)

salvage is a common measure of successful treatment of CLI, but what truly constitutes CLI is difficult to define. Although it is generally agreed that CLI has an adverse effect on quality of life, there are a few studies quantitatively assessing functional abilities in patients with CLI treated by revascularization. In this study the authors used the Katz index of independence and activities of daily living to assess the functional impact of revascularization in patients with CLI. The authors' findings that the Katz index did not improve following successful revascularization suggest that the functional impairment in patients with CLI is difficult to reverse with revascularization and it does not matter whether revascularization is by open or endovascular means (Fig 1). This study is consistent with the concept that treatment of CLI is much like treatment of an advanced malignancy. In patients with metastatic malignancy, frequently the goal is palliation, not cure. This also appears to be the case in many patients with CLI. Treatment of CLI may not cure the patient or improve functional status. However, one can hope successful treatment of CLI would at least slow the inevitable rate of decline in these patients.

G. L. Moneta, MD

Late outcomes of balloon angioplasty and angioplasty with selective stenting for superficial femoral-popliteal disease are equivalent
Nguyen B-N, Conrad MF, Guest JM, et al (Massachusetts General Hosp and Harvard Med School, Boston)
J Vasc Surg 54:1051-1057, 2011

Objective.—Several trials have reported early superior patency of stenting over isolated angioplasty (plain old balloon angioplasty [POBA]) for infra-inguinal occlusive disease, yet long-term data are sparse. The purpose of this study was to contrast long-term clinical outcomes and costs of angioplasty alone vs angioplasty with selective stenting in the treatment of femoropopliteal occlusive disease.

Methods.—Patients undergoing primary endovascular treatments of the native femoropopliteal arteries from 2002 to 2009 were divided into two groups, POBA alone or stenting based on final treatment received at their index procedure. Study end points included actuarial 5-year primary patency (using strict criteria of any hemodynamic deterioration or return of symptoms), 5-year limb salvage, and 5-year survival and hospital costs.

Results.—Eight hundred twenty-four primary procedures were performed during the study interval; 517 (63%) were POBA and 307 (37%) were stenting. The mean follow-up duration was 33 months (range, 0-98 months). The indication for intervention in the stenting group was claudication in 71% of the patients, whereas the remaining 29% had critical limb ischemia (CLI). In the POBA cohort, the indication for treatment was claudication in 59% of the patients and CLI in the remaining 41%. A higher percentage of POBA lesions were TransAtlantic Inter-Society Consensus (TASC) II A & B when compared to stenting (91% POBA vs 73% stenting; $P < .001$). There was no difference in overall 5-year primary patency (POBA 36% ± 3%; stenting 41% ± 4%; $P = .31$), nor was there a difference in patients with claudication (POBA 42% ± 4%; stenting 45% ± 4%; $P = .8$). In patients with CLI, the 4-year primary patency was 27% ± 5% (POBA) vs 36% ± 8% (stenting), $P = .22$; the 4-year limb salvage was 80% ± 4% (POBA) vs 90% ± 5% (stenting), $P = .18$. There was no difference in survival between the two groups (claudication: 83% ± 3% POBA vs 84% ± 4% stenting at 5 years ($P = .65$), CLI: 44% ± 4% POBA vs 49% ± 6% stenting at 4 years ($P = .40$). Subgroup analysis by lesion anatomy showed similar primary patency between POBA and stenting for TASC II A & B lesions, while the primary patency was significantly higher at 5 years after stenting of TASC II C & D lesions (34% ± 6% vs 12% ± 9%; $P < .05$). Stenting increased the procedural cost by 57% when compared to POBA ($P < .001$) regardless of treatment indication. In addition, stenting added 45% ($P < .001$) to the overall hospital cost of patients treated for claudication.

Conclusion.—Stenting resulted in equivalent long-term outcomes compared to POBA when stratified by indications. However, stenting yielded statistically better primary patency in patients with TASC II C & D lesions. The lack of improved clinical outcomes and significantly higher cost of stenting supports a posture of selective use of stents (especially in TASC II A & B) in the endovascular treatment of femoropopliteal occlusive disease.

▶ This study represents a large, single-center, multidisciplinary experience of endovascular treatment of superficial femoropopliteal occlusive disease and includes long-term follow-up outcome measures. While selective stenting resulted in equivalent outcomes as primary balloon angioplasty at 4 years based on Kaplan Meier analysis when stratified by clinical indications, selective stenting did show advantage for long-segment occlusive disease (TASC C & D lesions). However, to conclude that both are equivalent needs to be tempered by the retrospective design and selection bias. Decision to place a stent was left to the discretion of the interventional attending physician and was not based on any selective criteria. Also, although clinical follow-up was set at defined intervals and included ankle-brachial measurements only, duplex ultrasound and pulse volume recordings were obtained only on a discretionary basis. Furthermore, it is unclear from the study how strictly this follow-up was adhered to, with some degree of loss to follow-up noted on the Kaplan Meier life tables at 4 years. Without prospective randomized data collected at defined intervals or specific selection criteria for stenting defined, it is difficult to conclude that both balloon angioplasty with or without selective stenting are truly equivalent except with the caveats noted. Perhaps the most important retrospectively determined observation is that for patients undergoing endovascular treatment for critical limb ischemia or for TASC C & D lesions, stenting may be preferred, although whether stenting should still be selective or routine for this subset has yet to be defined.

M. A. Passman, MD

The combined ipsilateral antegrade-retrograde approach to insert an endoluminal femoropopliteal bypass

Lensvelt MMA, Zeebregts CJ, Stoer-Bouwman M, et al (Rijnstate Hosp, Arnhem, The Netherlands; Univ of Groningen, The Netherlands)
J Vasc Surg 54:1205-1207, 2011

The endoluminal femoropopliteal bypass is a minimally invasive treatment modality for occlusive superficial femoral artery disease. Technical failure of endovascular treatment of chronic total occlusions is often caused by the inability to re-enter the true lumen. Re-entry devices have a high technical success-rate, but increased procedural costs. We describe an alternative technique using an ipsilateral combined antegrade-retrograde approach to insert an endoluminal femoropopliteal bypass. In a supine position, with the leg elevated at 30 degrees, the popliteal artery is punctured and a 4F introducer sheath is introduced. The occlusion is crossed from distal to proximal and the wire is advanced through a 6F sheath that is positioned in the common femoral artery. The occlusion is predilated from proximal and the "re-entry" site is identified on an angiogram. The wire is then withdrawn into the balloon catheter and advanced intraluminally into one of the crural vessels. After confirming the intraluminal position of the wire, the 4F sheath is removed, and the endoluminal bypass is created in a standardized fashion. The ipsilateral antegrade-retrograde approach is a fast, inexpensive, and easy-to-learn technique, using standard materials only. The distal entry of the occlusion will lead to a minimization of the length of the endoluminal bypass, thereby possibly sparing collaterals and future surgical options.

▶ The value of this small series is as a technical note on an alternative for treating superficial femoropopliteal occlusion when antegrade crossing is unsuccessful. The technique describes obtaining percutaneous popliteal artery direct access for retrograde crossing of the occluded segment and recapture of the wire from an antegrade-directed femoral artery sheath. With a "body floss" wire and catheter exchange, an antegrade wire from the femoral sheath position can be then redirected across the occlusion and past the popliteal reentry access point into a tibial vessel. After popliteal sheath is removed, a standard heparin bonded ePTFE-covered stent (Gore Viabahn) is then deployed and balloon molded. Although only 4 patients are treated in this series, the technique described here certainly may be a useful adjunct for those difficult-to-cross occluded superficial femoral arteries and represents an expansion of current options in the tool box. However, to imply that this is an "endoluminal femoropopliteal bypass" or has any equivalence to a bypass graft is a bit confusing in that it falls more into an endoluminal-covered stent rather than bypass graft category. While this may represent another minimally invasive option in selected patients with acceptable anatomy, it is not a replacement for a well-performed femoropopliteal bypass in those patients who would benefit more from an operative approach.

M. A. Passman, MD

Sirolimus-eluting stents vs. bare-metal stents for treatment of focal lesions in infrapopliteal arteries: a double-blind, multi-centre, randomized clinical trial
Rastan A, Tepe G, Krankenberg H, et al (Herz-Zentrum Bad Krozingen, Germany; Eberhard-Karls-Universität, Tübingen, Germany; Universitäres Herz- und Gefäßzentrum Hamburg, Germany; et al)
Eur Heart J 32:2274-2281, 2011

Aims.—Preliminary reports indicate that sirolimus-eluting stents reduce the risk of restenosis after percutaneous infrapopliteal artery revascularization. We conducted a prospective, randomized, multi-centre, double-blind trial comparing a polymer-free sirolimus-eluting stent with a placebo-coated bare-metal stent in patients with either intermittent claudication or critical limb ischaemia who had a de-novo lesion in an infrapopliteal artery.

Methods and Results.—161 patients were included in this trial. The mean target lesion length was 31 ± 9 mm. The main study endpoint was the 1-year primary patency rate, defined as freedom from in-stent-restenosis (luminal narrowing of ≥50%) detected with duplex ultrasound if not appropriate with angiography. Secondary endpoints included the 6-month primary patency rate, secondary patency rate, and changes in Rutherford—Becker classification after 1 year. Twenty-five (15.5%) patients died during the follow-up period. One hundred and twenty-five patients reached the 1-year examinations. The 1-year primary patency rate was significantly higher in the sirolimus-eluting stent group (80.6%) than in the bare-metal stent group (55.6%, *P* = 0.004), and the 1-year secondary patency rates were 91.9 and 71.4% (*P* = 0.005), respectively. The median (interquartile range) change in Rutherford—Becker classification after 1 year was −2 (−3 to −1) in the sirolimus-eluting stent group and −1 (−2 to 0) in the bare-metal stent group, respectively (*P* = 0.004).

Conclusion.—Mid-term patency rates of focal infrapopliteal lesions are substantially improved with sirolimus-eluting stent compared with bare-metal stent. Corresponding to the technical results, the changes in Rutherford—Becker classification reveal a significant advantage for the sirolimus-eluting stent.

▶ In effect, this was a proof-of-concept study. Only very short lesions were included in the study. About half the patients had claudication. It is difficult to imagine the need for treatment of a short tibial artery lesion in a patient with claudication. The level of critical limb ischemia also did not appear to be critical. There was only 1 major limb amputation and 1 minor toe amputation in the sirolimus group (3.2%) and 2 major amputations and 2 toe amputations in the bare-metal stent group (6.4%). This, combined with an overall limb salvage rate of 98%, does not suggest a very critical ischemic group. The relevance of these data to treatment of patients with true limb threatening ischemia and patients with intermittent claudication is questionable. One must also question the use of duplex ultrasound to assess less than 50% stenosis in tibial arteries. There are really no data that this can be done with sufficient accuracy to serve as the basis of a primary endpoint in a clinical trial. Nevertheless, while the results here probably have little clinical significance, they do at least suggest the potential for use of drug-eluting stents to improve patency of focal arterial lesions following endovascular treatment of a stenotic infrapopliteal artery.

G. L. Moneta, MD

Trends in the national outcomes and costs for claudication and limb threatening ischemia: Angioplasty vs bypass graft
Sachs T, Pomposelli F, Hamdan A, et al (Beth Israel Deaconess Med Ctr, Harvard, MA)
J Vasc Surg 54:1021-1031, 2011

Purpose.—Debate exists as to the benefit of angioplasty vs bypass graft in the treatment of lower extremity peripheral vascular disease. The associated costs are poorly defined in the literature. We sought to determine national estimates for the costs, utilization, and outcomes of angioplasty and bypass graft for the treatment of both claudication and limb threat.

Methods.—We searched the Nationwide Inpatient Sample (NIS) database (1999-2007), identifying patients who had an identifiable International Classification of Disease (ICD)-9 diagnosis code of atherosclerotic disease (claudication [440.21] or limb threat [440.22-440.24]). Of these, only patients who underwent intervention of angioplasty ± stent (percutaneous transluminal angioplasty [PTA; 39.50-39.90]), peripheral bypass graft (BPG; 39.29) or aortofemoral bypass (ABF; 39.25) were included. We compared demographics, costs, and comorbidities, as well as multivariable-adjusted outcomes of in-hospital mortality and major amputation. Additionally, we used the New Jersey State Inpatient and Ambulatory databases in order to better understand the influence of outpatient procedures on current volume and trends.

Results.—There were 563,143 patients identified (PTA: 38%, BPG: 50%, ABF: 6%; 5.1%: multiple procedure codes). Patients who had PTA and BPG were similar in age (70.4 vs 69.5 years) but older than patients who had ABF (61.8 years, $P < .01$). Patients who underwent PTA were more often women (PTA: 46%, BPG: 42%, ABF: 45.2%; $P < .01$). Average costs for PTA increased over 60% for claudication between 2001 and 2007 ($8670 to $14,084) and limb threat ($13,903 to $23,196). For BPG, average costs increased 36% for both claudication ($9322 to $12,681) and limb threat ($16,795 to $22,910). In 2007, the average cost per procedure of PTA was higher than BPG for both claudication ($13,903 vs $12,681; $P = .02$) and limb threat ($23,196 vs $22,910; $P = .04$). The number of patients per year undergoing PTA increased threefold (15,903 to 46,138) for claudication and limb threat (6752 to 19,468). For BPG, procedures per year decreased approximately 40% for both claudication (13,625 to 9108) and limb threat (25,575 to 13,762). In-hospital mortality was similar for PTA and BPG groups for claudication (0.1% vs 0.2%; *P*=.04) and limb threat (2.1% vs 2.6%; *P* < .01). In-hospital amputation rates were significantly higher for patients who had PTA (7%) than BPG (3.9%, odds ratio [OR], 1.67 [1.49-1.85]; *P* < .01) or patients who underwent ABF (3.0%; OR, 2.32 [1.79, 3.03]; *P* < .01).

Conclusion.—PTA has altered the treatment paradigm for lower limb ischemia with an increase in costs and procedures. It is unclear if this represents an increase in patients or number of treatments per patient. Although mortality is slightly lower with PTA for all indications, amputation rates for limb-threat patients appear higher, as does the average cost. Longitudinal studies are necessary to determine the appropriateness of PTA in both claudication and limb-threat patients. The mortality benefit with PTA may be ultimately lost, and average costs elevated, if multiple interventions are performed on the same patients.

▶ I congratulate the authors for studying the impact of percutaneous endovascular revascularization and open revascularization on national outcomes and cost analysis. Clearly endovascular procedures are a primary treatment modality that we offer to many patients with a variety of vascular diseases. There are many factors for favoring endovascular procedures that include being less invasive, decreased complications, patient preference, provider preference, nonsurgical specialist providers performing endovascular, technology driven, and remunerative reasons for why percutaneous interventions are a primary modality before surgical revascularizations are considered. However, as we all know, there is a paucity of data studying the effectiveness and value of the procedure as it relates to outcomes and costs. This particular study uses the Nationwide Inpatient Sample database between 1999 and 2007. As expected, the number of patients per year undergoing percutaneous endovascular procedures for claudication and critical limb ischemia increased 3-fold, whereas the number of patients per year undergoing surgical bypass procedures decreased for claudication (33%) and critical limb ischemia (almost by 50%). Interestingly, the in-hospital mortality was just slightly lower for patients undergoing endovascular procedures than those undergoing bypass surgical procedures for claudication (0.1% vs 0.2%; *P* = .04) and critical limb ischemia (2.1% vs 2.6%; *P* < .01). However, in-hospital amputation rates were significantly higher for patients with critical limb ischemia (amputation rate for claudication was extremely low, no difference between endovascular and surgical bypass) who underwent percutaneous endovascular procedures (7%) than those who underwent surgical bypass (3.9%) (odds ratio [OR], 1.67; 95% confidence interval, 1.49-1.85; *P* < .01) or aortobifemoral bypass (3.0%) (OR, 2.32; 95% confidence interval, 1.79-3.03; *P* < .01). As one would surmise, the length of stay was lowest for patients undergoing percutaneous endovascular procedures (1.0 ± 0.02 days), followed by bypass surgery (4.52 ± 0.31 days) and aortobifemoral bypass surgery (5.88 ± 0.05 days; *P* < .01). Overall, the total costs for endovascular procedures are greater than that for surgical bypass. In 2007, the average cost per procedure for percutaneous endovascular procedures was higher than that for surgical bypass for both claudication ($13 903 vs

$12 681; $P = .02$) and critical limb ischemia ($23 196 vs $22 910; $P = .04$). In an era of cost containment, where providing durable and effective services in what matters to the patients (ie, able to walk, pain free, healed ulcer, quality of life, and freedom from reinterventions), it is incumbent upon vascular surgeons and vascular specialists to provide the best possible care to patients, given the resource, expertise, knowledge, and evidence-based practices possessed. Furthermore, it is important that we recognize how critical it is to educate and evaluate patients with systemic risk factors for peripheral arterial disease. Instituting early and preventative medical therapies will ultimately reduce complications and costs that are associated with the treatment of a disease that affects 12% of adults in the United States.

J. D. Raffetto, MD

A multicenter comparison between autologous saphenous vein and heparin-bonded expanded polytetrafluoroethylene (ePTFE) graft in the treatment of critical limb ischemia in diabetics

Dorigo W, on behalf of the Propaten Italian Registry Group (Univ of Florence, Italy; et al)
J Vasc Surg 54:1332-1338, 2011

Objectives.—The aim of this study was to evaluate early and follow-up results of below-knee bypasses performed using a bioactive heparin-treated expanded polytetrafluoroethylene (ePTFE) graft in diabetic patients with critical limb ischemia (CLI) in a multicenter retrospective registry involving seven Italian vascular centers and to compare them with those obtained in patients operated on with autologous saphenous vein (ASV) in the same centers in the same period of time.

Methods.—Over an 8-year period, ending in 2009, a heparin-bonded prosthetic graft (Propaten Gore-Tex; W. L. Gore & Associates Inc, Flagstaff, Ariz) was implanted in 180 diabetic patients undergoing below-knee revascularization for CLI in seven Italian hospitals (group 1). In the same period in these seven centers, 133 below-knee bypasses with ipsilateral ASV in diabetics with CLI were performed (group 2). Data concerning these interventions were retrospectively collected in a multicenter registry with a dedicated database. Early (<30 days) results were analyzed in terms of graft patency, major amputation rates, and mortality. Follow-up results were analyzed in terms of primary and secondary graft patency, limb salvage, and survival.

Results.—The interventions consisted of below-knee bypasses in 132 cases in group 1 (73%) and in 45 cases in group 2 (33%; $P < .001$); 48 patients in group 1 (27%) and 88 patients in group 2 (67%; $P < .001$) had distal tibial anastomosis. Patients in group 1 had more frequently adjunctive procedures performed at distal anastomotic sites to improve run-off status. Postoperative and long-term medical treatment consisted of single antiplatelet therapy in 93 cases (52%) in group 1 and in 64 cases (48%, $P = $ns) in group 2, of double antiplatelet therapy in 18 cases (10%) in group 1 and in four cases (3%; $P = .05$) in group 2 and of oral anticoagulants in 69 patients in group 1 (38%) and in 65 (49%; $P = .02$) in group 2. Mean duration of follow-up was 28.3 ± 21.4 months; 308 patients (98%) had at least one postoperative clinical and ultrasonographic examination and 228 (72%) reached at least a 1-year follow-up. Estimated 48-month survival rates were 76.6% in group 1 and 72.7% in group 2 ($P = > .9$, log-rank 0.08). Primary patency rate at 48 months was significantly better in group 2 (63.5%) than in group 1 (46.3%; $P = .03$, log-rank 4.1). Assisted primary patency rates at 48 months were 47.3% (SE 0.05) in group 1 and 69% (SE 0.05) in group 2 ($P = .01$, log-rank 6.3). The rates of secondary patency at 48 months were 57.5% in group 1 and 69.6% in group 2 ($P = .1$, log-rank 2.3); the corresponding values in terms of limb salvage and amputation free-survival rates were 75.4% and 82.4% ($P = .3$, log-rank 1), and 59.9% and 64.4% ($P = .3$, log-rank 0.9), respectively.

Conclusions.—Data from this large, retrospective registry confirmed that the indexed heparin-bonded ePTFE graft provides satisfactory early and midterm results in diabetic patients undergoing surgical treatment of CLI. While autologous saphenous vein maintains its superiority in terms of primary patency, secondary patency rates are not statistically different, even in the presence of a trend for improved secondary patency with vein graft; and also limb salvage rates are comparable.

▶ This multicenter comparison between autologous saphenous vein (ASV) and heparin-bonded expanded polytetrafluoroethylene (ePTFE) used for infrapopliteal and tibial bypass in diabetics with critical limb ischemia confirms superiority of primary patency for ASV, no statistical difference for secondary patency through trend favored ASV, and comparable limb salvage rates. However, these results should be tempered by the retrospective study design and the subanalysis of a larger multicenter registry of heparin-bonded ePTFE grafts used for bypass grafting in diabetics and nondiabetics, and comparison with a control group of bypass grafts using ASV from the same institutions over the same period, which were not part of the original registry design or were statistically matched in any way for analysis. This leads to discrepancy in the sample population with more femoral below-knee bypass grafts in the heparin-bonded ePTFE group (132 of 180, 73%) versus more tibial reconstructions in the ASV group (88 of 133, 67%); worse comorbidities in the heparin-bonded ePTFE group (tobacco use, hyperlipidemia, hypertension, and coronary artery disease), which may have led to a higher trend for observed perioperative mortality in the heparin-bonded ePTFE group; and differences in distribution of antiplatelet and anticoagulation adjuvant medication use, which makes influence of these factors variable and can affect long-term outcome data. With these inconsistencies, any conclusions of equivalence for heparin-bonded PTFE should be qualified by the option of using heparin-bonded ePTFE only if autologous vein is unsuitable or absent.

M. A. Passman, MD

Thrombolysis for lower extremity bypass graft occlusion

Koraen L, Kuoppala M, Acosta S, et al (Karolinska Univ Hosp, Stockholm, Sweden; Malmö Univ Hosp, Sweden)
J Vasc Surg 54:1339-1344, 2011

Background.—Thrombolysis is a common method in the treatment of lower extremity bypass graft occlusion. The purpose of this study was to investigate the results of thrombolytic therapy in the management of acute bypass graft occlusion and to identify risk factors for technical failure and amputation.

Methods.—All patients at two tertiary referral centers undergoing thrombolysis for acute graft occlusion in the lower limb between January 1, 2000 and December 31, 2008 were retrospectively reviewed. Factors associated with technical failure of thrombolytic therapy, major amputation, and mortality were determined with multivariate analysis, and long-term outcomes were assessed with the Kaplan-Meier method and log-rank test.

Results.—During the study period, 123 patients underwent thrombolysis for acute bypass graft occlusion. Mean age was 69 years (range, 27-91 years); 38% were women. Sixty-seven percent had synthetic grafts. Acute critical leg ischemia (74%) was the dominating symptom preceding thrombolytic treatment. In 29% of cases, no adjunctive interventions were required, whereas 21% underwent open surgery, 39% endovascular intervention, and 11% underwent a hybrid procedure. Technical failure of thrombolysis occurred in 18 patients. Presence of ischemic heart disease ($P = .013$), older grafts ($P = .014$), and synthetic grafts (trend; $P = .092$) were associated with success of thrombolysis, and ischemic heart disease remained as an independent factor in the multivariate analysis for technical success of thrombolysis ($P = .04$; odds ratio 4.0; 95% confidence interval [CI; 1.1-15.1]), whereas there was a trend for older grafts ($P = .089$). Mean follow-up was 38 months (range, 0-119 months). The major amputation rate was 11% (14/123) at 1 month and 25% (31/122) at 1 year. In a Cox regression model, technical failure ($P = .031$; hazard ratio [HR] 2.58, 95% CI [1.0-6.08]), higher age ($P = .004$; HR 1.06, 95% CI [1.02-1.10]), and synthetic graft as opposed to vein graft ($P = .050$; HR 2.63, 95% CI [1.0-6.9]) remained as independent factors associated with major amputation. The amputation-free survival rate was 89% and 75% at 1 and 12 months, respectively. Higher age ($P < .001$; HR 1.06, 95% CI [1.03-1.09]) and acute limb ischemia ($P = .007$; HR 2.40, 95% CI [1.26-4.56]) remained as independent adverse factors associated with amputation-free survival.

Conclusions.—Our findings support the use of thrombolysis in the treatment of acute bypass graft occlusion in the lower limb given its acceptable short- and long-term amputation-free survival rates. Technical failure and higher age were factors associated with major amputation. Synthetic grafts appeared to have a somewhat increased likelihood of technically successful thrombolysis compared with vein grafts, but on the other hand, they exhibited an increased risk of amputation during follow-up.

▶ Graft failure leading to acute graft thrombosis of a lower extremity bypass can have significant consequences if not appropriately treated. Thrombolysis is a therapy that has been used for several decades. The authors in this study retrospectively review a series from 2 hospitals undergoing thrombolysis for acute graft occlusion in the lower limb between January 2000 and December 2008. Factors associated with technical failure of thrombolytic therapy, major amputation, and mortality were determined with multivariate analysis, and long-term outcomes were evaluated. There were 123 patients identified who underwent thrombolysis, and 67% had synthetic grafts. Importantly, 71% required either a surgical, endovascular, or hybrid combination procedure to correct the underlying problem and restore flow. The mean follow-up was 38 months, and at 12 months, 25.4% of patients required a major amputation. Some interesting findings were that technical failure, higher age, and synthetic graft (as opposed to vein graft) remained as independent factors associated with major amputation. A major concern with thrombolysis is hemorrhagic stroke, which occurred at a rate of 1.6% in this series with a 50% fatality rate. In addition, major hemorrhage occurred in 13% of patients. Importantly, the mortality rate at 12 months was 13%, and in the Cox regression model, higher age, presence of acute limb ischemia, and major amputation remained as independent factors associated with mortality, likely reflecting the significant systemic disease and comorbid conditions that these patients present. It is clear from this study that acute graft thrombosis can be treated by thrombolysis; however, major amputation and mortality occurs at a high rate within the first year, and complication from thrombolysis must be carefully weighed when considering this form of therapy. Given that in this series nearly three-quarter of the patients had synthetic grafts, it is important to keep in mind that in certain patients, when prosthetic material thromboses, it can lead to critical limb ischemia, and as this study demonstrated, prosthetic material (suprainguinal proximal anastomoses and infrainguinal bypass grafts) was an independent risk factor for amputation in patients presenting with acute limb ischemia from graft occlusion.

J. D. Raffetto, MD

Limb Salvage Using Bypass to the Perigeniculate Arteries

De Luccia N, Sassaki P, Durazzo A, et al (Hospital das Clínicas Faculdade de Medicina Universidade de São Paulo, Brazil; Hospital Guilherme Álvaro, Santos, Brazil; et al)
Eur J Vasc Endovasc Surg 42:374-378, 2011

Objective.—To describe bypass to perigeniculate vessels for limb salvage.
Design.—Retrospective cohort study.
Material and Methods.—Between 1995 and 2009, 47 bypass procedures to perigeniculate collateral arteries were performed in 46 patients (15

women, 31 men; median age, 68 years). All patients presented with critical ischaemia (tissue loss in 87.5%, rest pain in 12.5%). Mean ankle brachial index was 0.27 ± 0.17. The site of distal anastomosis was the descending genicular artery (DGA) in 23 bypasses (1 bilateral) and the medial sural artery (MSA) in 24. Proximal anastomosis was to the external iliac artery in 2 cases, common femoral artery in 23 cases, superficial femoral artery in 8 cases, deep femoral artery in 8 cases, above-knee poplitaeal artery in 2 cases, and previous graft in 4 cases.

Results.—There were four deaths during the immediate postoperative period. Mean follow-up duration was 27 months. Ten patients required major amputation. Mean ankle brachial index post-operatively was 0.60 ± 0.21. At 3 years, primary patency was 74.7 ± 7%, secondary patency was 83.4 ± 8%, and the limb salvage and survival rates were 73.5 ± 7% and 77.4 ± 7%, respectively.

Conclusion.—Bypass to perigeniculate arteries is a viable treatment option for critical limb ischaemia in selected patients (Figs 1 and 4).

▶ Limb salvage continues to be one of the most challenging problems we face in vascular surgery. As the dictum for a successful bypass procedure historically mandated adequate inflow, outflow, and conduit, portions of this theory have been challenged and the outcomes have not fared as well. It is not difficult to find an inflow vessel, but the more proximal location requires longer length of conduit. Various conduits have been used, but autogenous single-segment saphenous vein has fared the best. The outflow vessel has also been challenged, and if a named tibial artery is continuous to the foot, a more proximal bypass to this artery is acceptable for critical limb ischemia. Bypass to discontinuous named vessels has also been attempted. A femoral artery bypass to an isolated popliteal artery segment, initially described by Mannick et al,[1] was noted to have acceptable rates of limb salvage. Further studies by Veith et al[2] described outcomes over 10 years in 207 patients with a femoral to isolated popliteal artery segment and found the 5-year primary graft patency to be 59% (reversed

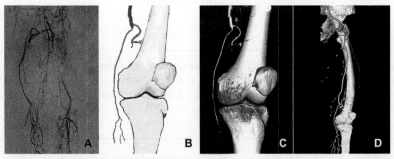

FIGURE 1.—A: Pre-operative arteriography. B: Illustration shows a bypass (blue) to the descending genicular artery (red). C, D: Postoperative angioCT showing the bypass. For interpretation of the references to colour in this figure legend, the reader is referred to the web version of this article. (Reprinted from European Journal of Vascular and Endovascular Surgery, De Luccia N, Sassaki P, Durazzo A, et al. Limb salvage using bypass to the perigeniculate arteries. *Eur J Vasc Endovasc Surg.* 2011;42:374-378. Copyright 2011, with permission from the European Society for Vascular Surgery.)

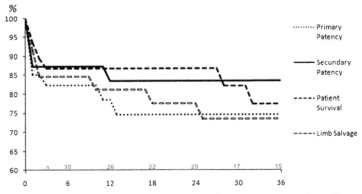

FIGURE 4.—Patient survival, limb salvage, and actuarial patency (primary and secondary patency) curves, in months. (Reprinted from European Journal of Vascular and Endovascular Surgery, De Luccia N, Sassaki P, Durazzo A, et al. Limb salvage using bypass to the perigeniculate arteries. *Eur J Vasc Endovasc Surg.* 2011;42:374-378. Copyright 2011, with permission from the European Society for Vascular Surgery.)

saphenous vein, 74% and polytetrafluoroethylene [PTFE] 55%), and 5-year limb salvage rate was 78% with either conduit. Subsequent sequential extension of the bypass to a more distal artery was required in 20% of patients.

The authors of this study describe their experience with bypass to the perigeniculate arteries (the descending genicular artery and medial sural artery) in 47 patients with critical limb ischemia over a 15-year time course. The proximal anastomosis emanated from the external iliac artery, common femoral artery, superficial femoral artery, and profunda femoris artery. Saphenous vein was used as a conduit in 28 patients, an arm vein in 18 patients, and PTFE in 1 patient. The estimated 3-year survival rate was 77.4 plus or minus 7%, and the 3-year primary patency was 74.7 plus or minus 7%. Ten patients underwent a major amputation, and the estimated 3-year limb salvage rate was 73.5 plus or minus 7%. The primary patency rate and limb salvage rate were nearly identical to that described for bypass to the isolated popliteal segment with saphenous vein in the series by Veith et al.

This technique is yet another option in limb salvage surgery, but it must also be tempered with the frailty of this patient population, as this series had 4 deaths prior to discharge and another 5 during the follow-up period. As endovascular techniques evolve and more aggressive attempts at recanalization of these occluded vessels occur, it will be interesting to see if surgeons attempt these unconventional bypasses for limb salvage.

N. Singh, MD

References

1. Mannick JA, Jackson BT, Coffman JD, Hume DM. Success of bypass vein grafts in patients with isolated popliteal artery segments. *Surgery.* 1967;61:17-25.
2. Kram HB, Gupta SK, Veith FJ, Wengertner KR, Panetta TF, Nwosisi C. Late results of two hundred seventeen femoropopliteal bypasses to isolated popliteal artery segments. *J Vasc Surg.* 1991;14:386-390.

Infrainguinal bypass is associated with lower perioperative mortality than major amputation in high-risk surgical candidates

Barshes NR, Menard MT, Nguyen LL, et al (Brigham and Women's Hosp, Boston, MA)
J Vasc Surg 53:1251-1259, 2011

Background.—Major amputation is often selected over infrainguinal bypass in patients with severe systemic comorbidities because it is assumed to have lower perioperative risks, yet this assumption is unproven and largely unexamined.

Methods.—The 2005 to 2008 National Surgical Quality Improvement Project (NSQIP) database was used to identify all patients undergoing either infrainguinal bypass or major amputation using procedural codes. Patients with systemic or local infections were excluded. A subset of high-risk patients were then defined as American Society of Anesthesiologists (ASA) class 4 or 5, or ASA class 3 with renal failure, dyspnea at rest, ventilator dependence, recent congestive heart failure, or recent myocardial infarct. Propensity score matching was used to obtain two high-risk patient groups matched for preoperative characteristics.

Results.—No significant differences in demographic, preoperative, or anesthetic variables were found between the matched, high-risk amputation or bypass groups (792 and 780 patients, respectively). Bypass was associated with a lower 30-day postoperative mortality than amputation (6.54% vs 9.97%; $P = .0147$). Amputation was associated with higher rates of pulmonary embolism (0.9% vs 0% for amputation vs bypass groups, respectively; $P = .009$) and urinary tract infection (5.2% vs 2.7%; $P = .01$), while bypass was associated with higher rates of return to the operating room (14.1% vs 27.6%; $P < .001$) and a trend toward higher postoperative transfusion requirements (0.9% vs 2.1%; $P = .054$). The postoperative time to discharge did not differ between the two groups.

Conclusion.—The decision to perform an infrainguinal bypass or amputation should depend on well-established predictors of graft patency and functional success rather than presumptions about different perioperative risks between the two procedures (Fig 1).

▶ Major amputation is usually reserved for patients who have significant tissue loss and gangrene or intractable rest pain and no available options for revascularization. However, in certain patients, major amputation is offered instead of a major surgical revascularization since an amputation requires less time in the operating room than a bypass and therefore would pose less risk to the patient in postoperative complications and death. This is a poorly studied area in vascular surgery, and I commend the authors for this important study. The authors investigate the question, does amputation (above knee or below knee) performed in patients with high risks (American Society of Anesthesiologists classes 4 and 5, or class 3 with renal insufficiency, dyspnea, ventilator dependence, recent congestive heart failure, or recent myocardial infarction) have lower perioperative complications than performing lower extremity surgical revascularization? In fact

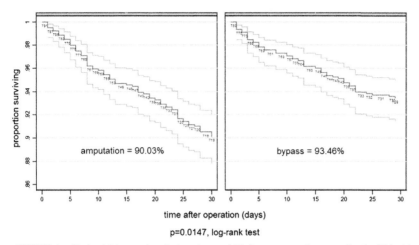

time after operation (days)

p=0.0147, log-rank test

FIGURE 1.—Kaplan-Meier product-limit estimate of 30-day postoperative mortality for high-risk, propensity score-matched patients undergoing major amputation (n = 792) or infrainguinal bypass (n = 780). (Reprinted from the Journal of Vascular Surgery, Barshes NR, Menard MT, Nguyen LL, et al. Infrainguinal bypass is associated with lower perioperative mortality than major amputation in high-risk surgical candidates. *J Vasc Surg.* 2011;53:1251-1259. Copyright 2011, with permission from The Society for Vascular Surgery.)

the opposite was found in this study about survival and several important complications. The study uses the American College of Surgeons National Surgical Quality Improvement Project database from the private sector from 2005 to 2008. Following propensity matching, scoring resulted in 2 matched cohorts of 792 patients who had a major amputation and 781 patients who had an infrainguinal bypass. The findings were the following: (1) Baseline demographics, characteristics, and risk factors did not differ between the 2 propensity matched groups. (2) Infrainguinal bypass was associated with a significantly better 30-day survival than major amputation in high-risk surgical candidates (93.46% vs 90.03%; P = .0147; Fig 1). (3) Amputation was associated with significantly higher rates of pulmonary embolism (0.9% vs 0%; P = .009) and urinary tract infection (5.2% vs 2.7%, respectively; P = .01). (4) Compared to amputation, bypass was associated with significantly higher rates of return to the operating room (14.1% vs 27.6%; P < .001). From this study one can conclude that major amputation seems no safer than revascularization in high-risk patients, and the presence of severe systemic comorbidities alone should not preclude patients from an attempt at surgical revascularization. Although there are limitations with a retrospective study, informed decisions regarding revascularization versus amputation in a high-risk population with critical limb ischemia should be based on patient preference, functional outcome, and quality of life.

J. D. Raffetto, MD

11 Upper Extremity Ischemia/Dialysis Access

A comparison between one- and two-stage brachiobasilic arteriovenous fistulas

Reynolds TS, Zayed M, Kim KM, et al (Harbor-UCLA Med Ctr, Torrance; Stanford Univ Med Ctr, Stanford, CA)

J Vasc Surg 53:1632-1639, 2011

Objectives.—Brachiobasilic arteriovenous fistulas (BBAVF) can be performed in one or two stages. We compared primary failure rates, as well as primary and secondary patency rates of one- and two-stage BBAVF at two institutions.

Methods.—Patients undergoing one- and two-stage BBAVF at two institutions were compared retrospectively with respect to age, sex, body mass index, use of preoperative venous duplex ultrasound, diabetes, hypertension, and cause of end-stage renal disease. Categorical variables were compared using chi-square and Fisher's exact test, whereas the Wilcoxon rank-sum test was used to compare continuous variables. Patency rates were assessed using the Kaplan-Meier survival analysis and the Cox proportional hazards model with propensity analysis to determine hazard ratios.

Results.—Ninety patients (60 one-stage and 30 two-stage) were identified. Mean follow-up was 14.2 months and the mean time interval between the first and second stage was 11.2 weeks. Although no significant difference in early failure existed (one-stage, 22.9% vs two-stage, 9.1%; $P = .20$), the two-stage BBAVF showed significantly improved primary functional patency at 1 year at 88% vs 61% ($P = .047$) (hazard ratio, 0.2; 95% confidence interval [CI], 0.04-0.80; $P = .03$). Patency for one-stage BBAVF markedly decreased to 34% at 2 years compared with 88% for the two-stage procedure ($P = .047$). Median primary functional patency for one-stage BBAVF was 31 weeks (interquartile range [IQR], 1154) vs 79 weeks (IQR, 29131 weeks) for the two-stage procedure, respectively ($P = .0015$). Two-year secondary functional patencies for one- and two-stage procedures were 41% and 94%, respectively ($P = .015$).

Conclusions.—Primary and secondary patency at 1 and 2 years as well as functional patency is improved with the two-stage BBAVF when compared with the one-stage procedure. Lower primary failure rates prior to dialysis with the two-stage procedure approached, but did not reach statistical significance. While reasons for these finding are unclear, certain technical aspects of the procedure may play a role.

▶ While brachiobasilic arteriovenous fistula (BBAVF) is an autologous option for hemodialysis access in patients who are not candidates for radial- or brachial-cephalic arteriovenous fistula and is preferred over prosthetic grafts, whether to perform as a 1- or 2-stage operation is under debate. As a 1-stage operation, the basilic vein is mobilized and moved to a subcutaneous position prior to basilic vein to brachial artery anastomosis, thereby carrying the advantage of single operation with potential earlier functioning. As a 2-stage operation, basilic vein to brachial artery anastomosis is performed in the first operation followed by superficialization of the arterialized basilic vein in the second operation. While the 2-stage approach has the disadvantage of a second operation and delayed functional use of the fistula, mobilization of the thicker arterialized conduit is less susceptible to injury and may avoid a second extended incision if the conduit fails early. In this study, improved primary, secondary, and functional patency at 2 years, and a trend toward decreased failure rate was observed in the 2-stage group. While these conclusions should be tempered by the retrospective study design, selection bias, and disparate sample size between the 2 groups, this study does add to a small body of evidence suggesting preference of the 2-stage approach, but to date there are few comparative studies and only limited randomized data available.

M. A. Passman, MD

Arteriovenous Graft Placement in Predialysis Patients: A Potential Catheter-Sparing Strategy

Shingarev R, Maya ID, Barker-Finkel J, et al (Univ of Alabama at Birmingham; Montana State Univ, Bozeman)
Am J Kidney Dis 58:243-247, 2011

Background.—When predialysis patients are deemed unsuitable candidates for an arteriovenous fistula, current guidelines recommend waiting until just before or after initiation of dialysis therapy before placing a graft. This strategy may increase catheter use when these patients start dialysis therapy. We compared the outcomes of patients whose grafts were placed before and after dialysis therapy initiation.

Study Design.—Retrospective analysis of a prospective computerized vascular access database.

Setting & Participants.—Patients with chronic kidney disease receiving their first arteriovenous graft (n = 248) at a large medical center.

Predictor.—Timing of graft placement (before or after initiation of dialysis therapy).

Outcome & Measurements.—Primary graft failure, cumulative graft survival, catheter dependence, and catheter-related bacteremia.

Results.—The first graft was placed predialysis in 62 patients and post-dialysis in 186 patients. Primary graft failure was similar for pre- and post-dialysis grafts (20% vs 24%; $P = 0.5$). Median cumulative graft survival was similar for pre- and postdialysis grafts (365 vs 414 days; HR, 1.22; 95% CI, 0.81-1.98; $P = 0.3$). Median duration of catheter dependence after graft placement in the postdialysis group was 48 days and was associated with 0.63 (95% CI, 0.48-0.79) episodes of catheter-related bacteremia per patient.

Limitations.—Retrospective analysis, single medical center.

Conclusion.—Grafts placed predialysis have primary failure rates and cumulative survival similar to those placed after starting dialysis therapy. However, postdialysis graft placement is associated with prolonged catheter dependence and frequent bacteremia. Predialysis graft placement may decrease catheter dependence and bacteremia in selected patients (Fig 1).

▶ The fistula first initiative (www.fistulafirst.org) strongly encourages patients with chronic kidney disease to receive dialysis access via arteriovenous fistulas rather than a graft whenever possible. Some patients, however, have vasculature that is more suitable for creation of a graft. In such cases, the National Kidney Foundation Kidney Disease Outcomes Quality Initiative suggests grafts be placed 3 to 6 weeks prior to the need for dialysis therapy. It is, however, extremely difficult to predict the onset of time for the need of dialysis in the patient who is not yet undergoing renal replacement therapy. Therefore, some surgeons postpone graft creation until after the initiation of hemodialysis, reasoning that placement of the graft prior to initiation of dialysis therapy may result in diminished time to graft failure once the patient has begun renal replacement therapy. However, postponing initiation of graft placement until after beginning of dialysis therapy exposes the patient to the risk of dialysis via a venous catheter and complications

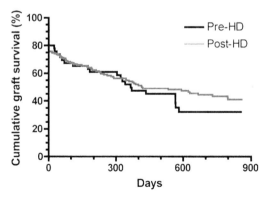

FIGURE 1.—Cumulative survival of grafts placed predialysis (black line) and after initiation of dialysis therapy (gray line). $P = 0.3$. Analysis is restricted to patients receiving their first arteriovenous graft. Graft survival in predialysis patients was calculated from the initiation of hemodialysis (HD) therapy. Graft survival was considered to be 0 days in patients with primary graft failure. (Reprinted from American Journal of Kidney Diseases, Shingarev R, Maya ID, Barker-Finkel J, et al. Arteriovenous graft placement in predialysis patients: a potential catheter-sparing strategy. *Am J Kidney Dis.* 2011;58:243-247. Copyright 2011, with permission from the National Kidney Foundation.)

of catheter related bacteremia, central vein stenosis, and decreased overall survival. This study shows similar graft-related outcomes between grafts placed for hemodialysis access predialysis and those created after the initiation of renal replacement therapy (Fig 1). The results indicate that predialysis graft placement is a reasonable strategy in selected patients even if there are occasional long delays before the need for dialysis initiation. In this study, in fact, 86% of predialysis patients started hemodialysis therapy with a permanent access. In contrast, when a graft was placed after initiation of dialysis therapy, catheter dependence was for a mean of 4 months. Given all the problems with venous catheters, the placement of arteriovenous grafts in selected patients prior to initiation of hemodialysis therapy should be considered a valuable catheter-sparing strategy. In addition, perhaps predialysis patients at high risk of fistula nonmaturation should have placement of a graft rather than an attempt to create an arteriovenous fistula that has little chance of maturing.

G. L. Moneta, MD

Vascular Access for Haemodialysis in Patients with Central Vein Thrombosis
Jakimowicz T, Galazka Z, Grochowiecki T, et al (Vascular and Transplant Surgery Med Univ of Warsaw, Poland)
Eur J Vasc Endovasc Surg 42:842-849, 2011

Objectives.—Dialysis-dependent patients often have central venous drainage complications. In patients with functioning arm arteriovenous fistula, this may result in venous hypertension, arm oedema and vascular access failure. Percutaneous angioplasty and stent implantation might be inadequate to resolve these issues. In these cases, new access can potentially be created with anastomosis to the subclavian vein, iliac vein or vena cava or by making a veno-venous graft to bypass the thrombosis.

The aim of this study was to assess the utility of unusual bypasses in vascular access in patients with the central vein thrombosis.

Materials.—A total of 49 patients were treated. The mean number of previous vascular access surgery procedures was 7.6 (3—17). We performed 19 axillo—iliac, 14 axillo—axillary bypasses and 16 conduits from the arm fistula to the jugular (nine conduits) or subclavian (seven conduits) vein for haemodialysis purposes.

Results.—All fistulas except one were used for haemodialysis. One patient died before the first use of the fistula. At 12 months, the primary, primary assisted and secondary patency rates were 85.4%, 89.6% and 95.8%, respectively. The follow-up period ranged from 1 to 84 months.

Conclusion.—Unusual grafts are an efficient option as a permanent vascular access for haemodialysis purposes in patients with central vein occlusion (Figs 3, 4 and 6).

▶ Maintaining vascular access is a persistent problem for any surgeon who deals with hemodialysis (HD) patients. Guidelines recommend the creation of

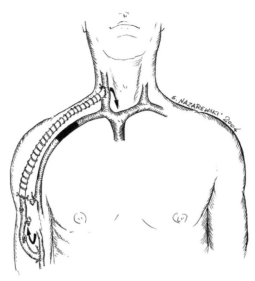

FIGURE 3.—PTFE bypass of the thrombosed proximal subclavian vein with spared native vessel fistula (9 patients). (Reprinted from European Journal of Vascular and Endovascular Surgery, Jakimowicz T, Galazka Z, Grochowiecki T, et al. Vascular access for haemodialysis in patients with central vein thrombosis. *Eur J Vasc Endovasc Surg.* 2011;42:842-849. Copyright 2011, with permission from the European Society for Vascular Surgery.)

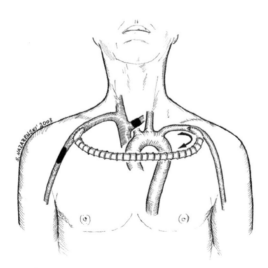

FIGURE 4.—Necklace graft – subcutaneous PTFE bridge from the subclavian artery to the contralateral subclavian vein (14 patients). (Reprinted from European Journal of Vascular and Endovascular Surgery, Jakimowicz T, Galazka Z, Grochowiecki T, et al. Vascular access for haemodialysis in patients with central vein thrombosis. *Eur J Vasc Endovasc Surg.* 2011;42:842-849. Copyright 2011, with permission from the European Society for Vascular Surgery.)

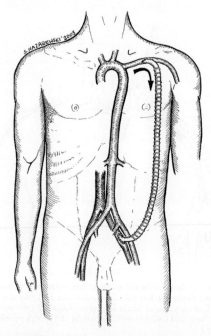

FIGURE 6.—Subcutaneous PTFE conduit from the subclavian artery to the external iliac vein (prosthetic axillary-femoral body wall access —19 patients). (Reprinted from European Journal of Vascular and Endovascular Surgery, Jakimowicz T, Galazka Z, Grochowiecki T, et al. Vascular access for haemodialysis in patients with central vein thrombosis. *Eur J Vasc Endovasc Surg*. 2011;42:842-849. Copyright 2011, with permission from the European Society for Vascular Surgery.)

autogenous access, but in clinical practice many patients present with a tunneled catheter in place that has been replaced or treated for dysfunction and with no extremity veins suitable for access. As the authors of this retrospective review of 49 patients with central venous occlusion over 20 years point out, prior central vein access, particularly subclavian access, is the usual culprit (28 patients). When faced with patients with multiple failed HD access procedures and central venous occlusion, the second tier of access procedures begins. This includes aggressive endovascular procedures with stenting of central venous occlusions, if necessary, as well as unconventional access to bypass the occluded central veins. An early portion of this study examines the time before endovascular techniques were commonly used. Numerous surgical revisions have since been initiated, which serve as a good review for the modern surgeon in the setting of failed endovascular attempts. The authors describe several bypass techniques (Figs 3, 4, and 6) to avoid the centrally occluded vein and, during their follow-up, noted that significant venous stenosis was found in 4 patients; 3 of these were treated with angioplasty, while 12 patients required graft thrombectomy; and 2 grafts were lost to infection. For the surgeon who performs significant HD access procedures, these numbers sound all too familiar, and although the authors describe several exotic techniques, many surgeons would likely opt for a permanent tunneled femoral line (if available) or counsel the patient for peritoneal dialysis.

N. Singh, MD

Secondary interventions in patients with autologous arteriovenous fistulas strongly improve patency rates

Ayez N, Fioole B, Aarts RA, et al (Maasstad Hosp, Rotterdam, The Netherlands)
J Vasc Surg 54:1095-1099, 2011

Background.—Nowadays, as a result of more liberal selection criteria, dialysis-dependent patients have become substantially older, more likely to be female and diabetic, and have more comorbidity. The 1-year primary patency rates of arteriovenous fistulas (AVFs) are poor. To improve these results, several secondary interventions can be performed. The aim of this study was to evaluate the results after secondary interventions in patients with an upper extremity AVF.

Methods.—Between January 2000 and December 2008, all consecutive patients who underwent construction of an autologous upper extremity AVF were included. Patient characteristics were collected retrospectively from digital patient files and a prospectively recorded database on hemodialysis patients.

Results.—Between January 2000 and December 2008, 736 hemodialysis access procedures were performed. A total of 347 autologous arteriovenous fistulas (AVFs) were created in 294 patients. The mean age was 62.1 ± 14.7 years, and the majority (66%) of the patients was male. Mean follow-up of all 347 fistulas was 21.9 ± 21.6 months. During follow-up, failure occurred in 209 (60%) of the AVFs. A total of 133 of these failures were followed by a secondary intervention, of which 78 (59%) were endovascular interventions. Twenty-nine patients developed a third failure, and 25 of these patients underwent another intervention, of which 22 were percutaneous transluminal angioplasty for stenosis. Fifteen patients developed a fourth failure, and all of them underwent an intervention. One patient had 11 interventions. The 1- and 2-year primary patency rates were 46% and 36.8%, respectively. The 1- and 2-year primary assisted patency rates were 74.6% and 71.2%, respectively. The 1- and 2-year secondary patency rates were 79.2% and 77.8%, respectively.

Conclusion.—The primary patency rate of AVFs is disappointing. However, due to mostly endovascular secondary interventions, 2-year primary assisted and secondary patency rates of more than 70% can be obtained.

▶ The National Kidney Foundation Dialysis Outcome and Quality Initiative and European Best Practice Guidelines on Vascular Access both recommend use of upper extremity arteriovenous fistula (AVF) first over prosthetic hemodialysis graft. However, with more liberal selection criteria for dialysis, patients undergoing dialysis access operations are becoming older with more comorbid risk factors and poorer vessel criteria, leading to a wider range of more recently reported primary patency for AVFs falling below those referenced in these guidelines. As noted in this study, overall primary patency was 46% at 1 year and 36% at 2 years, which is disappointingly low, but it highlights the need for intense surveillance and low threshold for secondary interventions with improved overall secondary patency to 79% at 1 year and 78% at 2 years. Patency was rather evenly distributed based on AVF fistula type, and only a few needed more than 1 secondary intervention representing more of an outlier on the data curve. Most of these secondary interventions were endovascular and were performed for stenosis (35%), and few were performed for thrombosis (12%). Although the fistula first approach is still supported by standard evidence-based guidelines, perhaps this perceived shift in dialysis patient profiles and impact on primary patency means that aggressive surveillance and secondary intervention is even more important for maintenance and durability of valued autogenous hemodialysis access resources.

M. A. Passman, MD

Duplex Guided Dialysis Access Interventions can be Performed Safely in the Office Setting: Techniques and Early Results
Fox D, Amador F, Clarke D, et al (Lenox Hill Hosp, NY; Norstar Imaging, NY; et al)
Eur J Vasc Endovasc Surg 42:833-841, 2011

Objective.—To determine the utility of duplex guided angioplasty for hemodialysis access maturation and maintenance.

Design/Materials/Methods.—Between January 2008 and June 2009, 223 office-based duplex-guided hemodialysis access angioplasty procedures were performed in 125 patients. Two hundred eight of the accesses were autogenous. The most common indication for intervention was maturation failure (104 cases). Other indications included pulsatility, low access flow, decreased flow and infiltration. Procedures were performed in the office using topical and local anesthesia. Volume flow (VF) was recorded prior to introducer insertion (baseline) and post intervention.

Results.—Technical success was achieved in 219 cases (98.2%). Minor complications occurred in 21 cases (9.4%). Immature autogenous AV accesses had a median baseline VF of 210 mL/min. Median final VF for these autogenous AV accesses was 485 mL/min. The VF increased by 131%. Dysfunctional autogenous AV accesses and nonautogenous AV accesses had a median baseline VF of 472 mL/min. Median final VF was 950 mL/min. The VF increased by 101%.

Conclusions.—Duplex guided dialysis access angioplasty can be performed safely and effectively in the office setting. It offers the advantage of treating the patient without radiation or contrast as well as the assessment of the hemodynamic effects of intervention (Fig 1, Table 4).

▶ The concept of office-based procedures in vascular surgery has evolved from sclerotherapy of spider veins to percutaneous laser and radiofrequency ablation of superficial veins over the last decade. Much of this advancement has been because of the increased reimbursement of these procedures in this setting. The result has been numerous outpatient "vein centers." The authors of this study have taken the office-based procedure to another commonly encountered problem we face: maintenance of dialysis access. Since it was described by

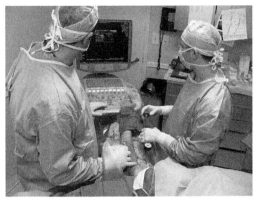

FIGURE 1.—Procedure room setup for duplex guided AV access intervention. The patient's right arm is seen in the middle of the figure. The duplex scanner is in the background. (Reprinted from European Journal of Vascular and Endovascular Surgery, Fox D, Amador F, Clarke D, et al. Duplex guided dialysis access interventions can be performed safely in the office setting: techniques and early results. *Eur J Vasc Endovasc Surg.* 2011;42:833-841. Copyright 2011, with permission from the European Society for Vascular Surgery.)

TABLE 4.—Volume Flow Measurements (VF)

Procedure Type	n	Mean	SD[a]	Range	Median	25% IQR[b]	75% IQR	P[c]
Maintenance + maturation (All cases)								
VF Pre (mL/min)	205	447	421	12−3265	340	168	556	
VF Post (mL/min)	205	820	600	116−4475	663	444	1001	
% Increase in VF		84%			95%			<.001
Maintenance PTA (All cases)								
VF Pre (mL/min)	98	639	506	110−3265	472	300	806	
VF Post (mL/min)	98	1146	684	200−4475	950	721	1404	
% Increase in VF		79%			101%			<.001
Maintenance PTA (Successful cases)								
VF Pre (mL/min)	94	616	437	110−2537	451	300	806	
VF Post (mL/min)	94	1143	652	286−4475	955	727	1404	
% Increase in VF		85%			112%			<.001
Maturation PTA (All)								
VF Pre (mL/min)	107	271	201	12−1030	210	108	397	
VF Post (mL/min)	107	522	272	116−1410	485	292	658	
% Increase in VF		93%			131%			<.001

[a]SD, Standard deviation.
[b]IQR, Inter-quartile ratio.
[c]Wilcoxon signed rank test.

Ascher, the concept of duplex-guided balloon angioplasty to preserve or assist in maintaining dialysis access has become more popular.[1] In addition to patient convenience and decreasing exposure of both the patient and the surgeon to radiation, the technique appears to be fairly straightforward. The technical success and increase in median volume flow (Table 4) are remarkable. Obviously, as stated in the study, ensuring the absence of a central venous stenosis and identifying patients who can tolerate this procedure without sedation are keys to their success. In addition, having the allotted space and personnel (Fig 1) to perform these procedures makes this office-based procedure a very efficient and attractive option for both the patient and physician.

N. Singh, MD

Reference

1. Ascher E, Hingorani A, Marks N. Duplex-guided balloon angioplasty of failing or nonmaturing arterio-venous fistulae for hemodialysis: a new office-based procedure. *J Vasc Surg.* 2009;50:594-599.

Treatment strategies of arterial steal after arteriovenous access
Gupta NY, Yuo TH, Konig G IV, et al (North Shore Univ Health System, Skokie, IL; Univ of Pittsburgh School of Medicine, PA)
J Vasc Surg 54:162-167, 2011

Introduction.—Ischemic steal syndrome (ISS) associated with arteriovenous (AV) access is rare but can result in severe complications. Multiple techniques have been described to treat ISS with varying degrees of success. This study compares the management and success associated with these techniques.

Methods.—Patients with ISS between June 2003 and June of 2008 at the University of Pittsburgh Medical Center were retrospectively reviewed. Demographics, type of AV access, management technique, and success of intervention were recorded. Success was defined as resolution of ISS symptoms while preserving access function. One hundred consecutive AV access procedures were reviewed for comparison. Data were analyzed using χ^2 test, Fisher's exact test, and Student's t test. The study was approved by our institutional review board.

Results.—A total of 114 patients with ISS had a mean age of 65 years (range, 20-90 years), were predominantly female (66%), diabetic (61%), and with a brachial origin fistula (69%). Risk factors for ISS included coronary artery disease (CAD; $P < .001$), hypertension ($P < .001$), and tobacco use ($P = .048$). Women were noted to have a brachial origin access more frequently than men (odds ratio [OR], 3.1; $P = .009$). Forty-four patients with mild steal were observed. Seventy patients underwent 87 procedures. Procedures performed included ligation (n = 27), banding (n = 22), distal revascularization and interval ligation (DRIL; n = 21), improvement of proximal inflow (n = 9), revision using distal inflow (RUDI; n = 4), and proximalization of arterial inflow (PAI; n = 3). Early procedures (<30 days from the index fistula) were mostly ligation (50%) or banding (38%), while DRIL was the most frequent choice for late interventions (41%). Banding had a high failure rate (62%) and was the most common reason for reintervention (8 of 11, 73%) and DRIL had a better success rate than banding ($P \leq .05$).

In our current practice, 18% of patients had an AV fistula with the proximal radial artery (PRA) as the inflow source, while this type of fistula accounted for only 2% of all ISS patients. Ligation resolved symptoms in all patients, but the AV access was lost.

Conclusions.—Risk factors for development of ISS include CAD, diabetes, female gender, hypertension, and tobacco use. Among various options to treat ISS, banding has a low success rate and high likelihood for reintervention, while DRIL is particularly effective although not uniformly. Less invasive treatment options such as RUDI and PAI may be quite effective in treating ISS. Use of the PRA as the inflow source may decrease the incidence of ISS.

▶ Identified risk factors for development of ischemic steal syndrome (ISS) from this study, including coronary artery disease, diabetes, female gender, hypertension, and tobacco use, and their clinical significance, are unclear based on study design and statistical analysis. Essentially, a group of patients with ISS (N = 114) is compared with a retrospectively determined control group made up of consecutive arteriovenous access patients (N = 100) during the same time period without matching. However, the more useful portion of this study includes the distribution and outcomes of various surgical options for treatment of ISS. Although it is acknowledged that with the retrospective design and absence of hemodynamic data that some patients with ISS may have been missed, overall the lack of effectiveness and need for additional interventions for patients undergoing banding should put to rest any need to perform restriction of flow-type operation. Procedures that reroute arterial flow through distal revascularization interval ligation (DRIL), improvement of proximal flow, revision using distal inflow, or proximalization of arterial inflow are preferred. As a retrospective study, DRIL was most frequently used, whereas other options were less common, so any difference between these options is not differentiated based on sample size power. And until better comparative effectiveness type studies supports one approach over another, any of these options are appropriate. Overall, some options may be better for certain situations than others, and experience with several different techniques applied based on clinical pattern of ISS will allow for most the optimal goal of reducing steal while maintaining access.

M. A. Passman, MD

Stent graft treatment for hemodialysis access aneurysms

Shemesh D, Goldin I, Zaghal I, et al (Shaare Zedek Med Ctr, Jerusalem, Israel)
J Vasc Surg 54:1088-1094, 2011

Background.—Aneurysms that develop in arteriovenous accesses as a result of repeated punctures are sometimes complicated by infection or ischemia causing sloughing of the overlying skin, which may endanger the access and risk major bleeding and other complications. Surgical revision may necessitate the temporary use of a central venous catheter until dialysis can be resumed via the access. We used stent grafts in selected patients for the exclusion of access aneurysms.

Methods.—Twenty of 63 patients requiring access revision for complication of an aneurysm from February 2005 to December 2009 underwent ambulatory endovascular stent graft deployment. Indications included signs of impending rupture, questionable viability of overlying skin, pain, infection, and limitation of cannulation sites by the size or number of the aneurysms. Endovascular treatment always included angioplasty of associated outflow or central vein stenoses at the same ambulatory session.

Results.—Twenty patients with complicated access aneurysms were treated by endovascular stent graft exclusion at an average of 4.8 ± 4.3 years (range, 0.2 to 16.1 years) after access construction: nine graft pseudoaneurysms, nine native vein aneurysms, and two acute iatrogenic pseudoaneurysms. Six patients had skin erosion over the aneurysm, and 12 had painful aneurysms and clinical signs of compromised blood supply to the skin. Another two patients with an acute giant false aneurysm occurring during endovascular procedures were treated in the same interventional session by the stenting technique to control bleeding. All the aneurysms underwent endovascular exclusion without complications. Only one infected puncture site failed to heal within 2 months of stenting and was closed surgically 10 months later due to persistent localized graft infection, but with no further bleeding episodes. Only one aneurysm did not reabsorb within 3 months. Patients with painful skin ischemia had immediate pain relief. All patients also had stenosis in the draining veins necessitating additional percutaneous transluminal angioplasty. Only one patient required hospitalization (for intravenous antibiotic treatment of staphylococcal sepsis). No patients required a central catheter for hemodialysis. One access occluded due to cephalic arch stenosis in a noncompliant patient. Functional patency was 87% at 12 months, with a median follow-up of 15 months (range, 6.3 to 55.5 months).

Conclusion.—Endovascular treatment with stent grafts in complicated access aneurysms is a simple, safe and rapid ambulatory procedure that enables treatment of both the aneurysm and its accompanying draining vein stenosis. It enables continued cannulation of the existing access and avoids the use of central catheters.

► Hemodialysis access aneurysms are associated with significant problems of expansion, skin necrosis, rupture, and potential infection, and they pose difficult challenges for management, balancing preservation of current access over using up potential future dialysis access points. Experience with endovascular stent graft treatment of hemodialysis access aneurysms is described in this retrospective series of 20 patients (11 native fistula; 9 graft aneurysms) over 5 years at a regional referral dialysis center. All patients had concomitant treatment of central vein outflow obstruction at the same time. It is important to note that this is a selected group, and although some cases involved infection, it was usually confined to the skin and did not involve overt infection of the shunt. Most patients had resolution of aneurysm-related symptoms or complications, and functional patency of 87% at 1 year was reasonable, thereby preserving access. Furthermore, although the commercially available stent grafts used in this study were not specifically designed for hemodialysis venipuncture, early use for uninterrupted dialysis occurred and stent graft patency seemed to be maintained despite repeated venipuncture. Although this study represents adaptation of current endovascular technology to solve hemodialysis access issues, wider dissemination of these techniques should be reserved for selected situations.

M. A. Passman, MD

Analysis of Infection Risk following Covered Stent Exclusion of Pseudoaneurysms in Prosthetic Arteriovenous Hemodialysis Access Grafts
Kim CY, Guevara CJ, Engstrom BI, et al (Duke Univ Med Ctr, Durham, NC)
J Vasc Interv Radiol 23:69-74, 2012

Purpose.—To determine whether exclusion of pseudoaneurysms with the use of a covered stent in prosthetic arteriovenous (AV) hemodialysis access grafts impacts the incidence of eventual AV graft infection.

Materials and Methods.—Review of an interventional radiology database for prosthetic AV graft interventions involving stent deployment anywhere within the AV graft circuit revealed 235 interventions in 174 patients between November 2004 and December 2008. Incidence of AV graft infection was analyzed based on stent type (bare metal vs covered), location, and indication for stent deployment on a per-stent, per-procedure, and per-graft basis.

Results.—A total of 16.3% of the stent-implanted AV grafts were eventually surgically excised as a result of graft infection. Covered stents used to treat an intragraft pseudoaneurysm were more commonly associated with subsequent graft infection compared with bare or covered stents deployed within the graft for other reasons: 42.1% versus 18.2% ($P=.011$). Stents deployed in an intragraft location were also associated with a higher incidence of graft infection compared with those deployed at the venous anastomosis or outflow vein: 26.9% versus 6.9% ($P<.001$). No significant difference was identified in infection rates between bare and covered stents.

Conclusions.—Covered stent exclusion of intragraft pseudoaneurysms demonstrated a significant correlation with eventual prosthetic AV graft infection.

▶ Patients with end-stage renal disease (ESRD) appear to be at increased risk of infection. Even when stratified for age, sex, and diabetes, ESRD patients have a 100- to 300-fold higher risk of death caused by sepsis.[1] Prosthetic arteriovenous (AV) grafts are prone to developing pseudoaneurysms thought to be related to graft material degeneration related to repeat cannulation at specific sites. Such pseudoaneurysms may be particularly prone to forming in patients with outflow obstruction. Endovascular treatment has been used by some to treat prosthetic AV graft pseudoaneurysms. There have been reports of high technical success and acceptable patency rates.[2,3] It was, however, these authors' anecdotal impression that incorporating this technique into their practice resulted in a higher incidence of prosthetic AV graft infection. The need for stent deployment in a hemodialysis access graft was relatively uncommon. In this series, less than 8% of hemodialysis access procedures performed involved stent deployment inside a prosthetic AV graft. Nevertheless, the consequences of an AV graft infection are profound with loss of access and the necessity of open wounds to heal by secondary intention. The data here are complicated by the fact that there is no comparison of infection rates of stent graft–treated AV graft pseudoaneurysms versus those treated by surgical excision. However, the high rate of infection of stent graft treatment of AV graft pseudoaneurysms in this series suggests that surgical excision of AV graft pseudoaneurysms should be strongly considered as preferred treatment. Stent graft intervention for AV graft pseudoaneurysms should be reserved for patients felt to be at high risk of operation.

G. L. Moneta, MD

References

1. Sarnak MJ, Jaber BL. Mortality caused by sepsis in patients with end-stage renal disease compared with the general population. *Kidney Int.* 2000;58:1758-1764.
2. Vesely TM. Use of stent grafts to repair hemodialysis graft-related pseudoaneurysms. *J Vasc Interv Radiol.* 2005;16:1301-1307.
3. Najibi S, Bush RL, Terramani TT, et al. Covered stent exclusion of dialysis access pseudoaneurysms. *J Surg Res.* 2002;106:15-19.

Angioplasty of Below-the-elbow Arteries in Critical Hand Ischaemia

Ferraresi R, Palloshi A, Aprigliano G, et al (Istituto Clinico Città Studi, Milan, Italy; et al)
Eur J Vasc Endovasc Surg 43:73-80, 2012

Background.—Critical hand ischaemia (CHI) due to pure below-the-elbow (BTE) artery obstruction is a disabling disease and there is still no consensus concerning the most appropriate revascularisation strategy. The aim of this study was to assess the feasibility, safety and outcomes of percutaneous transluminal angioplasty (PTA) in the treatment of CHI due to pure BTE artery disease.

Methods and Results.—Twenty-eight patients (age 62 ± 11 years; three females) with a total of 34 hands affected by CHI (one pain at rest; 18 non-healing ulcer; 15 gangrene) due to pure BTE artery disease underwent PTA. Most of the patients were males with a long history of diabetes mellitus, end-stage renal disease (ESRD) on haemodialysis and systemic atherosclerosis. The interosseous artery was free of disease in all cases, whereas the radial and ulnar arteries were simultaneously involved in 31/34 hands with long stenosis/occlusions (91%; mean length 155 ± 64 mm). The technical success rate was 82% (28/34), with only three minor complications. In the three cases with a functioning radial arteriovenous fistula, we successfully treated the ulnar artery. PTA was unsuccessful in 18% (6/34) hands due to inability to cross severely calcified lesions. The hand-healing rate was 65% (22/34). The predictors of hand healing were PTA technical success (odds ratio (OR) 0.5, confidence interval (CI) 0.28–0.88; $p \leq 0.0001$) and digital run-off (OR 0.37, CI 0.19–0.71; $p \leq 0.003$).

The mean follow-up period was 13 ± 9 months. Six patients (18%) underwent secondary procedures due to symptomatic restenosis. In all these cases, a successful re-PTA was performed at a mean 6 months after the index procedure, and there were no major procedure-related events. Ten patients (36%) died during follow-up.

Conclusions.—Angioplasty of BTE vessels for CHI is a feasible and safe procedure with acceptable rates of technical success and hand healing. Poor digital run-off due to obstructive disease of the digital vessels can reduce the hand-healing rate after a successful PTA. Pure isolated BTE vessel disease seems to characterise patients with ESRD and diabetes mellitus (Figs 1 and 3).

▶ Not unexpectedly, the authors found that critical hand ischemia (CLI) is associated with long-standing renal failure and diabetes, poor patient survival, and frequent digital artery occlusive disease. Interestingly, there appears to be a subgroup of patients who were primarily affected at the level of the forearm arteries with relative preservation of digital arteries (Figs 1 and 3). In such patients, opening of the forearm vessels with the angioplasty techniques described makes reasonable sense and can result in sufficient short-term patency to allow healing of digital gangrene or digital ulceration. The overall hand-healing incidence, however, was still only 65% in this series. This, coupled with the fact that only patients who were treated were included in this report, makes it difficult to judge the impact of below-the-elbow angioplasty on all patients with CLI secondary to long-standing diabetes or renal failure. In addition, there probably should be considerations of which fingers are involved with the ischemic process, the extent of the ischemic process, and whether the ischemic process is in the dominant or nondominant hand in considering whether to proceed with attempted angioplasty or simply primary amputation of the digit. Nevertheless, the fact

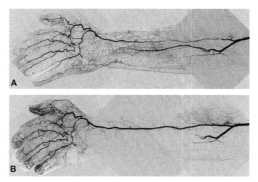

FIGURE 1.—Successful angioplasty with good digital run-off. Patient FN: 69-year-old male with ESRD on HD. A: Baseline angiogram: occlusion of the ulnar artery, diffuse disease with short occlusion of dominant radial artery; good patency of hand vessels. B: Final angiogram: eight patent digital vessels. (Reprinted from European Journal of Vascular and Endovascular Surgery, Ferraresi R, Palloshi A, Aprigliano G, et al. Angioplasty of below-the-elbow arteries in critical hand ischaemia. *Eur J Vasc Endovasc Surg.* 2012;43:73-80. Copyright 2012, with permission from the European Society for Vascular Surgery.)

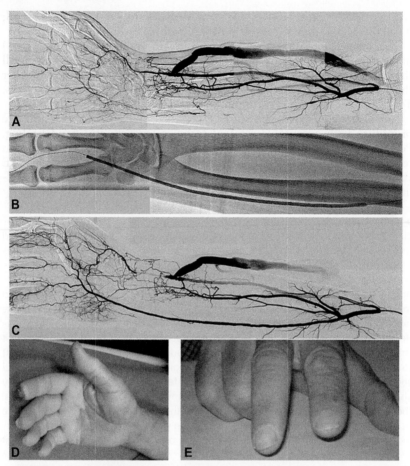

FIGURE 3.—Successful angioplasty of the non AVF-related artery. Patient AL: 52-year-old male with type 1 diabetes and ESRD on HD. A: Baseline angiogram: occlusion of the ulnar artery, patent radial artery with functioning distal AVF. B: Balloon inflation (Anphirion Deep, Medtronic Invatec): diameter 2.5–3.0, conic, 21 cm long, 15 atm. C: Final angiogram: eight patent digital vessels. D: Baseline lesion: second finger apical necrosis. E: Three months later: complete healing. (Reprinted from European Journal of Vascular and Endovascular Surgery, Ferraresi R, Palloshi A, Aprigliano G, et al. Angioplasty of below-the-elbow arteries in critical hand ischaemia. *Eur J Vasc Endovasc Surg.* 2012;43:73-80. Copyright 2012, with permission from the European Society for Vascular Surgery.)

that this procedure can be technically successful and can be associated with at least temporary resolution of the symptoms of hand ischemia is important information, given the limited survival of this patient cohort. With the increasing prevalence of obesity, diabetes, and resulting renal failure, there are going to be more patients with critical upper-extremity digital ischemia in the future. Based on the extent of the digital gangrene, which fingers are involved, and whether the fingers involved are on the dominant or nondominant hand, angiography and angioplasty of stenotic or occluded forearm arteries should be considered in the subset of patients with diabetes, end-stage renal disease, and digital gangrene.

G. L. Moneta, MD

12 Carotid and Cerebrovascular Disease

Silent cerebral events in asymptomatic carotid stenosis

Jayasooriya G, Thapar A, Shalhoub J, et al (Imperial College London, UK)
J Vasc Surg 54:227-236, 2011

Background.—Approximately 20% of strokes are attributable to carotid stenosis. However, the number of asymptomatic patients needed to prevent one stroke or death with endarterectomy is high at 17 to 32. There is a clear need to identify asymptomatic individuals at high risk of developing future ischemic events to improve the cost-effectiveness of surgery. Our aim was to examine the evidence for subclinical microembolization and silent brain infarction in the prediction of stroke in asymptomatic carotid stenosis using transcranial Doppler (TCD), computed tomography (CT), and magnetic resonance imaging (MRI).

Methods.—The review was conducted according to the preferred reporting items for systematic reviews and meta-analyses (PRISMA) guidelines. Articles regarding humans between 1966 and 2010 were identified through systematic searches of Pubmed, MEDLINE, and EMBASE electronic databases using a predetermined search algorithm.

Results.—Fifty-eight full text articles met the inclusion criteria. A median of 28% of microemboli positive patients experienced a stroke or transient ischemic attack during follow-up compared with 2% of microemboli negative patients ($P = .001$). The same was true for the end point of stroke alone with a median of 10% of microemboli positive patients experiencing a stroke vs 1% of microemboli negative patients ($P = .004$). A specific pattern of silent CT infarctions was related to future stroke risk (odds ratio [OR] = 4.6; confidence interval [CI] = 3.0-7.2; $P < .0001$). There are no prospective MRI studies linking silent infarction and stroke risk.

Conclusions.—There is level 1 evidence for the use of TCD to detect microembolization as a risk stratification tool. However, this technique requires further investigation as a stroke prevention tool and would be complemented by improvements in carotid plaque imaging.

▶ While there is benefit in carotid revascularization for patients with asymptomatic carotid occlusive disease, differentiating those patients at most risk for cerebral ischemic events has been under intense investigation. As a systemic review using meta-analysis methods, this article focuses on identifying evidence for subclinical microembolization and silent brain infarction as a predictor of stroke in patients with asymptomatic carotid stenosis. While findings of this study are dependent on search strategy and methodology, limitations exist in the absence of randomized controlled trials, inclusion of cross-sectional observational studies, existing reviews and other meta-analysis, and exclusion of case reports. Regardless of these constraints, detection of microemboli by transcranial Doppler in patients with asymptomatic carotid occlusive disease seems to be predictive of potential future stroke. However, what is missing from this analysis is any correlation to carotid plaque morphology. Until this connection is made, better identification of asymptomatic patients vulnerable to stroke who would potentially benefit from carotid revascularization awaits further investigation.

M. A. Passman, MD

Carotid stenosis as predictor of stroke after transient ischemic attacks
Bonifati DM, Lorenzi A, Ermani M, et al (Santa Chiara Hosp, Trento, Italy; Univ of Padua, Italy)
J Neurol Sci 303:85-89, 2011

ABCD2 score identifies high-risk TIAs but its validity in different countries and hospitals is unknown. Doubts remain also about the role of diagnostic work up for patients with TIAs in the emergency department. The present study was undertaken to confirm the usefulness of ABCD2 score in the emergency department of Trento Hospital and to evaluate if other exams (carotid ultrasound or CT scan) commonly performed in TIA patients are helpful. We retrospectively analysed discharge diagnosis of around 120,000 patients seen at the first aid of Trento Hospital over a 28 month period. ABCD2 score, carotid ultrasound and CT scan were recorded and were correlated with recurrence of stroke at different time points (mean follow-up period of 11.4 months) in all patients with TIA. We identified 965 patients with focal neurologic deficit and 502 could be classified as TIA. An ischemic stroke recurred in 30 patients at the end of the follow-up (30% in the first two days). ABCD2 score confirmed its value. A significant carotid stenosis (> 70%) was an independent risk factor for stroke at any time point. Our study confirms the role of ABCD2 in a large Italian cohort of TIA patients but also suggests the importance of performing a carotid ultrasound as soon as possible (Fig 1).

▶ After a first transient ischemic attack (TIA), between 4% and 20% of patients will have a stroke within 90 days, and half of these occur within the first 2 days of

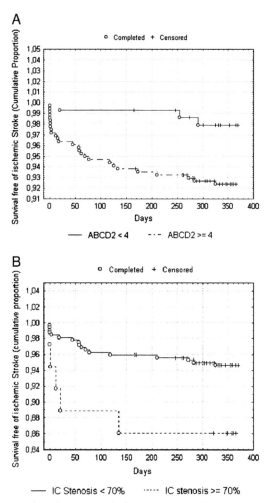

FIGURE 1.—Survival free of ischemic stroke for ABCD2 score below and above 4 (panel A) and for internal carotid (IC) stenosis below and above 70% (panel B). (Reprinted from Bonifati DM, Lorenzi A, Ermani M, et al. Carotid stenosis as predictor of stroke after transient ischemic attacks. *J Neurol Sci.* 2011;303:85-89. Copyright 2011, with permission from Elsevier.)

the TIA.[1,2] To stratify the risk of stroke following TIA, different scoring systems have been developed. Most recently, a unified risk score involving the California and ABCD scores was developed and called the ABCD2 score. It is based on 5 factors: age, blood pressure, clinical features, duration, and diabetes. It appears able to distinguish high-risk patients for stroke with recent TIA from lower-risk patients with higher scores having a 2-day stroke risk of 8.1% and lower scores a 2-day stroke risk of 1%. In addition, data from the NASCET study showed a risk of stroke as high as 25% at 90 days in patients with a hemispheric TIA associated with a 70% or greater carotid stenosis.[3] In this study, the authors sought to confirm the usefulness of the ABCD2 score in a cohort of TIA patients and to explore whether CT scanning or carotid ultrasound might also be useful in stratifying risk of stroke following TIA. The data underline the potential importance of ABCD2 scores, carotid ultrasound, and CT scanning in stratifying risk for stroke following TIA (Fig 1). The practical point is that physicians may use a combination of a carotid ultrasound, CT scan, and ABCD2 score to help stratify the urgency of treatment in patients with a recent TIA. Patients with high-grade carotid stenosis, CT scans indicative of previous infarct, and high ABCD2 scores should be considered for an urgent admission to the hospital and urgent intervention. Patients with negative CT findings, lower ABCD2 scores, and lesser degrees of carotid stenosis perhaps can be considered for more elective therapy.

G. L. Moneta, MD

References

1. Johnston SC, Gress DR, Browner WS, Sidney S. Short-term prognosis after emergency department diagnosis of TIA. *JAMA*. 2000;284:2901-2906.
2. Lovett JK, Dennis MS, Sandercock PA, Bamford J, Warlow CP, Rothwell PM. Very early risk of stroke after a first transient ischemic attack. *Stroke*. 2003;34:e138-e140.
3. Streifler JY, Eliasziw M, Benavente OR, et al. The risk of stroke in patients with first-ever retinal vs hemispheric transient ischemic attacks and high-grade carotid stenosis. North American Symptomatic Carotid Endarterectomy Trial. *Arch Neurol*. 1995;52:246-249.

Combination oral antiplatelet therapy may increase the risk of hemorrhagic complications in patients with acute ischemic stroke caused by large artery disease
Itabashi R, Mori E, Furui E, et al (Kohnan Hosp, Sendai, Miyagi, Japan; Tohoku Univ Graduate School of Medicine, Sendai, Miyagi, Japan)
Thromb Res 128:541-546, 2011

Introduction.—The association between the frequency or severity of bleeding complications and combination antiplatelet therapy for acute stroke treatment is not understood in detail. This retrospective study investigated whether combination oral antiplatelet therapy for cases with acute ischemic stroke due to large artery disease increased the incidence of hemorrhagic complications.

Materials and Methods.—We reviewed 1335 consecutive patients who were admitted to our department within 7 days of the onset of an ischemic stroke or transient ischemic attack between April 2005 and November 2009. We enrolled 167 patients with >50% stenosis or occlusion in culprit major vessels and who were administered oral antiplatelet agents within 48 hours of admission. Hemorrhagic complications were classified according to the bleeding severity index. We studied the association between the incidence and severity of hemorrhagic complications during hospitalization and the clinical characteristics, including antiplatelet therapy.

Results.—Fifty-nine and 108 patients were treated with only 1 antiplatelet agent and combination antiplatelet agents, respectively. Fourteen patients developed bleeds (3 major and 11 minor), and all of the major bleeds occurred in those given combination agents. The proportion of patients receiving combination agents was significantly higher in those with significant bleeds. Multivariate logistic regression analysis revealed that being older and receiving combination agents were independent predictors for significant bleeds during hospitalization.

Conclusions.—Despite the retrospective nature of this study, our findings suggest that the incidence of hemorrhagic complications increases in patients with acute ischemic stroke treated with combination antiplatelet agents (Fig 1).

▶ It is recommended that oral antiplatelet therapy be administered immediately after acute ischemic stroke to prevent recurrence and progression of stroke as well as other vascular events. It is known that monotherapy with aspirin does not reduce stroke progression.[1] However, it is thought that combination antiplatelet therapy such as that provided by clopidogrel and aspirin may have a role in

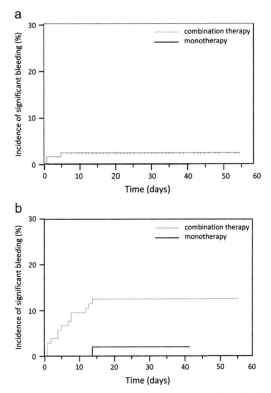

FIGURE 1.—Kaplan-Meier survival plots for the major (a) or significant bleeds (b) (Log rank test, p = 0.198 and p = 0.023, respectively). (Reprinted from Thrombosis Research, Itabashi R, Mori E, Furui E, et al. Combination oral antiplatelet therapy may increase the risk of hemorrhagic complications in patients with acute ischemic stroke caused by large artery disease. *Thromb Res.* 2011;128:541-546. Copyright 2011, with permission from Elsevier.)

reducing stroke progression in patients with stroke secondary to large artery disease.[2,3] It is known, however, that there is an increased risk of hemorrhagic complications with long-term secondary preventative therapy with combination antiplatelet agents.[4,5] The risk, however, of dual antiplatelet therapy in the short-term treatment of acute stroke is not well understood. The current study was designed to evaluate the risk of bleeding complications associated with aggressive antiplatelet therapy in patients with ischemic stroke and felt to be at high risk for stroke recurrence or progression. This study has a number of limitations, including its retrospective design, the fact that it was not randomized, there was no standard outcomes assessment, and the relatively small sample size. In addition, although the data were derived from the prospectively collected database, the retrospective nature of the study potentially underestimates the true number of bleeding complications. Nevertheless, the data presented here suggest that the administration of dual antiplatelet agents in patients with acute stroke, secondary to large artery disease, likely increases the risk of hemorrhagic complications (Fig 1). Unfortunately, the relative effects of combination versus mono-antiplatelet therapy in improving neurologic outcome, when balanced with hemorrhagic risk, cannot be assessed with the data presented here.

G. L. Moneta, MD

References

1. Markus HS, Droste DW, Kaps M, et al. Dual antiplatelet therapy with clopidogrel and aspirin in symptomatic carotid stenosis evaluated using Doppler embolic signal detection: the Clopidogrel and Aspirin for Reduction of Emboli in Symptomatic Carotid Stenosis (CARESS) trial. *Circulation.* 2005;111:2233-2240.
2. Wong KS, Chen C, Fu J, et al. Clopidogrel plus aspirin versus aspirin alone for reducing embolisation in patients with acute symptomatic cerebral or carotid artery stenosis (CLAIR study): a randomised, open-label, blinded-endpoint trial. *Lancet Neurol.* 2010;9:489-497.
3. Diener HC, Bogousslavsky J, Brass LM, et al; MATCH Investigators. Aspirin and clopidogrel compared with clopidogrel alone after recent ischaemic stroke or transient ischaemic attack in high-risk patients (MATCH): randomised, double-blind, placebo-controlled trial. *Lancet.* 2004;364:331-337.
4. Bhatt DL, Fox KA, Hacke W, et al. Clopidogrel and aspirin versus aspirin alone for the prevention of atherothrombotic events. *N Engl J Med.* 2006;354:1706-1717.
5. Gasparyan AY, Watson T, Lip GY. The role of aspirin in cardiovascular prevention: implications of aspirin resistance1. *J Am Coll Cardiol.* 2008;51:1829-1843.

Short-Term Outcomes After Symptomatic Internal Carotid Artery Occlusion
Burke MJ, on behalf of the Investigators of the Registry of the Canadian Stroke Network (Univ of Toronto, Canada; et al)
Stroke 42:2419-2424, 2011

Background and Purpose.—Previous studies concerning internal carotid artery (ICA) occlusion have focused on long-term prognosis. The purpose of the present study was to evaluate short-term outcomes of patients with symptomatic ICA occlusion.

Methods.—We used data from the Registry of the Canadian Stroke Network on consecutive patients presenting to 11 stroke centers in Ontario. We included patients with noncardioembolic ischemic stroke or transient ischemic attack within the anterior circulation. The resulting cohort was divided into 4 groups based on vascular imaging of the ipsilateral extracranial ICA: occlusion, severe stenosis, moderate stenosis, and mild/no stenosis. Logistic regression modeling was used to evaluate the association between the degree of stenosis/occlusion of the symptomatic ICA and a series of short-term outcome measures.

Results.—Of the 4144 patients who met study criteria, 283 patients had a symptomatic ICA occlusion. Compared with patients with ICA occlusion, patients with all other degrees of stenosis had a lower risk of in-hospital death, neurological worsening, and poor functional outcome. Particularly, severe stenosis was associated with a lower risk of in-hospital death (adjusted OR, 0.40; 95% CI, 0.20 to 0.79), neurological worsening (adjusted OR, 0.52; 95% CI, 0.34 to 0.78), and poor functional outcome (adjusted OR, 0.62; 95% CI, 0.41 to 0.94) compared with the ICA occlusion group.

Conclusions.—The results of our study showed that patients with symptomatic ICA occlusion are at a high risk of adverse outcomes that is as severe, if not worse, than any other degree of ICA stenosis in the short term. Thus, more aggressive management may be warranted for patients with acute, symptomatic ICA occlusion.

▶ It is known that patients presenting with symptomatic occluded ipsilateral internal carotid arteries (ICA) have poor long-term prognosis.[1] For example, patients with ICA occlusion who present with minor stroke or transient ischemic attacks have a subsequent stroke risk of 5% to 7% per year with an annual mortality of 6%. For patients with more severe strokes, recurrent stroke is 10%, and mortality is 45% after an average follow-up of 1.2 years.[2] Surprisingly, short-term prognosis of patients with symptomatic ICA occlusion is less frequently reported. It is unclear whether ICA occlusion acts as an independent predicator of future stroke recurrence, neurologic worsening, or adverse functional outcome. The authors sought to evaluate short-term outcomes of patients presenting with symptomatic ICA occlusion and compared these patients with other patients with symptomatic carotid disease of various degrees of ICA stenosis. In this cohort of 283 patients with symptomatic ICA occlusion, recurrent in-hospital stroke occurred in 6.7%, myocardial infarction in 2.5%, mortality in 12%, with an average length of stay of 18 days. The optimal medical management of patients with symptomatic ICA occlusion remains unknown. The authors' data did not capture the timing of initiation of antiplatelet use or the indications for warfarin use in these patients. It is known that early initiation of antiplatelet agents reduces risk of recurrent stroke, death, and dependency.[3] In addition, it is unknown whether the patients presented with acute or chronic ICA occlusion, and the database did not capture information on intracranial vascular stenosis or the location of recurrent stroke events. Finally, patients with mild or no stenosis might have included a number of stroke etiologies other than carotid artery disease. The study basically indicates patients with symptomatic ICA occlusions do not do well in the short term. Additional studies will be needed to determine whether this adverse prognosis can be favorably influenced by various combinations of medical and interventional management.

G. L. Moneta, MD

References

1. Klijn CJ, van Buren PA, Kappelle LJ, et al. Outcome in patients with symptomatic occlusion of the internal carotid artery. *Eur J Vasc Endovasc Surg.* 2000;19: 579-586.
2. Paciaroni M, Caso V, Venti M, et al. Outcome in patients with stroke associated with internal carotid artery occlusion. *Cerebrovasc Dis.* 2005;20:108-113.
3. CAST: randomised placebo-controlled trial of early aspirin use in 20,000 patients with acute ischaemic stroke. CAST (Chinese Acute Stroke Trial) Collaborative Group. *Lancet.* 1997;349:1641-1649.

Symptomatic internal carotid artery occlusion: a long-term follow-up study
Persoon S, Luitse MJA, de Borst GJ, et al (Univ Med Centre Utrecht, The Netherlands)
J Neurol Neurosurg Psychiatry 82:521-526, 2011

Background.—Information on outcome of patients with occlusion of the internal carotid artery (ICA) is limited by the short duration of follow-up and lack of haemodynamic studies on the brain.

Methods.—The authors prospectively investigated 117 consecutive patients with transient or moderately disabling cerebral or retinal ischaemia associated with ICA occlusion between September 1995 and July 1998, and followed them until June 2008. The authors determined the risk of recurrent ischaemic stroke and other vascular events and prognostic factors, including collateral pathways and transcranial Doppler CO_2 reactivity.

Results.—Patients (mean age 61 ± 9 years; 80% male) were followed for a median time of 10.2 years; 22 patients underwent endarterectomy for contralateral ICA stenosis and 16 extracranial/intracranial bypass surgery. Recurrent ischaemic stroke occurred in 23 patients, resulting in an annual rate of 2.4% (95% CI 1.5 to 3.6). Risk factors for recurrent ischaemic stroke were age (HR 1.07, 1.02 to 1.13), cerebral rather than retinal symptoms (HR 8.0, 1.1 to 60), recurrent symptoms after documented occlusion (HR 4.4, 1.6 to 12), limb-shaking transient ischaemic attacks at presentation (HR 7.5, 2.6 to 22), history of stroke (HR 2.8, 1.2 to 6.7) and leptomeningeal collaterals (HR 5.2, 1.5 to 17) but not CO_2 reactivity (HR 1.01, 0.99 to 1.02). The composite event of any vascular event occurred in 57 patients, resulting in an annual rate of 6.4% (95% CI 4.9 to 8.2).

Conclusion.—The prognosis of patients with transient ischaemic attack or minor stroke and ICA occlusion depends on age, several clinical factors

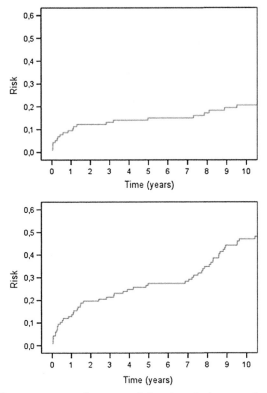

FIGURE 1.—Time-to-event curves for recurrent ischaemic stroke (upper part) and for any stroke, myocardial infarction or vascular death (lower part) in patients with symptomatic internal carotid artery occlusion (n=117). (Reprinted from Persoon S, Luitse MJA, de Borst GJ, et al. Symptomatic internal carotid artery occlusion: a long-term follow-up study. *J Neurol Neurosurg Psychiatry.* 2011;82:521-526. Copyright 2011, with permission from Elsevier.)

and the presence of leptomeningeal collaterals. The long-term risk of recurrent ischaemic stroke is much lower than that of other vascular events (Fig 1).

▶ Information on long-term outcomes in patients with symptomatic internal carotid artery (ICA) occlusion is scant. In the short- to medium-term, patients with transient ischemic attack (TIA) or stroke associated with occlusion of the ICA appear to have a risk of recurrent stroke of approximately 5% per year.[1] This risk may be doubled in individuals with a compromised hemodynamic state of the brain.[2] The authors have previously reported short-term data on prognosis of patients with symptomatic ICA occlusion with respect to hemodynamic compromise of the ICA distribution.[3] The current study represents long-term data of this original cohort with respect to hemodynamic characteristics of the brain and risk of ischemic stroke in long-term follow-up. The medical arm of the external carotid/internal carotid (EC/IC) bypass trial (EC/IC bypass study group)[4] has been the largest cohort of medically treated patients with symptomatic ICA occlusion. Follow-up in that study was 4.5 years, and the mean annual risk of ischemic stroke was 6.3% (Fig 1). The current study provides longer-term data and data with respect to measures of collateral circulation within the brain. The lower risk observed of recurrent ischemic stroke may be related to better medical management of cerebrovascular disease now than existed in the 1980s. Also, the inclusion of a larger percentage of patients with retinal symptoms than in the EC/IC bypass trial may have lowered overall risk in this study. The high rate of other vascular events in patients with ICA occlusion argues for aggressive management of atherosclerotic risk factors. Finally, while leptomeningeal collaterals appear predictive of recurrent ischemic stroke, it is not suggested that patients with ICA occlusion undergo routine angiography. Whether EC/IC bypass surgery will prevent stroke in patients with hemodynamic compromise is currently being investigated by the ongoing carotid occlusion surgery study.[5]

G. L. Moneta, MD

References

1. Klijn CJ, Kappelle LJ, Algra A, van Gijn J. Outcome in patients with symptomatic occlusion of the internal carotid artery or intracranial arterial lesions: a meta-analysis of the role of baseline characteristics and type of antithrombotic treatment. *Cerebrovasc Dis.* 2001;12:228-234.
2. Grubb RL Jr, Derdeyn CP, Fritsch SM, et al. Importance of hemodynamic factors in the prognosis of symptomatic carotid occlusion. *JAMA.* 1998;280:1055-1060.
3. Klijn CJ, Kappelle LJ, van Huffelen AC, et al. Recurrent ischemia in symptomatic carotid occlusion: prognostic value of hemodynamic factors. *Neurology.* 2000;55: 1806-1812.
4. Failure of extracranial-intracranial arterial bypass to reduce the risk of ischemic stroke. Results of an international randomized trial. The EC/IC Bypass Study Group. *N Engl J Med.* 1985;313:1191-1200.
5. Grubb RL Jr, Powers WJ, Derdeyn CP, Adams HP Jr, Clarke WR. The carotid occlusion surgery study. *Neurosurg Focus.* 2003;14:e9.

Cilostazol Versus Aspirin for Secondary Prevention of Vascular Events After Stroke of Arterial Origin

Kamal AK, Naqvi I, Husain MR, et al (Aga Khan Univ Hosp, Karachi, Pakistan)
Stroke 42:e382-e384, 2011

For the secondary prevention of stroke of arterial origin, aspirin is the most widely studied and prescribed agent the world over. Cilostazol is both an antiplatelet and vasodilating agent. This agent has been used mainly in Asian populations with noncardioembolic stroke and no clinically evident cardiac disease.

Methods.—Objectives: The objective of this review was to determine the relative effectiveness and safety of cilostazol compared directly with aspirin in the prevention of stroke and other serious vascular events in patients at high vascular risk for subsequent stroke, those with previous transient ischemic attack, or ischemic stroke of arterial origin.

Search Strategy: We searched the Cochrane Stroke Group Trials Register (last searched September 2010), the Cochrane Central Register of Controlled

Trials (CENTRAL; The Cochrane Library 2009, Issue 4), MEDLINE (1950 to May 2010), and EMBASE (1980 to May 2010). In an effort to identify further published, ongoing, and unpublished studies, we searched journals, conference proceedings, and ongoing trial registers; scanned reference lists from relevant studies; and contacted trialists and Otsuka Pharmaceutical Co Ltd.

Selection Criteria: We selected all randomized controlled trials comparing cilostazol with aspirin in which participants were treated for at least 1 month and followed systematically for development of vascular events (stroke, myocardial infarction, or vascular death).

Data Collection and Analysis: Two review authors independently selected trials for inclusion, extracted the data, and assessed trial quality. We calculated the treatment effect for each outcome in terms of risk ratio by using the Mantel-Haenszel method.

Results.—We included 2 trials from Japan and China, which included a total of 3477 participants with a history of ischemic stroke of arterial origin. These trials were of good quality. Compared with aspirin, cilostazol was associated with a significantly lower risk of composite outcome of vascular events (stroke, myocardial infarction, or vascular death; relative risk, 0.72; 95% CI, 0.57 to 0.91; Figure). The proportional benefit of cilostazol over aspirin on the outcome of "strokes of any type (ischemic or hemorrhagic)" was 33% (95% CI, 14% to 48%) compared with aspirin.

In relation to hemorrhagic stroke during follow-up, cilostazol was associated with a risk reduction of 74% (95% CI, 45% to 87%) compared with aspirin. In safety analyses, aspirin overall caused more bleeds with extracranial hemorrhage significantly higher in patients on aspirin compared with cilostazol (relative risk, 0.74; 95% CI, 0.61 to 0.90). Cilostazol was significantly associated with minor adverse effects, namely headache, gastrointestinal intolerance, palpitation, dizziness, tachycardia, angina, and cardiac failure.

Conclusions.—This review of the available trials in the Asian population shows cilostazol to be superior to aspirin in the secondary prevention of vascular events (stroke, myocardial infarction, or vascular death), strokes of all type (ischemic or hemorrhagic), and hemorrhagic stroke subtype alone after stroke of arterial origin. Cilostazol is associated with fewer major bleeding events than aspirin.

Implications for Practice: Cilostazol is a useful agent for the secondary prevention of stroke of arterial origin in Asians who do not have significant overt cardiac disease. It has a favorable major side effect profile (lower risk of intracranial hemorrhage compared with aspirin). This must be balanced against the daily cost of cilostazol, which is more expensive than aspirin, an important consideration when prescribing lifelong medications in low and middle-income country patients.

Implications for Research: Future randomized trials in patients with ischemic stroke are needed to determine whether the benefit observed in reduction of vascular events after stroke applies in non-Asian populations as well and across all ischemic stroke subtypes.

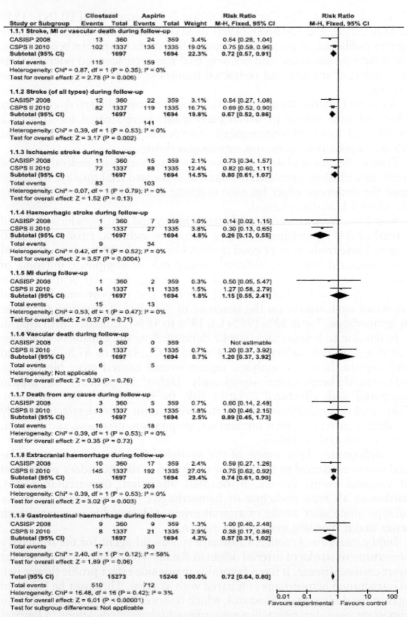

FIGURE.—Meta-analysis of randomized trials comparing aspirin versus cilostazol in patients with ischemic stroke of arterial origin. Results are expressed as Mantel-Haenszel risk ratios and 95% CI with fixed-effects model. Relative risk <1 suggests that cilostazol was better that aspirin. From Kamal AK, Naqvi I, Husain MR, Khealani BA. Cilostazol versus aspirin for secondary prevention of vascular events after stroke of arterial origin. *Cochrane Database Syst Rev.* 2011;1:CD008076. Reproduced with permission from John Wiley & Sons, Ltd. CASISP indicates Cilostazol vs Aspirin for Secondary Ischemic Stroke Prevention; CSPS II, Cilostazol Stroke Prevention Study 2; MI, myocardial infarction. (Reprinted from Kamal AK, Naqvi I, Husain MR, et al. Cilostazol versus aspirin for secondary prevention of vascular events after stroke of arterial origin. *Stroke.* 2011;42:e382-e384. © American Heart Association, Inc.)

Disclosures.—None (Fig).

▶ This is a summary of a Cochrane review that is based on the fact that aspirin for secondary prevention following a stroke of arterial origin has been both widely studied and widely prescribed. Cilostazol, a vasodilating agent with antiplatelet properties, has been used in Asian populations with noncardioembolic stroke and no clinically evident cardiac disease. The purpose of this review was to determine the relative effectiveness and safety of cilostazol compared directly with aspirin in the prevention of stroke and other vascular events in patients with a previous transient ischemic attack (TIA) or ischemic stroke of arterial origin. In the Asian population, at least those from China and Japan that were studied, cilostazol appeared to be superior to aspirin in secondary prevention of vascular events following a TIA or stroke (Fig). The results were even more dramatic in preventing secondary stroke secondary to intracranial hemorrhage. Better prevention of subsequent stroke with cilostazol was also associated with fewer major bleeding events than with aspirin (Fig). Based on this study, one should conclude cilostazol is the preferred agent for secondary prevention of vascular events following a stroke of arterial origin in Asian patients who do not have overt cardiac disease.

G. L. Moneta, MD

Age and Outcomes After Carotid Stenting and Endarterectomy: The Carotid Revascularization Endarterectomy Versus Stenting Trial

Voeks JH, for the CREST Investigators (Univ of Alabama at Birmingham; et al)
Stroke 42:3484-3490, 2011

Background and Purpose.—High stroke event rates among carotid artery stenting (CAS)-treated patients in the Carotid Revascularization Endarterectomy Versus Stenting Trial (CREST) lead-in registry generated an a priori hypothesis that age may modify the relative efficacy of CAS versus carotid endarterectomy (CEA). In the primary CREST report, we previously noted significant effect modification by age. Here we extend this investigation by examining the relative efficacy of the components of the primary end point, the treatment-specific impact of age, and contributors to the increasing risk in CAS-treated patients at older ages.

Methods.—Among 2502 CREST patients with high-grade carotid stenosis, proportional hazards models were used to examine the impact of age on the CAS-to-CEA relative efficacy, and the impact of age on risk within CAS-treated and CEA-treated patients.

Results.—Age acted as a treatment effect modifier for the primary end point (*P interaction*=0.02), with the efficacy of CAS and CEA approximately equal at age 70 years. For CAS, risk for the primary end point increased with age (P<0.0001) by 1.77-times (95% confidence interval, 1.38–2.28) per 10-year increment; however, there was no evidence of increased risk for CEA-treated patients (P=0.27). Stroke events were the primary contributor to the overall effect modification (*P interaction*=0.033), with equal risk at ≈ 64 years. The treatment-by-age interaction for CAS and CEA was not altered by symptomatic status (*P*=0.96) or by sex (*P*=0.45).

Conclusions.—Outcomes after CAS versus CEA were related to patient age, attributable to increasing risk for stroke after CAS at older ages. Patient age should be an important consideration when choosing between the 2 procedures for treating carotid stenosis.

Clinical Trial Registration.—URL: http://www.clinicaltrials.gov. Unique identifier: NCT00004732 (Fig 3).

▶ In 1997, when the protocol for the Carotid Revascularization Endarterectomy Versus Stenting Trial (CREST) trial was developed, it was not well recognized that age and vascular anatomy acted as predictors of complications of carotid artery stenting (CAS). Some had even thought that CAS might be safer than carotid endarterectomy (CEA) in older patients. However, the lead-in phase of

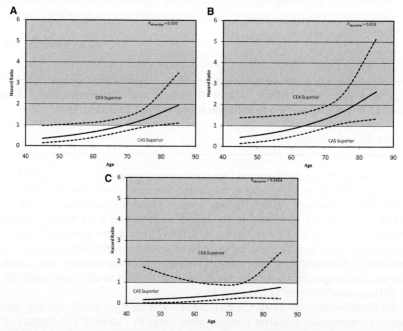

FIGURE 3.—The impact of age on the relative efficacy of carotid artery stenting (CAS) vs carotid endarterectomy (CEA). A, Hazard for the primary end point of any stroke, death, or myocardial infarction (MI) during the periprocedural period, plus ipsilateral strokes over the subsequent 4-year period. Progressively better outcomes were seen with CAS in patients younger than 70 years and with CEA in those older than 70 years. B, Hazard as a function of age for the stroke component of the primary end point (any stroke during the periprocedural period plus ipsilateral stroke over the subsequent 4-year period). Progressively better outcomes were seen with CAS in patients younger than 64 years, and with CEA in those older than 64 years. C, Hazard for the MI component of the primary end point (MI during the periprocedural period). The third component, deaths during the periprocedural period, is not provided because of the relatively small number of death events. (Reprinted from Voeks JH, for the CREST Investigators. Age and outcomes after carotid stenting and endarterectomy: the carotid revascularization endarterectomy versus stenting trial. *Stroke.* 2011;42:3484-3490. © American Heart Association, Inc.)

CREST demonstrated a high risk of stroke events in older CAS-treated patients. Octogenarians were therefore excluded from the lead-in phase of CREST. They were, however, continued in the randomized phase in an attempt to determine if equivalent risks were present for CEA-treated patients. CREST investigators then committed to a preplanned formal assessment of age on relative efficacy of CEA versus CAS. This article demonstrates a differential efficacy of CAS compared with CEA across the age spectrum that is primarily attributed to stroke events (Fig 3). Lower relative risk in the CAS group at younger ages and higher relative risk at older ages is driven by increased risk of stroke in older patients treated by CAS. Interestingly, the risk of stroke for CEA was constant across the age spectrum. The data indicated that patient age should be an important factor in selecting the treatment option for carotid stenosis. It is widely believed that CAS results in more postprocedure strokes in older ages because of anatomic factors affecting CAS, such as tortuosity of extracranial vessels, calcification of extracranial vessels, and higher prevalence of type II and type III aortic arches in older patients. The authors also noted longer fluoroscopy times in their older CAS patients. This suggests that indeed anatomic factors may be significantly contributing to the increase risk of stroke in older CAS-treated patients.

G. L. Moneta, MD

Health-Related Quality of Life After Carotid Stenting Versus Carotid Endarterectomy: Results From CREST (Carotid Revascularization Endarterectomy Versus Stenting Trial)
Cohen DJ, on behalf of the CREST Investigators (Saint Luke's Mid America Heart and Vascular Inst, Kansas City, MO; et al)
J Am Coll Cardiol 58:1557-1565, 2011

Objectives.—The purpose of this study was to compare health-related quality of life (HRQOL) outcomes in patients treated with carotid artery stenting (CAS) versus carotid endarterectomy (CEA).

Background.—In CREST (Carotid Revascularization Endarterectomy versus Stenting Trial), the largest randomized trial of carotid revascularization to date, there was no significant difference in the primary composite endpoint, but rates of stroke and myocardial infarction (MI) differed between CAS and CEA. To help guide individualized clinical decision making, we compared HRQOL among patients enrolled in the CREST study. We also performed exploratory analyses to evaluate the association between periprocedural complications and HRQOL.

Methods.—We measured HRQOL at baseline, and after 2 weeks, 1 month, and 1 year among 2,502 patients randomly assigned to either CAS or CEA in the CREST study. The HRQOL was assessed using the Medical Outcomes Study Short-Form 36 (SF-36) and 6 disease-specific scales designed to study HRQOL in patients undergoing carotid revascularization.

Results.—At both 2 weeks and 1 month, CAS patients had better outcomes for multiple components of the SF-36, with large differences for role physical function, pain, and the physical component summary scale (all p < 0.01). On the disease-specific scales, CAS patients reported less difficulty with driving, eating/swallowing, neck pain, and headaches but more difficulty with walking and leg pain (all p < 0.05). However, by 1 year, there were no differences in any HRQOL measure between CAS and CEA. In the exploratory analyses, periprocedural stroke was associated with poorer 1-year HRQOL across all SF-36 domains, but periprocedural MI or cranial nerve palsy were not.

Conclusions.—Among patients undergoing carotid revascularization, CAS is associated with better HRQOL during the early recovery period as compared with CEA—particularly with regard to physical limitations and pain—but these differences diminish over time and are not evident after 1 year. Although CAS and CEA are associated with similar overall HRQOL at 1 year, event-specific analyses confirm that stroke has a greater and more sustained impact on HRQOL than MI. (Carotid Revascularization Endarterectomy versus Stenting Trial [CREST]; NCT00004732).

▶ The Carotid Revascularization Endarterectomy versus Stenting Trial (CREST) compared carotid artery stenting (CAS) with carotid endarterectomy (CEA) in patients at low risk of surgical complications for carotid intervention. There were no differences in the primary composite endpoint of stroke, myocardial infarction (MI), or death within 4 years of follow-up. However, individual endpoints varied between treatment groups with patients assigned to CAS having higher rates of stroke and patients assigned to CEA having higher rates of MI. Previous studies have suggested less patient impairment during early recovery after CAS compared with CEA. However, differences were brief and limited to highly sensitive disease-specific outcomes and physical role limitation.[1] Previous studies addressing this question have also been limited in that they are small or they enrolled highly selected patients. The current article is a prospectively planned analysis of health-related quality of life (HRQOL) among patients randomly assigned to CAS or CEA in the CREST study. Overall HRQOL at 1 year in CEA versus CAS patients was not different. Because complications of MI and stroke were relatively infrequent, the effects of complications on HRQOL are mitigated by the number of patients who did not have complications. Basically what this study says is that the effects of stroke as a complication are worse for the patient than the effect of an MI or cranial nerve injury. Most of the strokes in CREST were so-called minor strokes as assessed by physician evaluators. Apparently, however, as assessed by patients, minor strokes may not be all that minor.

G. L. Moneta, MD

Reference

1. Stolker JM, Mahoney EM, Safley DM, Pomposelli FB Jr, Yadav JS, Cohen DJ. Health-related quality of life following carotid stenting versus endarterectomy: results from the SAPPHIRE (Stenting and Angioplasty with Protection in Patients at High Risk for Endarterectomy) trial. *JACC Cardiovasc Interv.* 2010;3:515-523.

Myocardial Infarction After Carotid Stenting and Endarterectomy: Results From the Carotid Revascularization Endarterectomy Versus Stenting Trial

Blackshear JL, for the CREST Investigators (Mayo Clinic, Jacksonville, FL; et al)

Circulation 123:2571-2578, 2011

Background.—The Carotid Revascularization Endarterectomy Versus Stenting Trial (CREST) found a higher risk of stroke after carotid artery stenting and a higher risk of myocardial infarction (MI) after carotid endarterectomy.

Methods and Results.—Cardiac biomarkers and ECGs were performed before and 6 to 8 hours after either procedure and if there was clinical evidence of ischemia. In CREST, MI was defined as biomarker elevation plus either chest pain or ECG evidence of ischemia. An additional category of biomarker elevation with neither chest pain nor ECG abnormality was prespecified (biomarker+ only). Crude mortality and risk-adjusted mortality for MI and biomarker+ only were assessed during follow-up. Among 2502 patients, 14 MIs occurred in carotid artery stenting and 28 MIs in carotid endarterectomy (hazard ratio, 0.50; 95% confidence interval, 0.26 to 0.94; $P = 0.032$) with a median biomarker ratio of 40 times the upper limit of normal. An additional 8 carotid artery stenting and 12 carotid endarterectomy patients had biomarker+ only (hazard ratio, 0.66; 95% confidence interval, 0.27 to 1.61; $P = 0.36$), and their median biomarker ratio was 14 times the upper limit of normal. Compared with patients without biomarker elevation, mortality was higher over 4 years for those with MI (hazard ratio, 3.40; 95% confidence interval, 1.67 to 6.92) or biomarker+ only (hazard ratio, 3.57; 95% confidence interval, 1.46 to 8.68). After adjustment for baseline risk factors, both MI and biomarker+ only remained independently associated with increased mortality.

Conclusions.—In patients randomized to carotid endarterectomy versus carotid artery stenting, both MI and biomarker+ only were more common with carotid endarterectomy. Although the levels of biomarker elevation were modest, both events were independently associated with increased future mortality and remain an important consideration in choosing the mode of carotid revascularization or medical therapy.

Clinical Trial Registration.—URL: http://www.ClinicalTrials.gov. Unique identifier: NCT00004732 (Fig 2).

▶ It is known that small elevations of cardiac enzymes after a variety of noncardiac and cardiovascular procedures are associated with increased future mortality.[1-3] The authors sought to determine whether a similar situation exists in patients undergoing carotid artery revascularization. They performed a post hoc analysis of the Carotid Revascularization Endarterectomy Versus Stenting Trial (CREST) data and explored the prognostic importance of myocardial infarction (MI) and cardiac biomarker-only elevation in patients undergoing either carotid endarterectomy (CEA) or carotid artery stenting (CAS). The data confirm previous observations that even a small MI following noncardiac intervention is associated with

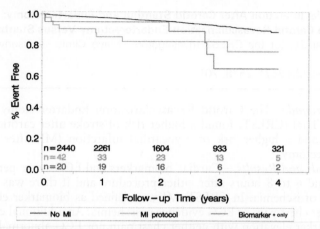

FIGURE 2.—Kaplan-Meier survival curves after randomized carotid revascularization in the Carotid Revascularization Endarterectomy Versus Stenting Trial (CREST). Groups represented include myocardial infarction (MI) patients, biomarker+ only patients, and patients with neither MI nor biomarker+ only. (Reprinted from Blackshear JL. for the CREST Investigators. Myocardial infarction after carotid stenting and endarterectomy: results from the carotid revascularization endarterectomy versus stenting trial. *Circulation*. 2011;123:2571-2578. © American Heart Association, Inc.)

increased late mortality (Fig 2). The data do not imply a cause-and-effect relationship. It is reasonable to postulate that periprocedure MI with biomarker-only elevation is likely a marker of more extensive atherosclerotic disease. One cannot determine from the CREST data whether an ischemic event itself, in relationship to performance of CEA or CAS, increases the late risk of this elevated atherosclerotic burden. The data do suggest that one should think twice about performing any form of revascularization of the carotid artery in patients felt to be at increased cardiac risk because of likely decreased long-term survival in such patients.

G. L. Moneta, MD

References

1. Kim LJ, Martinez EA, Faraday N, et al. Cardiac troponin I predicts short-term mortality in vascular surgery patients. *Circulation*. 2002;106:2366-2371.
2. Landesberg G, Shatz V, Akopnik I, et al. Association of cardiac troponin, CK-MB, and postoperative myocardial ischemia with long-term survival after major vascular surgery. *J Am Coll Cardiol*. 2003;42:1547-1554.
3. Bursi F, Babuin L, Barbieri A, et al. Vascular surgery patients: perioperative and long-term risk according to the ACC/AHA guidelines, the additive role of postoperative troponin elevation. *Eur Heart J*. 2005;26:2448-2456.

Cognition after carotid endarterectomy or stenting: A randomized comparison

Altinbas A, van Zandvoort MJE, van den Berg E, et al (Univ Med Ctr Utrecht, The Netherlands; et al)
Neurology 77:1084-1090, 2011

Objective.—To compare the effect on cognition of carotid artery stenting (CAS) and carotid endarterectomy (CEA) for symptomatic carotid artery stenosis.

Methods.—Patients randomized to CAS or CEA in the International Carotid Stenting Study (ICSS; ISRCTN25337470) at 2 participating centers underwent detailed neuropsychological examinations (NPE) before and 6 months after revascularization. Ischemic brain lesions were assessed with diffusion-weighted imaging before and within 3 days after revascularization. Cognitive test results were standardized into z scores, from which a cognitive sumscore was calculated. The primary outcome was the change in cognitive sumscore between baseline and follow-up.

Results.—Of the 1,713 patients included in ICSS, 177 were enrolled in the 2 centers during the substudy period, of whom 140 had an NPE at baseline and 120 at follow-up. One patient with an unreliable baseline NPE was excluded. CAS was associated with a larger decrease in cognition than CEA, but the between-group difference was not statistically significant: -0.17 (95% CI -0.38 to 0.03; $p = 0.092$). Eighty-nine patients had a pretreatment MRI and 64 within 3 days after revascularization. New ischemic lesions were found twice as often after CAS than after CEA (relative risk 2.1; 95% CI 1.0 to 4.4; $p = 0.041$).

Conclusions.—Differences between CAS and CEA in effect on cognition were not statistically significant, despite a substantially higher rate of new ischemic lesions after CAS than after CEA.

Classification of Evidence.—This study provides Class III evidence that any difference between the effects of CAS and CEA on cognition at 6 months after revascularization is small.

▶ Using diffusion-weighted imaging (DWI), new ischemic lesions are found 3 times as often following CAS than after CEA.[1] It is, however, known that in elderly people, free of dementia and baseline stroke, "silent" infarcts more than double the risk of dementia and are related to a steeper decline in cognitive function.[2] Given this background, the authors sought to compare the effects on cognition of CAS and CEA in patients with symptomatic carotid artery stenosis. A secondary goal was to compare the occurrence of new cerebral ischemic lesions on DWI-MRI in a subpopulation of these patients. The authors found that the demonstrated deterioration in cognitive functioning after CAS in this study supports concerns that even small and partially reversible DWI lesions may affect cognition in a population that is at risk for cognitive decline. However, it appears that at least within the limits of the sample size, the differences in cognitive decline following CAS and CEA are small and of uncertain clinical significance.

G. L. Moneta, MD

References

1. Schnaudigel S, Gröschel K, Pilgram SM, Kastrup A. New brain lesions after carotid stenting versus carotid endarterectomy: a systematic review of the literature. *Stroke.* 2008;39:1911-1919.
2. Vermeer SE, Prins ND, den Heijer T, Hofman A, Koudstaal PJ, Breteler MM. Silent brain infarcts and the risk of dementia and cognitive decline. *N Engl J Med.* 2003;348:1215-1222.

Comparison of Hospitalization Costs and Medicare Payments for Carotid Endarterectomy and Carotid Stenting in Asymptomatic Patients

McDonald RJ, Kallmes DF, Cloft HJ (Mayo Clinic, Rochester, MN)
AJNR Am J Neuroradiol 33:420-425, 2012

Background and Purpose.—Hospitals struggle to provide care for elderly patients based on Medicare payments. Amid concerns of inadequate reimbursement, we sought to evaluate the hospitalization costs for recipients of CEA and CAS placement, identify variables associated with increased costs, and compare these costs with Medicare reimbursements.

Materials and Methods.—All CEA and CAS procedures were extracted from the 2001–2008 NIS. Average CMS reimbursement rates for CEA and CAS were obtained from www.CMS.gov. Annual trends in hospital costs were analyzed by Sen slope analysis. Associations between LOS and hospital costs with respect to sex, age, discharge status, complication type, and comorbidity were analyzed by using the Wilcoxon rank sum test. Least-squares regression models were used to predict which variables had the greatest impact on LOS and hospital costs.

Results.—The 2001–2008 NIS contained 181,200 CEA and 12,485 CAS procedures. Age and sex were not predictive of costs for either procedure. Among favorable outcomes, CAS was associated with significantly higher costs compared with CEA ($P < .0001$). Average Medicare payments were $1,318 less than costs for CEA and $3,241 less than costs for CAS among favorable outcomes. Greater payment-to-cost disparities were noted for both CEA and CAS in patients who had unfavorable outcomes.

Conclusions.—The 2008 Medicare hospitalization payments were substantially less than median hospital costs for both CAS and CEA. Efforts to decrease hospitalization costs and/or increase payments will be necessary to make these carotid revascularization procedures economically viable for hospitals in the long term (Fig 1).

▶ There are, of course, multiple limitations to analyses of data from large databases that were never intended to be used in the manner many researchers use them. Coding errors, determining causal relationships of outcomes and isolation of procedural costs versus total hospital costs, and separating costs from charges are all difficult with these types of data. Nevertheless, some findings are likely valid here. First, there are a lot of procedures performed for asymptomatic carotid stenosis, but over the period of this study only a small percentage were carotid

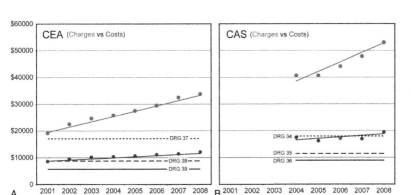

FIGURE 1.—Annual hospital charges and costs for CEA and CAS. Annual (mean ± SD) unadjusted hospital charges (red circles) and costs (blue circles) are shown for CEA (left) and CAS (right). Sen slope trend-lines are shown for each annual data series (colored lines). 2008 stratified CMS average payments, based upon DRG codes for CEA and CAS, are overlaid in A and B, respectively (Table 2, solid line: no complication or comorbidity; dashed line: minor complication or comorbidity; dotted line: major complication or comorbidity). For interpretation of the references to color in this figure legend, the reader is referred to web version of this article. (Reprinted from McDonald RJ, Kallmes DF, Cloft HJ. Comparison of hospitalization costs and Medicare payments for carotid endarterectomy and carotid stenting in asymptomatic patients. *AJNR Am J Neuroradiol.* 2012;33:420-425. Copyright by the American Society of Neuroradiology.)

stents. Second, as suggested by previous studies, carotid stenting is more expensive than carotid endarterectomy (Fig 1). Of course, there is considerable debate about the use of carotid intervention in the asymptomatic patient, and some might argue the best and least expensive procedure in most patients with asymptomatic carotid stenosis is no procedure at all.

G. L. Moneta, MD

Intracranial Hemorrhage Is Much More Common After Carotid Stenting Than After Endarterectomy: Evidence From the National Inpatient Sample

McDonald RJ, Cloft HJ, Kallmes DF (Mayo Clinic, Rochester, MN)
Stroke 42:2782-2787, 2011

Background and Purpose.—Intracranial hemorrhage (ICH) is a rare and devastating complication of carotid revascularization. We sought to determine the prevalence of, type of, and risk factors associated with ICH among recipients of carotid endarterectomy (CEA) and carotid angioplasty and stenting (CAS) within the National Inpatient Sample (NIS).

Methods.—Postoperative cases of ICH after CEA (International Classification of Disease 9th edition [ICD-9]: 38.12) or CAS (ICD-9: 00.63) were retrieved from the 2001 to 2008 NIS. Clinical presentation (asymptomatic versus symptomatic), discharge status, in-hospital mortality, demographics, and hospital characteristics were extracted from NIS data. Charlson indices of comorbidity were determined based on ICD-9 and clinical classification software codes. Multivariate regression was used to determine the impact of revascularization procedure type and symptom status on adverse outcomes, including ICH, in-hospital mortality, and unfavorable discharge status.

Results.—Among 57 663 486 NIS hospital admissions, 215 012 CEA and 13 884 CAS procedures were performed. Symptomatic presentations represented the minority of CEA (N=10 049; 5%) and CAS cases (N=1251; 10%). ICH occurred significantly more frequently after CAS than CEA in both symptomatic (4.4% versus 0.8%; *P*<0.0001) and asymptomatic presentations (0.5% versus 0.06%; *P*<0.0001). Multivariate regression suggested that symptomatic presentations (versus asymptomatic) and CAS procedures (versus CEA) were both independently predictive of 6-fold to 7-fold increases in the frequency of postoperative ICH. ICH was independently predictive in a 30-fold increased risk of mortality before discharge.

Conclusions.—CAS procedures are associated with elevated adverse outcomes, including ICH, in-hospital death, and unfavorable discharges, especially among symptomatic presentations.

▶ The prevalence of intracranial hemorrhage (ICH) after carotid revascularization is somewhere between 0.2% and 0.5%.[1] There is, however, little data, if any, to determine if intracranial hemorrhage (ICH) rates vary between specific revascularization procedures. Even large prospective studies such as CREST lack sufficient power to study relative rates of infrequent complications such as ICH. The national inpatient sample (NIS) is a sufficiently large database to investigate the occurrence of infrequent complications. It provides information with respect to approximately 20% of nonfederal hospitalizations in the United States. This represents more than 8 million annual hospitalizations. The authors used the NIS to determine prevalence of, type of, and risk factors associated with ICH among recipients of carotid angioplasty and stenting (CAS) and carotid endarterectomy (CEA). NIS is a sufficiently large database that can be used to investigate the relative frequencies of uncommon postprocedure complications. The NIS data do not allow independent diagnosis of hyperperfusion among cases of ICH, nor do they allow us to determine whether hyperperfusion was most predictive of ICH. In addition, the NIS clearly contains coding errors, but arguably such errors occur at random and not in a systemic manner to bias the data for or against one procedure or the other. The overall dramatic relative increase in ICH in CAS versus CEA patients, especially those who are symptomatic, is another bit of data arguing for preferential use of CEA in the symptomatic patient if one wishes to primarily minimize the risk of adverse neurologic outcome.

G. L. Moneta, MD

Reference

1. van Mook WN, Rennenberg RJ, Schurink GW, et al. Cerebral hyperperfusion syndrome. *Lancet Neurol.* 2005;4:877-888.

Microembolization During Carotid Artery Stenting in Patients With High-Risk, Lipid-Rich Plaque: A Randomized Trial of Proximal Versus Distal Cerebral Protection

Montorsi P, Caputi L, Galli S, et al (Univ of Milan, Italy; Fondazione IRCCS Istituto Neurologico C. Besta, Milan, Italy)

J Am Coll Cardiol 58:1656-1663, 2011

Objectives.—The goal of this study was to compare the rate of cerebral microembolization during carotid artery stenting (CAS) with proximal versus distal cerebral protection in patients with high-risk, lipid-rich plaque.

Background.—Cerebral protection with filters partially reduces the cerebral embolization rate during CAS. Proximal protection has been introduced to further decrease embolization risk.

Methods.—Fifty-three consecutive patients with carotid artery stenosis and lipid-rich plaque were randomized to undergo CAS with proximal protection (MO.MA system, n = 26) or distal protection with a filter (FilterWire EZ, n = 27). Microembolic signals (MES) were assessed by using transcranial Doppler during: 1) lesion wiring; 2) pre-dilation; 3) stent crossing; 4) stent deployment; 5) stent dilation; and 6) device retrieval/deflation. Diffusion-weighted magnetic resonance imaging was conducted before CAS, after 48 h, and after 30 days.

Results.—Patients in the MO.MA group had higher percentage diameter stenosis (89 ± 6% vs. 86 ± 5%, p = 0.027) and rate of ulcerated plaque (35% vs. 7.4%; p = 0.019). Compared with use of the FilterWire EZ, MO.MA significantly reduced mean MES counts (p < 0.0001) during lesion crossing (mean 18 [interquartile range (IQR): 11 to 30] vs. 2 [IQR: 0 to 4]), stent crossing (23 [IQR: 11 to 34] vs. 0 [IQR: 0 to 1]), stent deployment (30 [IQR: 9 to 35] vs. 0 [IQR: 0 to 1]), stent dilation (16 [IQR: 8 to 30] vs. 0 [IQR: 0 to 1]), and total MES (93 [IQR: 59 to 136] vs. 16 [IQR: 7 to 36]). The number of patients with MES was higher with the FilterWire EZ versus MO.MA in phases 3 to 5 (100% vs. 27%; p < 0.0001). By multivariate analysis, the type of brain protection was the only independent predictor of total MES number. No significant difference was found in the number of patients with new post-CAS embolic lesion in the MO.MA group (2 of 14, 14%) as compared with the FilterWire EZ group (9 of 21, 42.8%).

Conclusions.—In patients with high-risk, lipid-rich plaque undergoing CAS, MO.MA led to significantly lower microembolization as assessed by using MES counts. (Carotid Stenting in Patients With High Risk Carotid Stenosis ["Soft Plaque"] [MOMA]; NCT01274676) (Figs 2 and 3).

▶ It is well recognized that distal cerebral protection during carotid artery stenting (CAS) does not fully prevent embolic complications. There is at least a 37% mean rate of post-CAS of new embolic lesions, mainly silent, on post-CAS diffusion-weighted imaging (DWI) MRI.[1] The reasons for this are unclear, but may include crossing the lesion while unprotected, suboptimal apposition of the device to the arterial wall, the presence of emboli smaller than the filter porous size, and loss of debris after filter recapture. A strategy of proximal endovascular occlusion using

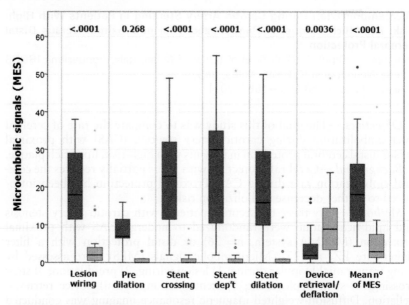

FIGURE 2.—MES Counts During Carotid Stenting Phases. The median and interquartile range of each phase microembolic signals (MES) count are reported in the MO.MA group (**green box plots**) and in the FilterWire EZ group (**red box plots**). Statistical significance is indicated for each phase. dep't = deployment. For interpretation of the references to color in this figure legend, the reader is referred to web version of this article. (Reprinted from the Journal of the American College of Cardiology, Montorsi P, Caputi L, Galli S, et al. Microembolization during carotid artery stenting in patients with high-risk, lipid-rich plaque: a randomized trial of proximal versus distal cerebral protection. *J Am Coll Cardiol.* 2011;58:1656-1663. Copyright 2011, with permission from American College of Cardiology.)

balloons to occlude both the external carotid artery and the common carotid artery, resulting in blood flow arrest in the internal carotid artery, may be a better technique for providing cerebral protection during CAS. Although the technique (Fig 3) has several potential drawbacks, including patient intolerance to occlusion, potential dissection of external carotid artery, and the need for a larger sheath (8-F or 9-F), the potential to decrease microembolic events during CAS is intriguing. Higher levels of microembolic signals (MES) detected with transcranial Doppler (TCD) have been associated with a greater prevalence of post-CAS DWI lesions. The significance of silent DWI-detected ischemic lesions following carotid intervention is unknown, but there is some indication they potentially could be associated with late cognitive decline, especially in patients at increased risk for cognitive decline. In addition, patients with lipid-rich plaque appear to be at higher risk, with an increased prevalence of post-CAS DWI-determined ischemic lesions. Compared to the FilterWire technique, the proximal cerebral protection device reduced the mean number of TCD-detected MES during all phases of stenting (Fig 2). The clinical impact and implications of cerebral microembolization during carotid interventions have not been established. Although there is evidence to suggest that cerebral microemboli may be involved in cognitive decline after cardiac surgery, carotid endarterectomy, and CAS, there are also multiple risk factors, including age, hypertension, and diabetes that may increase

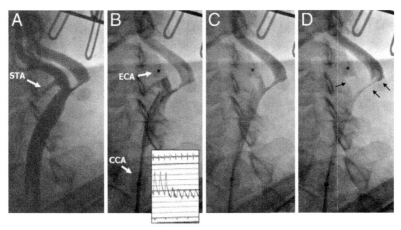

FIGURE 3.—Angiographic Sequence of Carotid Stenting Performed with MO.MA (patient #3). (A) Baseline angiography (**arrow** indicates superior thyroid artery [STA]). (B) Inflation of external carotid artery (ECA) and common carotid artery (CCA) balloons. Flow arrest is confirmed by blood pressure drop (frame) and contrast stagnation. Note that STA is still patent due to its origin close to ECA ostium. (**C and D**) Progressive contrast dilution indicating collateral flow from STA to ICA (**black arrows**). (Reprinted from the Journal of the American College of Cardiology, Montorsi P, Caputi L, Galli S, et al. Microembolization during carotid artery stenting in patients with high-risk, lipid-rich plaque: a randomized trial of proximal versus distal cerebral protection. *J Am Coll Cardiol.* 2011;58:1656-1663. Copyright 2011, with permission from American College of Cardiology.)

brain vulnerability to ischemic injury secondary to microemboli following a carotid intervention. Whereas it is unclear whether microemboli that occur during a carotid intervention are clinically important, it is extremely unlikely that such embolic techniques will help the patient.

G. L. Moneta, MD

Reference

1. Schnaudigel S, Gröschel K, Pilgram SM, Kastrup A. New brain lesions after carotid stenting versus carotid endarterectomy: a systematic review of the literature. *Stroke.* 2008;39:1911-1919.

Periprocedural Cilostazol Treatment and Restenosis after Carotid Artery Stenting: The Retrospective Study of In-Stent Restenosis after Carotid Artery Stenting (ReSISteR-CAS)
Yamagami H, Sakai N, Matsumaru Y, et al (Kobe City Hosp Organization, Chuo-ku, Japan; Toranomon Hosp, Tokyo, Japan; et al)
J Stroke Cerebrovasc Dis 21:193-199, 2012

Restenosis after carotid artery stenting (CAS) is a critical issue. Cilostazol can reduce restenosis after interventions in coronary or femoropopliteal arteries. We investigated whether periprocedural cilostazol treatment was related to the incidence of in-stent restenosis (ISR) or target vessel revascularization (TVR) after CAS. The study group comprised 553 of 580 patients who underwent CAS between April 2003 and August 2006 and were followed for 30 months after the procedure. ISR was defined as stenosis of at least 50% detected on angiography or ultrasonography. TVR was defined as revascularization of the treated carotid artery. During CAS, 207 patients (37.4%) were treated with cilostazol. Over 30 months, ISR occurred in 23 patients (4.2%), TVR occurred in 16 patients (2.9%), and either ISR or TVR occurred in 25 patients (4.5%). The incidence of ISR or TVR was significantly lower in the cilostazol-treated group than in the untreated group (1.4% vs 6.4%; log-rank $P = .006$). In a multivariate analysis, cilostazol treatment (hazard ratio [HR], 0.28; 95% confidence interval [CI], 0.08-0.95; $P = .041$) and stent diameter (HR, 0.73/1-mm increase; 95% CI, 0.54-0.99; $P = .044$) were independent factors for the occurrence of ISR or TVR. The incidence of a composite of events, including thromboembolism, hemorrhage, death, and TVR, tended to be lower in the cilostazol-treated group than in the untreated group (15.0% vs 19.9%; log-rank $P = .17$). Periprocedural cilostazol treatment was associated with lower rates of ISR and retreatment after CAS. A prospective randomized controlled trial is needed to clarify the effect of cilostazol on ISR after CAS (Fig 1).

▶ Reports of cilostazol reducing restenosis after various vascular procedures seem to be increasing. Most of the data appear to be coming from Asian centers where the drug seems to be more widely used than in the United States or Europe. This particular study was a retrospective study, and the patients treated with cilostazol

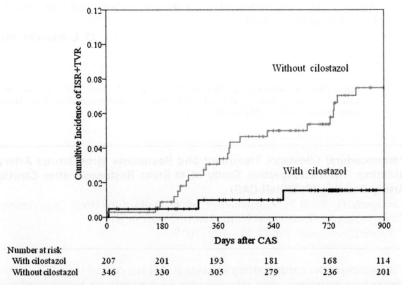

FIGURE 1.—Cumulative incidence of ISR or TVR according to periprocedural cilostazol use. (Reprinted from the Journal of Stroke and Cerebrovascular Diseases, Yamagami H, Sakai N, Matsumaru Y, et al. Periprocedural cilostazol treatment and restenosis after Carotid Artery Stenting: the Retrospective Study of In-Stent Restenosis after Carotid Artery Stenting (ReSISteR-CAS). *J Stroke Cerebrovasc Dis.* 2012;21:193-199. © 2012, with permission from the National Stroke Association.)

were apparently being treated with a variety of dosages for a mix of indications, not just to prevent restenosis following placement of the carotid stent. Nevertheless, the statistical analysis here is reasonable, and use of cilostazol was found to be an independent predictor of freedom from restenosis following carotid artery stenting (Fig 1). Cilostazol has a number of ill-defined effects that could possibly contribute to decreasing restenosis, including improvement in endothelial function and suppression of vascular smooth muscle cell proliferation. It is probably time to consider design of a proper trial with quantitative, blindly evaluated, prospectively determined endpoints to investigate whether cilostazol actually can be demonstrated to have a clinical benefit in reducing restenosis in a variety of patient populations. There have been enough hypothesis-seeking studies on this question—time to move on to the big leagues and do a proper study.

G. L. Moneta, MD

Carotid endarterectomy for treatment of in-stent restenosis after carotid angioplasty and stenting
Reichmann BL, van Laanen JHH, de Vries J-PPM, et al (Univ Med Ctr Utrecht, The Netherlands; Erasmus Med Ctr, Rotterdam, The Netherlands; St Antonius Hosp, Nieuwegein, The Netherlands)
J Vasc Surg 54:87-92, 2011

Objective.—Carotid angioplasty and stenting (CAS) has emerged as an alternative for carotid endarterectomy (CEA) in the prevention of stroke. The benefit of the procedure, however, is hampered by a suggested higher incidence of in-stent restenosis (ISR) for CAS relative to CEA during follow-up. ISR management remains a challenge for clinicians. In this observational retrospective analysis, we evaluated the operative management of ISR by standard CEA with stent removal, including midterm follow-up in 15 patients.

Methods.—The present analysis included 15 patients from three Dutch vascular centers who underwent CEA for symptomatic (n = 10) or hemodynamically significant ($\geq 80\%$) asymptomatic ISR (n = 5). Median time between CAS and CEA was 18.3 months (range, 0-51 months).

Results.—Standard CEA with stent removal was performed in all 15 patients. A Javid shunt was used in two procedures. One patient sustained an intraoperative minor ischemic stroke, with complete recovery during the first postoperative days. No neurologic complications occurred in the other 14 patients. Two patients required a reoperation to evacuate a neck hematoma. There were no peripheral nerve complications. After a median follow-up of 21 months (range, 3-100 months), all 15 patients remained asymptomatic and without recurrent restenosis ($\geq 50\%$) on duplex ultrasound imaging.

Conclusion.—CEA with stent explantation for ISR after CAS seems an effective and durable therapeutic option, albeit with potential cerebral and

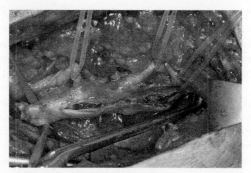

FIGURE 1.—Stent in situ. (Reprinted from the Journal of Vascular Surgery, Reichmann BL, van Laanen JHH, de Vries J-PPM, et al. Carotid endarterectomy for treatment of in-stent restenosis after carotid angioplasty and stenting. *J Vasc Surg.* 2011;54:87-92. Copyright 2011, with permission from The Society for Vascular Surgery.)

bleeding complications, as in this study. The optimal treatment for carotid ISR, however, has yet to be defined (Fig 1).

▶ Carotid artery stenting is a therapy that is offered as an alternative to carotid endarterectomy. The recent CREST trial has shown equivalence in the composite endpoints between carotid artery stenting and carotid endarterectomy; however, carotid artery stenting has increased risk of stroke after procedure, while carotid endarterectomy has increased risks of myocardial infarction after procedure. The durability and restenosis rates following carotid artery stenting are less well defined than for carotid endarterectomy. Most stents that are placed in the arterial system or, for that matter, in the venous system, are usually not removed after failure, but conventional surgical interventions are usually undertaken to restore arterial inflow or venous outflow. In this study, the authors report on a retrospective series of patients who underwent carotid artery stenting and had in-stent restenosis. There were a total of 15 patients, 10 of whom were symptomatic, and 5 were asymptomatic with greater than 80% stenosis of the carotid artery stent. An interesting aspect of this study is that there were 3 participating centers in the Netherlands, and patients with a symptomatic hemodynamically significant in-stent restenosis of 70% were evaluated by a multidisciplinary cerebrovascular committee that included vascular surgeons, interventional radiologists, neurologists, and clinical neurophysiologists discussing the need for reintervention. In asymptomatic patients, significant in-stent restenosis, contralateral occlusion of the internal carotid artery, or severe 4-vessel disease with critical cerebral perfusion through the stented internal carotid artery were indications for reintervention. Also interesting were the operative findings: (1) In some cases minimal edema/inflammation around the stented carotid artery was observed. (2) Adequate exposure of the entire carotid and distal internal carotid artery for clamping with mean stent length 40 mm was always possible without any other exposure maneuvers (eg, jaw subluxation, digastrics muscle division). The majority of the stents were placed across the carotid bifurcation. (3) In all cases, the operating team described intimal hyperplasia with no stent under expansion. (4) The stent and carotid plaque in all cases could be completely removed as one single complex, and there was no need to cut the stent (Fig 1). In the results, the study reports that in a 13-year period, there were 1700 carotid artery stents performed at the 3 centers, and there was a 20% restenosis rate of greater than 50%. Less than 3% of the patients with in-stent restenosis were treated by repeated percutaneous transluminal angioplasty. It is unclear if, of the 15 patients reported in this study, any underwent repeat percutaneous re-intervention before surgical removal of the stent with carotid endarterectomy. The average interval between carotid artery stenting and surgical intervention was 18.3 months. One patient had a postoperative neurologic event that resolved after 24 hours, and 2 patients required reoperation for neck hematomas, both of which were on dual antiplatelet therapy. At a mean follow-up of 21 months, all patients were asymptomatic with no restenosis. What is interesting about this study is that the restenosis lesions were all described by the operating surgeons as intimal hyperplasia. This would be expected given the time frame within 2 years and the known process of stent reaction intraarterially. What is somewhat perplexing is that two-thirds of the patients were symptomatic with this type of lesion, with symptoms comprising an ischemic stroke in 5, repetitive transient ischemic attacks in 4, and amaurosis fugax in 1 patient. It may be possible that the intimal hyperplasia that develops from a stent is different than that of surgical interventions, such as endarterectomies and anastomsis, lending to a more vulner-able plaque in the former. However, in this study, there are no data on microscopic analysis to further evaluate if the recurrent plaque had other features that could explain its potential for causing embolic events. The importance of this study is that it shows that recurrent stenosis following carotid artery stenting is a signifi-cant problem; however, only a small fraction of patients require reinterventions. Furthermore, long-term studies are required before we fully understand the re-intervention rates that will be required in restenosis following carotid artery stenting, but as this study demonstrates, in carefully selected patients, carotid endarterectomy with full removal of the intact stent with the atheromatous plaque is possible.

J. D. Raffetto, MD

Multicentric Retrospective Study of Endovascular Treatment for Restenosis after Open Carotid Surgery

Midy D, Association Universitaire de Recherche en Chirurgie Vasculaire (Bordeaux Univ Hosp, France; et al)
Eur J Vasc Endovasc Surg 42:742-750, 2011

Objectives.—To analyse perioperative and midterm outcomes of carotid artery stenting (CAS) for symptomatic >50% and asymptomatic >70% restenosis after open carotid surgery (OCS).

Design.—A multicentric retrospective study.

Methods.—Outcome measures 30-day death, neurologic and anatomic (thrombosis, restenosis) events. Univariant and multivariant logistic regres-sion analyses were performed to identify predictive factors for neurologic and anatomic events.

Results.—A total of 249 patients with a mean age of 69 years (range, 45—88) were treated for asymptomatic (86%) or symptomatic (14%) restenosis. The 30-day combined operative mortality and stroke morbidity was 2.8% in asymptomatic patients and 2.9% in symptomatic patients. Events during follow-up (mean duration, 29 months) included stroke in four cases, TIA in two, stent thrombosis in four and restenosis in 21. Kaplan—Meier estimates of overall survival, neurologic-event-free survival, anatomic-event-free survival and reintervention-free survival were 95.4%, 94.7%, 96.7% and 99.5%, respectively, at 1 year and 80.3%, 93.8%, 85.1% and 96%, respectively, at 4 years. Multivariant analysis showed that statin use was correlated with a lower risk of anatomic events (odds ratio (OR) = 0.15 (95% confidence interval (CI) 0.03—0.68), $p = 0.01$) and that bypass was associated with a higher risk of anatomic events than endarterectomy (OR = 5.0 (95% CI 1.6—16.6), $p = 0.009$).

Conclusion.—CAS is a feasible therapeutic alternative to OCS for carotid restenosis with acceptable risks in the perioperative period. Restenosis rate may be higher in patients treated after bypass.

▶ With the advancement in endovascular techniques and the introduction of low-profile delivery systems and embolic protection devices, carotid artery stenting (CAS) has become a very common procedure and the subject of much debate as a primary treatment modality in this disease process. One area in the last decade that has not been met with as much resistance is the treatment of carotid restenosis after carotid endarterectomy (CEA). The authors of this series describe their experience over 10 years at 20 Belgian and French centers for endovascular treatment of restenosis after CEA and demonstrate excellent results. In this series, 249 patients underwent CAS for restenosis, and the majority of patients were asymptomatic (86%). The mean degree of restenosis in the asymptomatic group was 82.4% ± 8% (60%-95%) and 82.4% ± 7% (70%-95%) in the symptomatic group. The mean interval of CAS after CEA was 43.4 months, with 48.6% undergoing CAS within 2 years. It is interesting that they did have a subgroup of 28 patients who experienced restenosis after bypass from the common carotid to internal carotid artery. The technical success rate was excellent at 99.6%. Nine ipsilateral neurologic events were noted in the short term (7 strokes and 2 transient ischemic attacks) in a single symptomatic patient and 8 asymptomatic patients. There were no myocardial infarctions noted in the short term. In longer-term follow-up (mean, 29 months), 6 neurologic events occurred, and in 3 of these patients, stent thrombosis was the cause. Repeated angioplasty was required in 6 asymptomatic patients with a restenosis of more than 70%. The Kaplan-Meier estimates of survival and neurologic-event-free survival were 95.4% and 94.7%, respectively, at 1 year.

The results of this study demonstrate the ability to achieve technical success after carotid restenosis with endovascular techniques, which is likely the more common procedure performed currently versus open reoperative surgery. When dealing with this process, we must be cautious with asymptomatic restenosis, as this entity is felt to be a benign process. A study by Healy et al[1] from the University of Washington noted that carotid restenosis (> 50%) by life-table analysis at 7 years occurred in 31% of their study patients with a regression of 10%, resulting in a restenosis rate of 21%. The idea that these lesions occur early and regress over a period and remain stable has been shown in other series and perhaps waiting to intervene in this population up to a certain threshold (ie, > 80%) is warranted.

N. Singh, MD

Reference

1. Healy DA, Zierler RE, Nicholls SC, et al. Long-term follow-up and clinical outcome of carotid restenosis. *J Vasc Surg.* 1989;10:662-669.

Structure of Delay in Carotid Surgery — An Observational Study
Vikatmaa P, Sairanen T, Lindholm J-M, et al (Helsinki Univ Central Hosp, Finland)
Eur J Vasc Endovasc Surg 42:273-279, 2011

Objectives and Design.—Undelayed investigation and surgical treatment of symptomatic carotid artery stenosis are recommended as per guidelines on stroke prevention. We evaluated patient referral pathways and delays from symptom to surgery in Helsinki University Central Hospital (HUCH) region.

Materials and Methods.—One hundred consecutive symptomatic patients scheduled for carotid endarterectomy (CEA) between August 2007 and September 2008 were identified and the delay between ischaemic index symptom and CEA was analysed.

Results.—The median time from the index symptom to surgery was 47 days (range: 3−688 days). The longest delay was surgery related with a median of 25 days (range: 2−202 days) from the consultation of the vascular surgeon to the operation. Only 11% of the patients were operated within the recommended 2 weeks' time. It was more likely that CEA was performed within 2 weeks if an emergent consultation to Meilahti Hospital neurologist on call did take place (odds ratio (OR) 12.6, 95% confidence interval (CI) 1.5−104, $p = 0.019$).

Conclusion.—Delays from symptom to surgery were generally too long and the in-hospital door-to-knife time (DKT) was long mostly due to waiting for the operation theatre. The investigation of all stroke, amaurosis fugax and transient ischaemic attack patients should be performed on an emergency basis and most optimally centralised to hospitals were carotid surgery is performed.

▶ The timing of carotid surgery after symptoms has been an ongoing source of debate in vascular surgery, but the one factor common is that the time to intervention has been shortened. The recommendation Blaisdell et al to delay surgery 6 to 8 weeks after the neurologic event to decrease the incidence of hemorrhagic conversion of an ischemic stroke has evolved.[1] The precursor to these recommendations was the extremely poor outcomes in patients who underwent carotid endarterectomy (CEA). However, over the last 20 years, numerous series have described shortening this interval to surgery within 2 to 4 weeks. The improved outcomes have been attributed to better imaging of the brain and classifying the degree of ischemia, better surgical techniques and patient selection, and more liberal use of intraluminal shunts. All these factors along with increase in technical expertise have shown that we should be performing CEA sooner in symptomatic patients.[2] The authors of this retrospective study describe their experience at a single center where all CEAs in their region are performed. Over a 1-year period, they examined 100 consecutive patients who were symptomatic, and among these patients, the presenting symptoms were amaurosis fugax (AFX) in 19%, transient ischemic attack (TIA) in 29%, and stroke in 46%. The degree of carotid stenosis was 50% to 70% in 57 patients and 70% to 99% in 43 patients. The timing of surgery was within 4 weeks of presenting symptoms in 32% of patients, and only 11% underwent a procedure within 2 weeks. The factors that were associated with earlier operation (< 2 weeks) were younger age and emergency consultation of the center's neurologist or vascular surgeon. The median time of surgery was 47 days, and the timing was shorter if the index symptom was a minor or major stroke (median, 34 and 22 days, respectively) versus AFX (median, 66 days) and TIA (median, 69 days). Other factors that shortened the delay to intervention were referral to the center as an emergency versus an elective referral, consultation of a vascular surgeon during the first admission, and urgent evaluation of the carotid artery. The authors describe lack of operating room availability as another major limiting factor to early intervention. During this delay, 105 of the patients had progression of their symptoms. Regarding the outcomes, 2 patients had perioperative strokes and 1 patient died.

This study reveals what most surgeons now accept as true: intervention should be performed earlier in symptomatic patients with carotid stenosis; however, the referral may not occur in an expeditious manner. Better understanding of the importance of early CEA in this population by the referring physicians may decrease time delay and lead to earlier intervention.

N. Singh, MD

References

1. Blaisdell WF, Clauss RH, Galbraith JG, Imparato AM, Wylie EJ. Joint study of extracranial arterial occlusion. IV. A review of surgical considerations. *JAMA.* 1969;209:1889-1895.
2. Paty PS, Darling RC 3rd, Feustel PJ, et al. Early carotid endarterectomy after acute stroke. *J Vasc Surg.* 2004;39:148-154.

Carotid Endarterectomy within Seven Days after the Neurological Index Event is Safe and Effective in Stroke Prevention
Rantner B, Kollerits B, Schmidauer C, et al (Innsbruck Med Univ, Austria)
Eur J Vasc Endovasc Surg 42:732-739, 2011

Background.—Timing of surgery remains a controversial subject with some concerns persisting that the benefit of early carotid endarterectomy

(CEA) offsets the perioperative risks. We investigated the neurological outcome of patients with symptomatic internal carotid artery (ICA) stenosis after surgery in relation to the timing of treatment.

Methods.—From January 2005 to June 2010, 468 patients ($n = 349$ male, 74.6%, median age 71 years) underwent CEA for symptomatic stenosis. Perioperative morbidity and mortality rates were assessed in the 30 days' follow-up.

Results.—The median time interval between index event and CEA was 7 days; the overall stroke and death rate reached 3.4%. There was no difference in the 30 days' rate of stroke /death rate, depending on the timing of surgery ($n = 5/241$, 2.1% in patients treated within 1 week vs. $n = 10/215$, 4.7% in patients treated thereafter, $p = 0.12$). Patients with a postoperative neurological deterioration had more often an ischaemic infarction on preoperative cerebral computed tomography (CCT) compared with those without deterioration ($n = 6/15$, 40.0% vs. $n = 39/441$, 9.0%, $p = 0.003$). Logistic regression analysis showed that patients with preoperative infarction on CCT had the highest risk for postoperative neurological deterioration.

Conclusion.—An infarction on the preoperative CCT leads to an increased risk for a postoperative deterioration after CEA. Patients should be treated at an early point in time with bland CCTs.

▶ Carotid artery surgery is the most commonly studied vascular procedure, and to that end, the timing of carotid endarterectomy after an ischemic event has now been found in several studies to be optimized if performed within 2 weeks of the initial event. The authors of this study again reveal that this is true and found that the postoperative stroke and death rate was 3.4% in the 468 patients treated and that there was no significant increase in occurrence if the procedure occurred within a week or later. The authors describe the vital role of preoperative imaging with either cerebral CT or MRI in all their patients including those with a transient ischemic attack or atrial fibrillation. The identification of a recent infarction on preoperative imaging was the most predictive factor of postoperative neurologic complication. On multiple logistic regression analysis, recent infarction was found to increase the risk of postoperative neurological deficit by almost 7-fold (odds ratio, 6.83; 95% confidence interval, 2.14-21.77; $P = .001$).

Obviously, bias can be inferred from the retrospective analysis, but the authors provide yet another study to establish the benefit of early carotid intervention after a neurological event. In addition, they provide another objective finding of preexisting morphological signs of cerebral infarction on preoperative cerebral CT that can alert the surgeon to increased risk of postoperative neurologic issues when contemplating a carotid endarterectomy. As in most instances, it is not the surgeon who delays surgery but often the timing of the referral, and the authors describe their method to obviate this by having an interdisciplinary conference composed of neurologists, interventional radiologists, and vascular surgeons that assesses the clinical findings as well as the imaging to decide on the timing of surgery. This factor is likely the most important method to achieve a median time of 7 days from the initial neurologic event to the procedure.

N. Singh, MD

Patients With Severe Asymptomatic Carotid Artery Stenosis Do Not Have a Higher Risk of Stroke and Mortality After Coronary Artery Bypass Surgery

Mahmoudi M, Hill PC, Xue Z, et al (Washington Hosp Ctr, DC)
Stroke 42:2801-2805, 2011

Background and Purpose.—Stroke development is a major concern in patients undergoing coronary artery bypass grafting (CABG). Whether asymptomatic severe carotid artery stenosis (CAS) contributes to the development of stroke and mortality in such patients remains uncertain.

Methods.—A retrospective analysis of 878 consecutive patients with documented carotid duplex ultrasound who underwent isolated CABG in our institution from January 2003 to December 2009 was performed. Patients with severe CAS (n = 117) were compared with those without severe CAS (n = 761) to assess the rates of stroke and mortality during hospitalization for CABG. The 30-day mortality rate was also assessed.

Results.—Patients with severe CAS were older and had a higher prevalence of peripheral arterial disease and heart failure. Patients with severe CAS had similar rates of in-hospital stroke (3.4% versus 3.6%; $P = 1.0$) and mortality (3.4% versus 4.2%; $P = 1.0$) compared with patients without severe CAS. The 30-day rate of mortality was also similar between the 2 cohorts (3.4% versus 2.9%; $P = 0.51$).

Conclusions.—Severe CAS alone is not a risk factor for stroke or mortality in patients undergoing CABG. The decision to perform carotid imaging and subsequent revascularization in association with CABG must be individualized and based on clinical judgment (Fig).

▶ There are multiple postulated mechanisms for stroke in association with coronary artery bypass grafting (CABG). Stroke may arise from hypoperfusion secondary to a severely stenotic carotid artery, embolization from an ulcerated plaque, introduction of air during the procedure, or calcific debris from a diseased

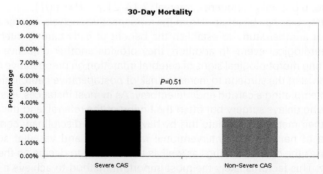

FIGURE.—Thirty-day mortality in patients with and without severe carotid artery stenosis (CAS). (Reprinted from Mahmoudi M, Hill PC, Xue Z, et al. Patients with severe asymptomatic carotid artery stenosis do not have a higher risk of stroke and mortality after coronary artery bypass surgery. *Stroke.* 2011;42:2801-2805, with permission from American Heart Association, Inc.)

valve or aorta. Stroke complicates CABG approximately 2% of the time.[1] Most of these strokes occur within 24 hours of operation, and mortality is up to 25%. There is significant controversy as to optimal management of patients undergoing CABG who have severe carotid artery stenosis, which may have a prevalence up to 20% in patients undergoing CABG.[2] The main finding of this study is that severe carotid artery stenosis was not associated with an increased risk of in-hospital stroke, in-hospital mortality, or 30-day mortality following CABG (Fig). Ricotta et al has found that major morbidity of combining carotid endarterectomy (CEA) with CABG relates to patient comorbidities rather than the CEA.[3] Others, however, have found, similar to this study, that the presence of severe carotid artery stenosis in itself does not significantly contribute to neurologic complication rates following CABG. It would seem that the preponderance of the data suggest that performance of CEA to facilitate safety of CABG is not justified. The decision to perform CEA must be made on individual patient merit irrespective of the need for coronary surgery. This comes on a background of increasing scrutiny and criticism regarding the merits of prophylactic carotid artery procedures.

G. L. Moneta, MD

References

1. Naylor AR, Mehta Z, Rothwell PM, Bell PR. Carotid artery disease and stroke during coronary artery bypass: a critical review of the literature. *Eur J Vas Endovasc Surg.* 2002;23:283-294.
2. Qureshi A, Alexandrov AV, Tegeler CH, et al. Guidelines for screening of extracranial carotid artery disease: a statement for healthcare professionals from the multidisciplinary practice guidelines committee of the American Society of Neuroimaging; cosponsored by the Society of Vascular and Interventional Neurology. *J Neuroimaging.* 2007;17:19-47.
3. Ricotta JJ, Wall LP, Blackstone E. The influence of concurrent carotid endarterectomy on coronary bypass: a case-controlled study. *J Vasc Surg.* 2005;41:397-401.

Staged Versus Synchronous Carotid Endarterectomy and Coronary Artery Bypass Grafting: Analysis of 10-Year Nationwide Outcomes

Gopaldas RR, Chu D, Dao TK, et al (Univ of Missouri-Columbia School of Medicine; Baylor College of Medicine, Houston, TX; The Michael E. DeBakey Veterans Affairs Med Ctr, Houston, TX; et al)
Ann Thorac Surg 91:1323-1329, 2011

Background.—The timing of operative interventions for patients with concurrent carotid and coronary artery disease is controversial. We evaluated nationwide data regarding staged or synchronous carotid endarterectomy (CEA) and coronary artery bypass grafting (CABG) and compared the two approaches' outcome profiles.

Methods.—From Nationwide Inpatient Sample database 1998 to 2007, we identified 6,153 (28.9%) patients who underwent CEA before or after CABG during the same hospital admission but not on the same day (STAGED) and 16,639 patients who underwent both procedures on the same day (SYNC). Hierarchic multivariable regression was used to assess the independent effect of operative strategy on mortality, neurologic and overall complications, and charges.

Results.—Mean age (69.5 ± 9.0 years) and Charlson-Deyo score (4.6 ± 1.5) were similar for both groups. Mortality (4.2% vs 4.5%) or neurologic complications (3.5% vs 3.9%) were similar between the STAGED and SYNC groups ($p > 0.7$ for both). The STAGED patients had higher morbidity (48.4% vs 42.6%; odds ratio [OR] 1.8; 95% confidence interval [CI], 1.5 to 2.2; $p < 0.001$) and more cardiac (OR, 1.5; 95% CI, 1.4 to 1.7; $p < 0.001$), wound (OR, 2.1; 95% CI, 1.8 to 2.4; $p < 0.001$), respiratory (OR, 1.2; 95% CI, 1.1 to 1.3; $p = 0.001$), and renal complications (OR, 1.2; 95% CI, 1.03 to 1.3; $p < 0.001$). In SYNC patients, on-pump CABG increased stroke rates (OR, 1.6; 95% CI, 1.3 to 1.9; $p < 0.001$). The STAGED procedures were independently associated with higher hospital charges by \$23,328 ($p < 0.001$).

Conclusions.—We identified no significant difference in mortality or neurologic complications between STAGED and SYNC approaches. Staged procedures were associated with a greater risk of overall complications and higher hospital charges than SYNC. On-pump CABG was associated with higher stroke rates in SYNC patients.

▶ There continues to be no definitive answer to the question of what to do with patients requiring both carotid endarterectomy (CEA) and coronary artery bypass grafting (CABG) in close proximity to each other. This study would favor a simultaneous procedure, in that hospital charges are higher with staged procedures, while neurologic complications and mortality were not significantly different in staged versus simultaneous procedures. However, the exact severity of the carotid or coronary disease is unknown in these patients. We do not know what proportion of patients underwent a so-called staged procedure to treat a complication of the initial procedure. Patients who had separate but temporarily close admissions for CABG and CEA are not identified by these studies but could in effect have undergone staged procedures. Finally, in about half the patients in this study, data on dates of admission, operation, or discharge were missing, thus preventing classifying operations as synchronous or staged. The best that one can conclude from this article is that it does not discredit the practice of simultaneous CEA and CABG. However, given the weaknesses of the article, it is also not strong evidence toward the performance of synchronous procedures.

G. L. Moneta, MD

Emergent Endovascular Recanalization for Cervical Internal Carotid Artery Occlusion in Patients Presenting With Acute Stroke
Hauck EF, Natarajan SK, Ohta H, et al (Univ at Buffalo, NY)
Neurosurgery 69:899-907, 2011

Background.—Acute proximal (cervical) internal carotid artery (ICA) occlusion may cause ischemia of an entire hemisphere or no ischemia at all, depending on the presence of intracranial collaterals.

Objective.—To retrospectively analyze the clinical results for emergent endovascular carotid recanalization in patients with acute proximal (cervical) ICA occlusion and to assess predictors of recanalization and clinical, neurological, and functional outcome.

Methods.—Emergent endovascular revascularization was attempted in 22 patients presenting with acute stroke secondary to complete cervical ICA occlusion. Patients with pseudo-occlusion were excluded. Recanalization was assessed with the Thrombolysis in Myocardial Ischemia (TIMI) system: grade 0 (no flow) to grade 3 (normal flow).

Results.—The median age of the patients was 65 years; mean admission National Institutes of Health Stroke Scale (NIHSS) score was 14. Recanalization (TIMI grade 2/3) occurred in 17 patients (77.3%). Ten patients (45.5%) demonstrated significant clinical improvement during hospitalization (NIHSS improved ≥4 points). Fifty percent of patients had good outcomes (modified Rankin Scale ≤2) after a median follow-up of 3 months. Patient age <70 years and successful recanalization (TIMI grade 2/3) predicted a good outcome ($P \leq .01$). Presence of atrial fibrillation, admission NIHSS score ≥20, and complete ICA occlusion at all levels (cervical, petrocavernous, and intracranial) were associated with poor outcomes ($P \leq .05$). Patients with complete cervical ICA occlusion but partial distal preservation of the vessel were most likely to benefit from the intervention (recanalization in 88.2%; good outcome in 64.7%).

Conclusion.—Attempts at emergent endovascular carotid recanalization for acute stroke are encouraged, particularly in younger patients with partial distal preservation of the ICA (Fig 2).

▶ There has been a recent surge of interest in endovascular intervention for acute carotid occlusion.[1-3] Authors have demonstrated better- than- expected successful recanalization rates (50%–65%) and an improvement in neurologic status in some patients. In 1 study, mortality was 30% with recanalization of the internal carotid artery (ICA), but mortality was 73% in the nonrecanalized patients.[4] In this clinical series, the authors present their results with emergent endovascular carotid recanalization in patients with acute proximal (cervical) ICA occlusion. The authors' technique involves initially advancing a platform guide catheter into the common carotid artery just proximal to the bifurcation. They would then explore the carotid artery bifurcation with a microcatheter and microwire with subsequent advancement of a microcatheter into the petrocavernous segment of the carotid artery. If distal patency could not be demonstrated, the procedure was aborted. If distal patency was present (Fig 2) or could be restored, they then attempted to restore flow in the cervical ICA. They sought to assess success rates, predictors of recanalization, and neurological and functional outcome. The results presented here are not "what dreams are made of," but they are arguably better than the natural history of the disease. The stakes are high, and it may be the patients who do the best would have done reasonably well even without interventional treatment. The approach advocated here must be tempered with knowledge of hemorrhage risk and considered in the context of pretreatment infarct size. Whereas 50% of the patients had a favorable outcome, all patients with initial

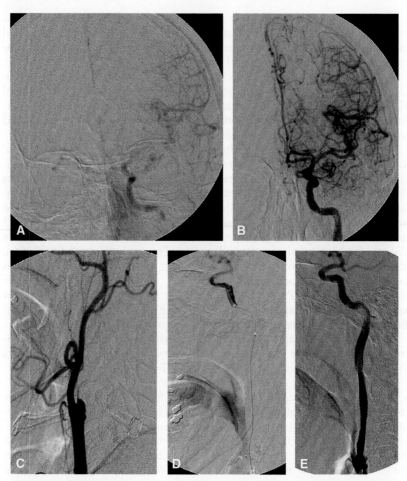

FIGURE 2.—Angiographic images of the same patient as in Figure 1. **A,** digital subtraction angiogram, anteroposterior projection, intracranial view, before intervention. Notice the reconstitution of the internal carotid artery (ICA) distal to the petrocavernous segment via external carotid artery collaterals. **B,** digital subtraction angiogram, anteroposterior intracranial view, after intervention. Extensive filling of the left anterior and middle cerebral artery branches consistent with hyperperfusion. **C,** digital subtraction angiogram, lateral cervical view, before intervention demonstrating complete proximal (cervical) ICA occlusion. **D,** working view, distal microinjection. Notice the 9F Concentric balloon catheter (Concentric Medical) at the level of the carotid bifurcation with the Nautica microcatheter (ev3) advanced into the petrous ICA segment. The microrun confirms distal patency, suggesting likely recanalization with carotid stenting. **E,** digital subtraction angiogram, lateral view after deployment of a Wallstent (Boston Scientific) for successful ICA revascularization. Proximal protection was provided with balloon occlusion of the common carotid artery and simultaneous suction/aspiration. (Reprinted from Hauck EF, Natarajan SK, Ohta H, et al. Emergent endovascular recanalization for cervical internal carotid artery occlusion in patients presenting with acute stroke. *Neurosurgery.* 2011;69:899-907.)

complete carotid artery occlusion, including the intracranial segments, either died or were severely disabled, suggesting this approach be limited to patients with partial carotid reconstitution above the level of the cervical ICA occlusion.

G. L. Moneta, MD

References

1. Zaidat OO, Alexander MJ, Suarez JI, et al. Early carotid artery stenting and angioplasty in patients with acute ischemic stroke. *Neurosurgery.* 2004;55:1237-1242.
2. Dabitz R, Triebe S, Leppmeier U, Ochs G, Vorwerk D. Percutaneous recanalization of acute internal carotid artery occlusions in patients with severe stroke. *Cardiovasc Intervent Radiol.* 2007;30:34-41.
3. Miyamoto N, Naito I, Takatama S, Shimizu T, Iwai T, Shimaguchi H. Urgent stenting for patients with acute stroke due to atherosclerotic occlusive lesions of the cervical internal carotid artery. *Neurol Med Chir (Tokyo).* 2008;48:49-55.
4. Flint AC, Duckwiler GR, Budzik RF, Liebeskind DS, Smith WS; MERCI and Multi MERCI Writing Committee. Mechanical thrombectomy of intracranial internal carotid occlusion: pooled results of the MERCI and Multi MERCI Part I trials. *Stroke.* 2007;38:1274-1280.

A Systematic Review of Stenting and Angioplasty of Symptomatic Extracranial Vertebral Artery Stenosis

Stayman AN, Nogueira RG, Gupta R (Vanderbilt Univ School of Medicine, Nashville, TN; Emory Univ School of Medicine, Atlanta, GA)
Stroke 42:2212-2216, 2011

Background and Purpose.—Extracranial vertebral artery stenosis (ECVAS) is common among patients with ischemic stroke. Despite the limited knowledge of the natural history of patients with symptomatic vertebral disease, endovascular revascularization techniques are now utilized in clinical practice. We sought to determine the risk of endovascular treatment for ECVAS with a systematic review of the literature.

Methods.—A search strategy was used using the terms "stenting," "vertebral," "ostium," "origin," and "extracranial" through Medline. All articles were reviewed along with their references to determine the risk and durability of endovascular treatment.

Results.—A total of 27 articles were identified that met inclusion criterion, with a total of 980 of 993 patients treated with stents. The majority of patients (56%) were noted to have contralateral vertebral artery stenosis or occlusion and 92% were symptomatic at the time of treatment. A total of 11 patients (1.1%) experienced a stroke and 8 (0.8%) experienced a transient ischemic attack within 30 days of the procedure. Drugeluting stents were associated with lower restenosis rates (11%) compared to bare metal stents (30%) at a mean of 24 months of follow-up.

Conclusions.—Stenting and angioplasty of ECVAS appear to have a low rate of periprocedural stroke or transient ischemic attack and restenosis rates that may not be as high as suspected. Given the frequency of ECVAS as an etiology for ischemic stroke, future studies aimed at determining efficacy of this treatment modality relative to medical therapy would be of benefit to clinicians caring for these patients.

▶ It is increasingly recognized that vertebral artery stenosis may be a more significant etiology for stroke than previously thought. Stenosis of the extracranial vertebral arteries is the second most common area of stenosis in the extracranial cerebrovascular circulation, second only to disease of the carotid bifurcation. Stroke registries suggest that strokes in the posterior circulation account for up to 25% of all ischemic cerebral vascular events.[1] Surgical reconstruction of the origin of the vertebral artery is infrequently performed in most centers. Therefore, placement of stents at the origin of the vertebral artery is potentially therapeutically useful in patients with vertebral artery stenosis should such stent placement be safe and reasonably durable. Despite the lack of high-level data supporting stenting of the vertebral arteries, it has become increasingly used in clinical practice. The authors sought to examine the available data on vertebral artery stenting through a systematic review of the available literature. The review used the bulk of available data on stenting of the extracranial vertebral arteries. There is clearly heterogeneity in clinical and angiographic follow-up, outcome measures, and patient selection, all of which limit the analysis of the data. Nevertheless, the data that are available suggest the feasibility and safety of stenting the vertebral artery origin is perhaps better than many would have thought. Technical success rates were 99.3% as evidenced by less than 20% residual stenosis at the conclusion of the procedure. The study did not focus on medical management used in conjunction with vertebral artery stenting prior to or after vertebral artery stenting. Clearly the question remains as to how the combination of optimal medical management and vertebral artery stenting will compare with optimal medical management alone in a long-term prevention of posterior circulation infarct.

G. L. Moneta, MD

Reference

1. Moulin T, Tatu L, Vuillier F, Berger E, Chavot D, Rumbach L. Role of a stroke data bank in evaluating cerebral infarction subtypes: patterns and outcome of 1,776 consecutive patients from the Besançon stroke registry. *Cerebrovasc Dis.* 2000;10:261-271.

Neurosonographic monitoring of 105 spontaneous cervical artery dissections: A prospective study
Baracchini C, Tonello S, Meneghetti G, et al (Univ of Padua, Padova, Italy)
Neurology 75:1864-1870, 2010

Objective.—To monitor the sonographic course of spontaneous cervical artery dissections (sCADs) and investigate their recanalization and recurrence rates.

Methods.—All consecutive patients with an MRI-proven sCAD were prospectively evaluated by neurovascular ultrasound (nUS) daily while in hospital, then monthly for the first 6 months after discharge and every 6 months thereafter, for a mean follow-up period of 58 months (range, 28–96 months).

Results.—A total of 105 sCADs were detected in 76 patients: 61 (58.1%) involved the internal carotid artery and 44 (41.9%) the vertebral artery, while multiple sCADs were found in 4 patients (5.3%). Follow-up was obtained in 74 patients (97.3%, 103 vessels). The complete and hemodynamically significant (<50% stenosis) recanalization rates were 51.4% (53/103) and 20.4% (21/103). All but one complete recanalization occurred within the first 9 months. There were early recurrences (while in hospital) in 20 previously unaffected arteries (26.3%) and late recurrences in 2 arteries (2.7%), site of a previous sCAD. All patients (n = 6) with a family history of arterial dissection had a sCAD recurrence (4 early and 2 late) as opposed to 16 (22.8%) among those with no known familial disease (*p* < 0.001).

Conclusions.—These results suggest that most lumen changes occur within the first few months after the initial event, but recanalization may occur even after 1 year. Early recurrence is not uncommon and usually involves arteries previously unaffected by dissection, while the risk of late recurrence is low. A family history of arterial dissection is strongly associated with sCAD recurrence (Fig 1).

▶ Spontaneous cervical artery dissections (sCADs) are a leading cause of stroke in young adults and result from an intramural hematoma of unknown origin. This hematoma may occur within the medial or adventitial layers. When it occurs within the medial layer, it frequently causes arterial stenosis or occlusion and leads to cerebral ischemia, most frequently secondary to embolization and less frequently from low flow. When the mural hematoma is subadventitial, the usual symptoms are pain secondary to compression of adjacent structures. Although cervical artery mural hematomas are best detected by cervical MRI with T1 fat suppression, vascular ultrasound, in reality, is the test most frequently used to follow patients with sCAD. In this study, the authors used consecutive patients with MRI-proven sCAD. Patients were prospectively followed by duplex ultrasound daily in the hospital, monthly for the first 6 months after discharge, and every 6 months thereafter. It is generally acknowledged that sCAD is a highly dynamic process following the initial event. Information on recanalization and

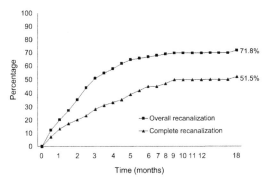

FIGURE 1.—Time to overall (diamonds) and complete (squares) recanalization. Percentages on the right represent the recanalization rates at 18 months for vessels with overall and complete recanalization. (Reprinted from Baracchini C, Tonello S, Meneghetti G, et al. Neurosonographic monitoring of 105 spontaneous cervical artery dissections: a prospective study. *Neurology.* 2010;75:1864-1870, with permission from AAN Enterprises, INC.)

recurrence rates in patients with sCAD is, however, limited, and the authors data help clarify recanalization rates of dissected cervical arteries (Fig 1). There are several other interesting points in the authors' data. First, although recurrence of sCAD is reasonably uncommon, it generally occurs early following the initial event and in a different cervical artery. The early recurrence rate reported here of 25% is considerably higher than previously suspected and may relate to the rigorous follow-up protocol used by the authors. The fact that late sCAD recurrence can happen in previously affected arteries suggests recurrence following sCAD in the early and late periods may have different pathologic mechanisms. Perhaps, as the authors point out, early recurrences are correlated with a transient arterial disorder such as a vasculitis, whereas late recurrences may be indicative of underlying persistent connective tissue weakness. The high early recurrence rate suggests that aggressive treatment of sCAD, perhaps including control of double product and lowering blood pressure within the constraints imposed by the neurologic pathology, should be implemented.

G. L. Moneta, MD

13 Vascular Trauma

Imaging vascular trauma

Patterson BO, on behalf of the London Vascular Injuries Working Group (St George's Univ of London, UK)
Br J Surg 99:494-505, 2012

Background.—Over the past 50 years the management of vascular trauma has changed from mandatory surgical exploration to selective non-operative treatment, where possible. Accurate, non-invasive, diagnostic imaging techniques are the key to this strategy. The purpose of this review was to define optimal first-line imaging in patients with suspected vascular injury in different anatomical regions.

Methods.—A systematic review was performed of literature relating to radiological diagnosis of vascular trauma over the past decade (2000–2010). Studies were included if the main focus was initial diagnosis of blunt or penetrating vascular injury and more than ten patients were included.

Results.—Of 1511 titles identified, 58 articles were incorporated in the systematic review. Most described the use of computed tomography angiography (CTA). The application of duplex ultrasonography, magnetic resonance imaging/angiography and transoesophageal echocardiography was described, but significant drawbacks were highlighted for each. CTA displayed acceptable sensitivity and specificity for diagnosing vascular trauma in blunt and penetrating vascular injury within the neck and extremity, as well as for blunt aortic injury.

Conclusion.—Based on the evidence available, CTA should be the first-line investigation for all patients with suspected vascular trauma and no indication for immediate operative intervention (Table 7).

▶ This article points out that the available literature currently suggests that computed tomography angiography (CTA) is the best first-line investigation

TABLE 7.—Potential Pitfalls in the Use of Computed Tomography Angiography for Assessment of Extremity Vascular Trauma (After Miller-Thomas et al.[92])

Venous injury may be missed if dual-phase imaging is not used
'Pseudothrombus' artefact may occur if the venous phase is too early
Patient movement artefacts are more common in trauma
Extravasation of contrast or failure of injection equipment can reduce opacification
Preset contrast bolus timings may be an underestimate in low cardiac output states

Editor's Note: Please refer to original journal article for full reference.

for all patients with suspected vascular trauma and no indication for immediate operative intervention. One actually would have to be living in a cave to not realize that over the last decade, CTA has emerged as the preferred imaging modality in patients with traumatic injuries. The important part of the article is not so much the final conclusion that CTA is the best imaging for screening for vascular injury but an analysis of the quality of the data on which this conclusion is based. The authors point out that the data are based on a mixture of prospective and retrospective studies without standard protocols for when CTAs should be performed. Much of the literature originates from level 1 trauma centers with a special interest in application of CTA in the evaluation of the trauma victim. The data from such centers may be subject to publication bias. In addition, earlier studies with less-sophisticated CT technology may have underestimated the accuracy of CTA. Close study of the tables in the article is suggested, and the tables indicate CTA is virtually 100% diagnostic in the evaluation of extremity arterial injury and penetrating cervical vascular injury. The data are a bit more mixed for the evaluation of blunt aortic injury and blunt cervical vascular injury. The article is also valuable in pointing out potential pitfalls in the use of CTA for diagnosis of vascular injury (Table 7). Overall, this is a good summary of the evidence of the accuracy of CTA in diagnosis of vascular injury.

G. L. Moneta, MD

A 5-year review of management of lower extremity arterial injuries at an urban level I trauma center

Franz RW, Shah KJ, Halaharvi D, et al (Vascular and Vein Ctr at Grant Med Ctr, Columbus, OH; Doctors Hosp, Columbus, OH; et al)
J Vasc Surg 53:1604-1610, 2011

Background.—The purpose of this study was to review the management of lower extremity arterial injuries to determine incidence, assess the current management strategy, and evaluate hospital outcome.

Methods.—This was a retrospective review, including trauma database query, and medical records review set in an urban level I trauma center. Sixty-five patients with 75 lower extremity arterial injuries were admitted between April 2005 and April 2010. The interventions were primary amputation, medical management, vascular surgical intervention, and subsequent amputation. The main outcome measures were age, gender, race, mechanism of injury, type of injury, associated lower extremity injuries, concomitant injuries, Injury Severity Score, Abbreviated Injury Scale, surgical procedures and interventions, limb salvage rate, mortality, length of stay, and discharge disposition.

Results.—During a 5-year period, 65 patients with 75 lower extremity arterial injuries were admitted to the hospital, yielding an incidence of 0.39% among trauma admissions. The study population was comprised primarily of young men, with a mean Injury Severity Score of 15.2 and a mean Abbreviated Injury Scale of 2.7 (moderate to severe injuries). The majority of patients (78.4%) suffered concomitant lower extremity injuries, most frequently bony or venous injuries, whereas 35.4% experienced associated injuries to other body regions. The most common injury mechanism was a gunshot wound (46.7%). Arterial injuries were categorized into 42 penetrating (56.0%) and 33 blunt mechanisms (44.0%). Involved arterial distribution was as follows: 4 common femoral (5.3%), 4 profunda femoris (5.3%), 24 superficial femoral (32.0%), 16 popliteal (21.3%), and 27 tibial (36.0%) arteries. The types of arterial injuries were as follows: 28 occlusion (37.3%), 23 transection (30.7%), 16 laceration (21.3%), and 8 dissection (10.7%). Orthopedic surgeons performed amputations as primary procedures in 3 patients (4.6%). The majority (76.8%) of injuries receiving vascular management underwent surgical intervention, with procedure distribution as follows: 26 bypass (49.1%); 13 primary repair (24.5%); 7 ligation (13.2%); 4 endovascular (7.5%); and 3 isolated thrombectomy (5.7%) procedures. Concomitant venous repair and fasciotomy were performed in 22.4% and 38.2% of cases, respectively. Medication was the primary strategy for 16 arterial injuries (23.2%). Subsequent major amputation was required for 3 patients (4.8%) who initially received vascular management. Three patients (4.6%) died during hospitalization.

Conclusion.—The current multidisciplinary team management approach, including use of computed tomographic or conventional angiography and prompt surgical management, resulted in successful outcomes after lower extremity arterial injuries and will continue to be utilized.

▶ Dr Franz and colleagues present their review of the management of civilian trauma from 2005 to 2010. In this review, the authors reach their stated goal of providing more specific detail on the incidence of lower extremity arterial injuries. They've found that tibial arteries are most frequently injured, most commonly the posterior tibial artery. I found it more interesting, however, to see how the civilian management of vascular trauma has learned from the lessons of the military during the previous 5 years in the wars in Iraq and Afghanistan. The use of computed tomography (CT) angiography has now become routine for the diagnosis of vascular injuries in patients without overt signs. In the young trauma patient population, CT angiography has little artifact and can be done rapidly with 150 mL of contrast with little morbidity. Once diagnosed, arterial injuries are repaired using standard techniques commonly used by both civilian and military surgeons. Some unique aspects, as pointed out in this article, include routing of grafts through clean tissue planes that sometimes require them to be extra anatomic, ensuring good graft coverage, which sometimes may require rotational muscle flaps. Preferred techniques of arterial repair include simple suture repair; end-to-end primary repair; interposition grafting with vein preferably, prosthetic if not possible; and finally, ligation. The use of endovascular methods of vascular injury repair was mentioned but without a large experience in this series. Techniques such as coil embolization and covered stent repair have been used successfully in several civilian and military series. In addition, the authors appropriately emphasize the importance of vein repair prior to arterial repair in most, with ligation used for those unstable patients. Fasciotomies should be performed liberally through extensile incisions and continually monitored for efficacy. The authors, however, did not mention the importance of obtaining proximal control of extremity vascular injuries. In the military experience, the application of tourniquets have been extremely successful in preserving life in these patients. Despite this success, junctional vascular injury control remains a morbid and often fatal event. Injuries at this location have taken on more importance, as they are responsible for one-third of soldiers being killed in action over the last 10 years. This is an area of extreme importance for the military and civilian communities alike and a current focus for Department of Defense research and investigation.

D. L. Gillespie, MD, FACS

Lower extremity vascular injuries: Increased mortality for minorities and the uninsured?
Crandall M, Sharp D, Brasel K, et al (Dept of Surgery at Northwestern Univ Feinberg School of Medicine, Chicago, IL; Dept of Surgery at the Med College of Wisconsin, Milwaukee; et al)
Surgery 150:656-664, 2011

Background.—There is increasing evidence to suggest that racial disparities exist in outcomes for trauma. Minorities and the uninsured have been found to have higher mortality rates for blunt and penetrating trauma. However, mechanisms for these disparities are incompletely understood. Limiting the inquiry to a homogenous group, those with lower extremity vascular injuries (LEVIs), may clarify these disparities.

Methods.—The National Trauma Data Bank (NTDB; version 7.0, American College of Surgeons) was used for this study. LEVIs were identified using codes from the International Classification of Diseases, 9th revision. Univariate and multivariate analyses were performed using Stata software (version 11; StataCorp, LP, College Station, TX).

Results.—Records were reviewed for 4,928 LEVI patients. The mechanism of injury was blunt in 2,452 (49.8%), penetrating in 2,452 (49.8%), and unknown in 24 cases (0.5%). Mortality was similar by mechanism (7.6% overall). Regression analysis using mechanism as a covariate revealed a significantly worse mortality for people of color (POC; odds ratio [OR], 1.45; 95% confidence interval [CI], 1.03–2.02; $P = .03$) and the uninsured (UN; OR, 1.62; 95% CI, 1.15–2.23; $P = .006$). However, when separate analyses were performed stratifying by mechanism, no significant mortality disparities were found for blunt trauma (POC OR, 1.28; 95% CI, 0.85–1.96; $P = .23$; UN OR, 1.33; 95% CI, 0.78–2.22; $P = .29$), but disparities remained for penetrating trauma (POC OR, 1.81; 95% CI, 0.93–3.57; $P = .08$; UN OR, 1.85; 95% CI, 1.18–2.94; $P = .009$).

Conclusion.—For patients with LEVI, mortality disparities based on race or insurance status were only observed for penetrating trauma. It is possible that injury heterogeneity or patient cohort differences may partly explain mortality disparities that have been observed between racial and socioeconomic groups.

▶ The US Department of Health and Human Services reported in 1985 that 60 000 excess deaths occur in minority populations each year.[1] Investigators have found that outcome disparities for Medicaid patients, people of color, and the uninsured may be partially attributable to differences in baseline health care characteristics or hospital performance.[2] The authors considered that among trauma patients, heterogeneity of injury, difficulties in injury measurement, and a lack of standardized pre- or postinjury care may contribute to potential disparities in trauma outcomes, including vascular injury. Their hypothesis was that mortality rate disparities by socioeconomic status and race could be potentially explained by injury heterogeneity. This study suggests injury heterogeneity may, at least partially, explain mortality disparities observed between racial and socioeconomic groups. Mechanism of injury may partially drive mortality because of facilities in which patients with penetrating injuries are treated, provider bias in treating patients with injuries caused by violence, or other unknown physiologic or sociologic confounders. Data here, however, clearly indicate race and insurance status influence mortality after penetrating lower extremity vascular injuries and that the magnitude of the association is large.

G. L. Moneta, MD

References

1. US Department of Health and Human Services. *Report of the Secretary's Task Force on Black and Minority Health: Volume I: Executive Summary.* GPO; 1985.
2. Osborne NH, Upchurch GR Jr, Mathur AK, Dimick JB. Explaining racial disparities in mortality after abdominal aortic aneurysm repair. *J Vasc Surg.* 2009;50: 709-713.

Embolisation for Vascular Injuries Complicating Elective Orthopaedic Surgery
Mavrogenis AF, Rossi G, Rimondi E, et al (Univ of Bologna, Italy; Istituto Ortopedico Rizzoli, Italy)
Eur J Vasc Endovasc Surg 42:676-683, 2011

Objectives.—The study aims to present the indications and emphasise the role of embolisation for vascular injuries in orthopaedic surgery.

Methods.—Thirty-one patients with vascular injuries complicating elective orthopaedic surgery had embolisation from 2003 to 2010. N-2-butyl cyano-acrylate (NBCA) was used as embolic agent in 28 patients, gelatin sponge in three and coil embolisation in addition to NBCA or gelatin sponge in two patients. The mean follow-up period was 37 months (range, 4—96 months).

Results.—The most common orthopaedic operations associated with vascular injuries amenable to embolisation were hip-joint procedures; and the most common injuries were arterial tears of branch vessels or non-critical

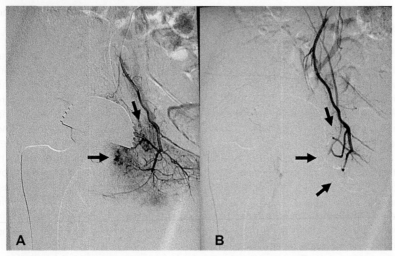

FIGURE 2.—AB. A 39-year-old woman with swelling and wound bleeding after right total hip arthroplasty (Patient 11). (A) Selective angiography and catheterization of the inferior glutaeal artery at 2 days after the operation shows contrast leakage (*arrows*). (B) Completion angiography after NBCA embolisation shows occlusion of the bleeding vessels (*arrows*). (Reprinted from European Journal of Vascular and Endovascular Surgery, Mavrogenis AF, Rossi G, Rimondi E, et al. Embolisation for vascular injuries complicating elective orthopaedic surgery. *Eur J Vasc Endovasc Surg*. 2011;42:676-683. Copyright 2011, with permission from the European Society for Vascular Surgery.)

axial vessels, most commonly of the superior glutaeal artery. In all cases, angiography showed the bleeding point, and a single embolisation session effectively stopped bleeding. Embolisation-related complications were not observed.

Conclusions.—Embolisation should be considered the treatment of choice for vascular injuries of branch vessels or non-critical axial vessels following elective orthopaedic surgery because of the advantages of minimally invasive therapy and the lack of complications (Fig 2).

▶ The incidence of vascular complications in orthopedic surgery is 0.005% to 0.5%.[1] The management of these injuries is by no means standard; however, more often than not they are currently being approached using minimally invasive techniques. Herein presented is the largest series to date (albeit still small) describing embolization for vascular injuries complicating elective orthopedic surgical operations.

Vascular injuries are most commonly associated with procedures involving the knee. These injuries are overwhelmingly managed by direct open surgical repair. In this series of 31 patients at a single institution, the most common orthopedic procedures associated with a vascular injury amenable to embolization were hip-joint procedures (Fig 2).

The embolic agent of choice was N-2 butyl cyanoacrylate. The most commonly embolized vessel was the superior gluteal artery. Technical points involving embolotherapy are described.

B. W. Starnes, MD

Reference

1. Wilson JS, Miranda A, Johnson B, Shames M. Vascular injuries associated with elective orthopedic procedures. *Ann Vasc Surg.* 2003;17:641-644.

Long-term Follow-up of Vascular Reconstructions after Supracondylar Humerus Fracture with Vascular Lesion in Childhood
Konstantiniuk P, Fritz G, Ott T, et al (Univ Hosp Graz, Austria; General Hosp Leoben, Austria)
Eur J Vasc Endovasc Surg 42:684-688, 2011

Introduction.—Supracondylar humerus fractures in childhood present with a pulseless but well-perfused hand in 2.6% of cases and with limb-threatening ischaemia in <1%. Conservative treatment is widely used in non-limb-threatening ischaemia, in particular if the child is very young (<2.5 years). It has been sufficiently proven that conservative treatment may retard growth. The aim of our study was to determine long-term patency rates after surgical reconstruction and growth impairment, if any, after surgical vascular reconstruction.

Patients and Methods.—Between June 1990 and June 2004, 12 children (mean age 6.6 years, eight boys and four girls) with supracondylar fracture with vascular lesions underwent surgical reconstruction at the Department of Vascular Surgery at the University Hospital, Graz. Patient files were reviewed retrospectively. All patients were recalled for physical (forearm length and volume) and ultrasonographic examinations (forearm blood flow) in 2005 and for ultrasonographic examinations (reconstructed vascular area) in 2011, with a final mean follow-up time of 14.0 years (range 6.8—20.9 years).

Results.—Twelve patients, 10 of whom had undergone growth measurements in 2005, were available for the latter examination. All were doing well, with patent vascular reconstructions. Seven reconstructed brachial arteries were enlarged, two of which with intramural calcifications, four did not show abnormalities and one presented with 45% thinning. There were no differences between affected and healthy forearms concerning volume, length and blood flow.

Conclusions.—Our data emphasise that surgical reconstruction is effective in terms of blood supply and growth. In cases with interposition of greater saphenous vein or venous patch plasty, we found a high risk for development of enlargements. We suggest that these patients be followed periodically, with ultrasound studies, to detect aneurysms and/or thrombotic changes as early as possible.

▶ Most pediatric fractures (75%) involve the upper extremity.[1] Fractures above the elbow, however, represent only about 8% of all upper extremity fractures in children, with supracondylar humerus fractures being the most common upper arm fracture in children. Of the children with supracondylar fractures, 2.6% will present with a pulseless, but well-perfused hand.[2] Conservative treatment is widely used in such cases of nonlimb-threatening ischemia.[3] However, there is concern that situations with reduced blood supply to the epiphyseal region and reduced muscular blood flow will retard growth. Growth retardation, however, may also be a result of sequelae of the fractures with disturbances of the epiphyseal cartilage. The authors sought to better understand potential growth changes of the upper extremity following supracondylar fracture complicated by arterial insufficiency with subsequent arterial repair. They also sought to describe changes in the repair site during follow-up. The data indicate that in these children with repaired arterial injury following supracondylar fracture, if the grafts remain patent, the forearm development is normal during follow-up. The authors did find, and this is of some concern, that the grafts placed for repair of the brachial artery appear to have a high risk for development of ectatic lesions. It is unknown whether these lesions will go on to be affected by partial thrombosis and a tendency to embolize distally into the hand. In light of these findings, the authors suggest children with arterial repairs necessitated by a supracondylar fracture be followed indefinably and their grafts undergo periodic ultrasound imaging.

G. L. Moneta, MD

References

1. Klimkiewicz JJ. In: DeLee D, ed. *Orthopedic Sports Medicine. Principles and Practice.* 2nd ed. Philadelphia, PA: Saunders; 2003.
2. Choi PD, Melikian R, Skaggs DL. Risk factors for vascular repair and compartment syndrome in the pulseless supracondylar humerus fracture in children. *J Pediatr Orthop.* 2010;30:50-56.
3. Lazarides MK, Georgiadis GS, Papas TT, Gardikis S, Maltezos C. Operative and nonoperative management of children aged 13 years or younger with arterial trauma of the extremities. *J Vasc Surg.* 2006;43:72-76.

Vascular Trauma in Geriatric Patients: A National Trauma Databank Review

Konstantinidis A, Inaba K, Dubose J, et al (Univ of Southern California, Los Angeles; Univ of Maryland Med Ctr, Baltimore)
J Trauma 71:909-916, 2011

Background.—The epidemiology of vascular injuries in the geriatric patient population has not been described. The purpose of this study was to examine nationwide data on vascular injuries in the geriatric patients and to compare this with the nongeriatric adult patients with respect to the incidence, injury mechanisms, and outcomes.

Methods.—Geriatric patients aged 65 or older with at least one traumatic vascular injury were compared with an adult cohort aged 16 years to 64 years with a vascular injury using the National Trauma Databank version 7.0.

Results.—During the study period, 29,736 (1.6%) patients with a vascular injury were identified. Of those, geriatric patients accounted for 7.6% (2,268) and the nongeriatric adult patients accounted for 83.1% (n = 24,703). Compared with the nongeriatric adult patients, the geriatric vascular patients

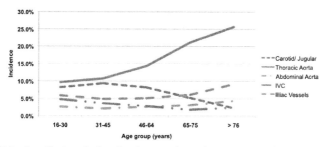

FIGURE 3.—Stratification of selected major truncal vascular injuries according to age groups. Iliac vessels include iliac arteries/veins. IVC, inferior vena cava. (Reprinted from Konstantinidis A, Inaba K, Dubose J, et al. Vascular trauma in geriatric patients: a national trauma databank review. *J Trauma.* 2011;71:909-916.)

had a significantly higher Injury Severity Score (26.6 ± 17.0 vs. 21.3 ± 16.7; $p < 0.001$) and less frequently sustained penetrating injuries (16.1% vs. 54.1%; $p < 0.001$). The most commonly injured vessels in the elderly were vessels of the chest (n = 637, 40.2%), including the thoracic aorta and innominate and subclavian vessels. The overall incidence of thoracic aorta injuries was significantly higher in geriatric patients (33.0% vs. 13.9%; $p < 0.001$) and increased linearly with progressing age. After adjusting for confounding factors, geriatric patients demonstrated a fourfold increase in mortality following vascular injuries (adjusted odds ratio, 3.9; 95% confidence interval, 3.32–4.58; $p < 0.001$).

Conclusion.—Vascular trauma is rare in the geriatric patient population. These injuries are predominantly blunt, with the thoracic aorta being the most commonly injured vessel. Although vascular injuries occur less frequently than in the nongeriatric cohort, in the geriatric patient, vascular injury is associated with a fourfold increase in adjusted mortality (Fig 3).

▶ There is relatively little literature on the epidemiology of vascular injuries in the geriatric patient population. There is also poor documentation of diagnosis, management, and outcome of these injuries. Most reports are single-center experiences with injuries in particular regions, such as intrathoracic injuries, intra-abdominal injuries, or peripheral vascular injuries. In this study, the authors used the National Trauma Data Bank (NTDB), the largest trauma registry in the United States, to determine the epidemiology of vascular injuries in geriatric patients and also to compare geriatric vascular injuries to vascular injuries in a younger adult population. Comparisons were made with respect to incidence of injury, injury mechanism, and outcome. The result is likely the largest comprehensive examination of the epidemiology of geriatric vascular trauma available. This study has the obvious limitations of being retrospective and dependent on individual reporting bias of more than 900 trauma centers participating in the NTDB. Nevertheless, we can conclude that vascular trauma in the elderly is relatively infrequent compared with the younger population, the mechanism of vascular trauma in the elderly is predominately blunt, the thoracic aorta is the most commonly injured vessel (Fig 3), and there is increased relative mortality of vascular injury in the elderly.

G. L. Moneta, MD

Role of conservative management in traumatic aortic injury: Comparison of long-term results of conservative, surgical, and endovascular treatment
Mosquera VX, Marini M, Lopez-Perez JM, et al (Complejo Hospitalario Universitario de A Coruña, Spain; et al)
J Thorac Cardiovasc Surg 142:614-621, 2011

Objective.—The purpose of this study is to compare early and long-term results in terms of survival and cardiovascular complications of patients with acute traumatic aortic injury who were conservatively managed with patients who underwent surgical or endovascular repair.

Methods.—From January 1980 to December 2009, 66 patients with acute traumatic aortic injury were divided into 3 groups according to treatment intention at admission: 37 patients in a conservative group, 22 patients in a surgical group, and 7 patients in an endovascular group. Groups were similar with regard to gender, age, Injury Severity Score, Revised Trauma Score, and Trauma Injury Severity Score.

Results.—In-hospital mortality was 21.6% in the conservative group, 22.7% in the surgical group, and 14.3% in the endovascular group ($P = .57$). In-hospital aortic-related complications occurred only in the conservative group. Median follow-up time was 75 months (range, 5–327 months). Conservative group survival was 75.6% at 1 year, 72.3% at 5 years, and 66.7% at 10 years. Surgical group survival remained at 77.2% at 1, 5, and 10 years, whereas survival in the endovascular group was 85.7% at 1 and 5 years ($P = .18$). No patient in the surgical or endovascular group required reintervention because of aortic-related complications, whereas 37.9% of the conservative group had an aortic-related complication that required surgery or caused the patient's death during the follow-up period. Cumulative survival free from aortic-related complications in the conservative group was 93% at 1 year, 88.5% at 5 years, and 51.2% at 10 years. Cox regression confirmed the initial type of aortic lesion (hazard ratio, 2.94; $P = .002$) and a Trauma Score-Injury Severity Score greater than 50% on admission (hazard ratio, 1.49; $P = .042$) as risk factors for the appearance of aortic-related complications. Two peaks in the complication rate of the conservative group were detected in the first week and between the first and third months after blunt thoracic trauma.

Conclusions.—The advent of thoracic aortic endografting has enabled a revolution in the management of acute traumatic aortic injury in patients with multisystem trauma with a low in-hospital morbimortality. Nonoperative management may be only a therapeutic option with acceptable survival in carefully selected patients. The natural history of these patients has revealed a marked trend of late aortic-related complications developing, which may justify an endovascular repair even in some low-risk patients.

▶ Traditional treatment of blunt thoracic aortic trauma is open surgical repair with graft interposition. Recently, endovascular repair of blunt thoracic injury has become a new defacto standard. However, limited studies of thoracic aortic trauma suggest that, at least in the short term, a conservative approach with medical management only of thoracic aortic trauma can be appropriate. Such studies have, however, focused on in-hospital mortality and morbidity with little long-term follow-up. The current study is based on 30 years of management of blunt thoracic injury. It reports results in terms of survival and cardiovascular complications of patients with acute thoracic aortic injury who were conservatively managed and those who underwent surgical or endovascular repair. The study does not really argue for or against conservative management of aortic injury. After all, overall survival rates in operative-managed patients and the conservative-managed patients were not statistically different. However, there are many more late complications with conservative management. The potential benefit of conservative management in selected patients is therefore dependent on close follow-up of the thoracic aorta, especially within the first several months after the injury. Whether this heightened diligence for potential aortic complications is necessary beyond 1 year in the patient treated conservatively for thoracic aortic blunt injury is a topic that clearly requires further study. Such a question will only likely be resolved from the pooling of data from many centers.

G. L. Moneta, MD

Incidence and Outcome of Pulmonary Embolism Following Popliteal Venous Repair in Trauma Cases

Tofigh AM, Karvandi M (Shahid Beheshti Univ of Med Sciences, Tehran, Iran)
Eur J Vasc Endovasc Surg 41:406-411, 2011

Objectives and Design.—Popliteal vein repair and ligation are the two main approaches to the treatment of the venous component of major, complex, knee injuries with vascular involvement. We have studied the incidence of pulmonary embolism following popliteal vein repair in trauma cases using computed tomography (CT) angiography and report the outcome.

Material and Methods.—From June 2006 to December 2009, 45 patients with popliteal vein injury were operated on in our vascular unit using lateral venorrhaphy, end-to-end anastomosis, a saphenous vein interposition graft and venous patch repair. All the patients were operated on using a medial approach to the knee. On the third postoperative day, all patients underwent a colour Doppler scan of the repaired popliteal vein to study patency, and pulmonary artery CT angiography using a 64-slice multidetector CT scan unit to establish the incidence of pulmonary embolism.

Results.—The number of patients treated by each method were: lateral venorrhaphy 20 (44%), end-to-end anastomosis 13 (29%), saphenous vein interposition graft 9 (20%) and venous patch repair three (7%). Two patients (4%) died because of sudden cardio-respiratory arrest the day after surgery with massive bilateral pulmonary artery embolism at autopsy. Popliteal colour duplex ultrasound imaging showed seven (16%) cases of complete vein thrombosis and seven (16%) cases of partial vein thrombosis. CT angiography showed pulmonary embolism in 11 (26%) patients. From seven patients with complete thrombosis three patients, and from seven patients with incomplete thrombosis five patients showed pulmonary embolism on

CT angiography. Other than two cases of early mortality, five (12%) patients developed clinical manifestations of pulmonary embolism and 11 (26%) patients had pulmonary embolism detected by CT angiography. Seven (16%) of our patients had mild-to-severe pulmonary embolism and 13 patients (29%) had proven pulmonary embolism. The total mortality rate was 7%.

Conclusion.—A surprisingly high incidence of pulmonary embolism was observed after popliteal vein repair in civil trauma patients. Additional prophylactic methods such as using higher doses of heparin and using inferior vena cava (IVC) filters might be needed to prevent this potentially fatal complication (Fig 1).

▶ Currently there is no accepted approach to the treatment of popliteal venous injuries. Some prefer repair of the vein and others ligation. Those preferring repair cite acceptable patency rates and potential reduced morbidity compared with ligation. Those advocating ligation argue that venous repair is complex and

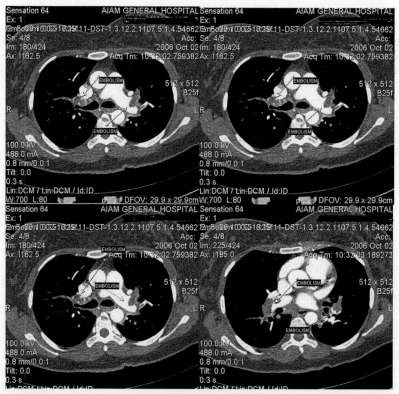

FIGURE 1.—Axial sections of a pulmonary CT angiography performed for a 38 year old patient, operated on using an interposition vein graft for acute venous trauma, showing bilateral pulmonary artery embolism. (Reprinted from Tofigh AM, Karvandi M. Incidence and outcome of pulmonary embolism following popliteal venous repair in trauma cases. *Eur J Vasc Endovasc Surg.* 2011;41:406-411. Copyright 2011, with permission from European Society for Vascular Surgery.)

potentially complicated by deep vein thrombosis (DVT) and pulmonary embolism (PE). Indeed, there are case reports of venous thromboembolism (VTE) after popliteal artery repair. The authors' study is the largest to date reporting the incidence of VTE complications following popliteal venous repair. The authors found a surprisingly high incidence of PE after popliteal vein repair in civilian trauma patients. They found that more complex methods of vein repair such as interposition grafts or patch repairs were associated with higher PE rates than simple lateral repair. Of particular importance was the total PE rate of 29% (Fig 1) and 2 cases of early mortality secondary to PE following popliteal vein repair. There were no patients who underwent vein ligation in this study, so it is unclear whether popliteal vein repair results in a higher incidence of venous thromboembolic complications than venous ligation. Given the high incidence of venous thromboembolic complications noted here, it may be reasonable to consider temporary placement of inferior vena cava filters in patients with popliteal vein repair following traumatic injury.

G. L. Moneta, MD

Nonoperative Management of Adult Blunt Splenic Injury With and Without Splenic Artery Embolotherapy: A Meta-Analysis

Requarth JA, D'Agostino RB Jr, Miller PR (Wake Forest Univ Baptist Med Ctr, Winston Salem, NC; Wake Forest Univ Health Sciences, Winston Salem, NC)
J Trauma 71:898-903, 2011

Background.—Observation and splenic artery embolotherapy (SAE) are nonoperative management (NOM) modalities for adult blunt splenic injury; however, they are quite different, inconsistently applied, and controversial. This meta-analysis compares the known outcomes data for observational management versus SAE by splenic injury grade cohort.

Methods.—Thirty-three blunt splenic injury outcomes articles, published between 1994 and 2009, comprising 24 unique data sets are identified. Of these, nine gave outcomes data by splenic injury grade for observational management and SAE separately. Failure rates were collected and analyzed using random effects estimates.

Results.—Overall, 68.4% of the 10,157 patients were managed nonoperatively. The overall failure rate estimate of NOM is 8.3% with a 95% confidence interval (CI) of 6.7% to 10.2%. The observational management failure rate estimate without SAE increases from 4.7% to 83.1% in splenic injury grade 1 to 5 patients. The overall failure rate estimate of SAE is 15.7% (95% CI, 10.4–23.2) and did not vary significantly from splenic injury grades 1 to 5 ($p = 0.413$). The failure rate of observational management without SAE is statistically higher than the failure rare estimate of SAE in splenic injury grade 4 and 5 injuries: 43.7% (95% CI, 25.5–63.8) versus 17.3% (95% CI, 7.8–34.1), $p = 0.035$ and 83.1% (95% CI, 45.2–96.7) versus 25.0% (95% CI, 8.7–53.8), $p = 0.016$, respectively.

Conclusions.—This meta-analysis synthesizes NOM outcomes data by modality and splenic injury grade. The failure rate of observational management increases with splenic injury grade, whereas the failure rate of SAE does not change significantly. SAE is associated with significantly higher splenic salvage rates in splenic injury grade 4 and 5 injuries.

▶ Most would agree that blunt splenic injury (BSI) in the hemodynamically unstable patient should be managed with immediate operation. For hemodynamically stable patients, nonoperative management of blunt splenic injury (BSI) is the standard of care in children[1] and is frequently used in adults as well. Nonoperative management of BSI can be purely observational management without splenic embolization or observational management with splenic embolization. Patients managed nonoperatively must be followed up carefully and will have a certain failure rate, with most failures occurring within 72 hours of injury.[2] The authors of this study have pointed out that observational management alone and splenic embolization are different methods of nonoperative management of patients with BSI, and that information can be lost when failure rates of the two methods are combined in a single analysis. The relative effectiveness of these two approaches stratified for grade of splenic injury is unknown. The American Association for the Surgery of Trauma classifies splenic injuries into 5 grades. Grade 1 injuries are subcapsular hematomas of less than 10% of the surface area or capsular tear of less than 1 cm in depth. This increases to grade 5 injuries, defined as a shattered spleen or hilar vascular injury. Previous studies of the effectiveness of splenic embolization for treatment of BSI are complicated by the fact that purely observational nonoperative management of BSI is frequently reported along with embolic therapy for splenic injury, but these are clearly different modes of treatment. This meta-analysis was performed to evaluate the failure rate of adults with BSI treated with observational management only versus splenic embolization in patients with comparable grades of injury to the spleen. The data suggest that patients with high-grade splenic injuries, grades 4 and 5, should be treated with embolization if nonoperative management of blunt splenic injury is chosen. Patients with grades 4 and 5 splenic injuries comprise only a small fraction (12.3%, 41 of 332 patients) of patients with BSI treated with nonoperative management. The data indicate that high failure rates of patients with BSI treated with nonoperative management and with grades 4 and 5 splenic injuries can be improved through the use of splenic embolization.

G. L. Moneta, MD

References

1. Davis KA, Fabian TC, Croce MA, et al. Improved success in nonoperative management of blunt splenic injuries: embolization of splenic artery pseudoaneurysms. *J Trauma*. 1998;44:1008-1013.
2. Peitzman AB, Heil B, Rivera L, et al. Blunt splenic injury in adults: Multi-institutional Study of the Eastern Association for the Surgery of Trauma. *J Trauma*. 2000;49: 177-187.

14 Nonatherosclerotic Conditions

Surgical Consideration of *In Situ* Prosthetic Replacement for Primary Infected Abdominal Aortic Aneurysms

Lai C-H, Luo C-Y, Lin P-Y, et al (Natl Cheng Kung Univ College of Medicine and Hosp, Tainan, Taiwan; et al)

Eur J Vasc Endovasc Surg 42:617-624, 2011

Objectives.—To review our surgical experience of primary infected abdominal aortic aneurysms, with the aim of assessing the safety and durability of *in situ* prosthetic replacement.

Design.—Retrospective study in a university hospital.

Materials and Methods.—Thirty-four patients who underwent surgery for primary infected abdominal aortic aneurysms over the past 18 years were reviewed. Operative details and outcomes were recorded for analysis.

Results.—There were six suprarenal and 28 infrarenal infections. *Salmonellae* (18 patients) were the most common pathogens. Thirty patients underwent *in situ* prosthetic replacement, two underwent extra-anatomic bypass and two underwent endovascular repair. The surgical mortality for overall patients was 18%, and for patients reconstructed *in situ*, 17%. Among the 30 patients reconstructed *in situ*, four patients who underwent concomitant gastrointestinal procedures (e.g., repair of the duodenal defect) died. By contrast, 25 of 26 patients without gastrointestinal involvement survived surgery. After a median follow-up period of 58 months, two discharged patients who underwent *in situ* reconstruction died of late graft infection.

Conclusions.—Our experience suggests that *in situ* prosthetic replacement can be performed safely with durable outcomes in the majority of patients with infected abdominal aortic aneurysms. Nevertheless, we advise caution when considering this technique with concomitant gastrointestinal procedures.

▶ Aortic infection is a formidable surgical problem. The patients are sick, operation is often technically difficult, and there is no agreed-upon consensus as to how to proceed. In recent years, there has been a tendency to perform in situ graft replacement for infected aortic aneurysm. Advocates of the procedure generally indicate that the degree of retroperitoneal sepsis and infection must not be too extensive. The concept of "not too extensive" is only useful at the extreme ends of the spectrum. In addition, one cannot really tell the true extent of retroperitoneal infection until the time of exposure at operation. Nevertheless, this article and others like it indicate that under some circumstances one can get away with in situ graft replacement for treatment of primary aortic infection. Indeed, for infection of the thoracic aorta, there is generally little choice but in situ placement. The authors' patients with infected aortas are not greatly different from anyone else's patients with infected aortas. The authors, however, do make 2 points worth considering. The first is that placement of an in situ graft for aortic infection in the setting of a concomitant gastrointestinal procedure has a poor outcome. If it is known that there is a duodenal defect preoperatively, the authors' data suggest these patients would be better served by extra-anatomic bypass and ligation of the infrarenal abdominal aorta. The second point is that if patients require in situ replacement of the abdominal aorta with a bifurcated graft, it makes sense to perform the distal anastomoses in the groin. This takes a site of potential anastomotic disruption out of the abdomen and turns a potentially fatal complication into one whose management is more likely to be successful.

G. L. Moneta, MD

Major arterial aneurysms and pseudoaneurysms in Behçet's disease: results from a single centre

Cho SB, Kim T, Cho S, et al (Yonsei Univ College of Medicine, Seoul, Korea)
Scand J Rheumatol 40:64-67, 2011

Objective.—Behçet's disease (BD) with arterial involvement is closely correlated with mortality and morbidity due to life-threatening complications such as arterial occlusion and aneurysm rupture. We aimed to determine the clinical characteristics of BD patients with aneurysms and pseudoaneurysms in the major arterial systems.

Methods.—Medical records of 30 BD patients diagnosed with aneurysms or pseudoaneurysms in the major arterial systems were reviewed to determine the clinical characteristics of BD, the sites and types of arterial aneurysms or pseudoaneurysms, laboratory test results, and response to treatment.

Results.—A total of 47 aneurysms and pseudoaneurysms (32 saccular aneurysms, eight fusiform aneurysms, and seven pseudoaneurysms) were detected in 30 patients. Most aneurysms and pseudoaneurysms (27 patients, 90%) had not ruptured. Symptomatic lesions presented in 21 patients (70%), and asymptomatic lesions were incidentally detected in nine (30%). Ten of the 30 patients (33.3%) presented two or more aneurysmal lesions. Recurrence was observed in five patients (16.7%) after treatment with stent graft (n = 3), graft interposition (n = 1), or graft embolization (n = 1).

Conclusion.—We suggest that BD patients diagnosed with major arterial aneurysms should be further evaluated to detect possible associated

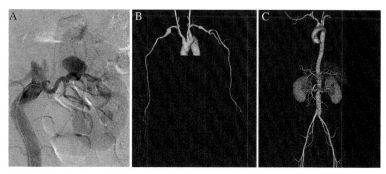

FIGURE 1.—(A) Digital subtraction angiography presenting three saccular aneurysmal lesions on the renal artery in a 57-year-old female BD patient. (B) A 43-year-old male BD patient with bilateral fusiform aneurisms on both subclavian arteries: three-dimensional (3D) reconstructed image of computed tomography angiography (CTA). (C) Recurring saccular aneurysm on the distal portion of the stent-grafted infrarenal abdominal aorta in a 52-year-old male BD patient: 3D reconstructed image of CTA. (Reprinted from Cho SB, Kim T, Cho S, et al. Major arterial aneurysms and pseudoaneurysms in Behçet's disease: results from a single centre. *Scand J Rheumatol.* 2011;40:64-67. Informa Healthcare © Scandinavian Society of Rheumatology.)

TABLE 1.—Sites, Numbers, and Types of Aneurysms and Pseudoaneurysms in Behçet's Disease (BD) Patients

Site	No. of Lesions in BD Patients		
	Aneurysm (Saccular/Fusiform)	Pseudoaneurysm	Sum
Intracranial artery	6/0	1	7
Infrarenal abdominal aorta	5/1	1	7
Popliteal artery	3/1	2	6
Common iliac artery	2/2	2	6
Common femoral artery	4/0	0	4
Subclavian artery	2/2	0	4
Renal artery	3/0	0	3
Thoracic aorta	1/1	1	3
Internal iliac artery	1/1	0	2
Superficial femoral artery	2/0	0	2
Superior mesenteric artery	1/0	0	1
Sinus of Valsalva	1/0	0	1
Pulmonary artery	1/0	0	1

venous or arterial thrombosis formations or aneurysmal lesions at other sites (Fig 1, Table 1).

▶ Behçet disease (BD) is a multisystem autoinflammatory vasculitis that can, in theory, affect all sizes and types of vessels.[1] The disease primarily affects veins, venules, and capillaries.[2] Major arterial involvement in BD is actually relatively infrequent and occurs in only approximately 1% to 7% of BD patients. However, it is the arterial involvement of BD that correlates closely with mortality and morbidity. Pathology is both arterial occlusions and aneurysm rupture. This report focuses on 30 BD patients from Korea diagnosed with aneurysms and pseudoaneurysms of major arteries. The article confirms the clinical impression of an apparent high rate of graft-related complications with treatment of BD aneurysms, perhaps related to ongoing inflammation in the Behçet patient. Of most interest is the fact that if you find an aneurysm in a patient with BD, when looking further, one-third of the time, you will find an additional aneurysm. Therefore, patients with BD and a discovered aneurysm essentially require visualization of their entire arterial system. BD arterial aneurysms can be found anywhere (Table 1 and Fig 1) from the aortic arch to the pulmonary circulation, as well as in intracranial arteries and the tibial arteries.

G. L. Moneta, MD

References

1. Cocco G, Gasparyan AY. Behçet's disease: an insight from a cardiologist's point of view. *Open Cardiovasc Med J.* 2010;4:63-70.
2. Alpagut U, Ugurlucan M, Dayioglu E. Major arterial involvement and review of Behcet's disease. *Ann Vasc Surg.* 2007;21:232-239.

Clinical Outcome After Extended Endovascular Recanalization in Buerger's Disease in 20 Consecutive Cases
Graziani L, Morelli L, Parini F, et al (Istituto Clinico Cittá di Brescia, Italy; Calderon Guardia Hosp, San Jose, Costa Rica; Univ of Brescia Med School, Italy; et al)
Ann Vasc Surg 26:387-395, 2012

Background.—To present our experience of extended endovascular management for thromboangiitis obliterans (Buerger's disease) patients with critical limb ischemia (CLI).

Methods.—Between January 2005 and July 2010, a consecutive series of 17 Buerger's disease patients with CLI in 20 limbs were admitted and the diagnosis confirmed. The mean age of the patients was 41.5 years (standard error: ± 1.7). All patients presented with history of smoking, one patient presented with hypertension, and eight patients presented with dyslipidemia. According to Rutherford classification, all patients were found to be between grades 3 and 5. Ultrasonography first, and angiography examination later, confirmed a severe arterial disease involving almost exclusively below-the-knee and foot arteries in all cases. A new approach for revascularization, defined as extended angioplasty of each tibial and foot artery obstruction, was performed to achieve direct perfusion of at least one foot artery.

Results.—An extensive endovascular treatment was intended in all patients with success in 19 of 20 limbs, achieving a technical success in 95%. No mortality or complication related to the procedure was observed. During a mean follow-up of 23 months (standard error: ±4.05), amputation-free survival with no need of major amputation in any case and sustained clinical improvement was achieved in 16 of the 19 limbs (84.2%) successfully treated, resulting in a 100% limb salvage rate (19/19).

Conclusion.—In this first experience, in patients with thromboangiitis obliterans, extended endovascular intervention was a feasible and effective revascularization procedure in case of CLI. High technical success, amputation-free survival, and sustained clinical improvement rates were achieved at midterm follow-up was achieved (Fig 1, Table 1).

▶ The authors report on an aggressive approach to endovascular treatment of tibial and pedal artery occlusive disease in a consecutive series of patients with presumed Buerger disease. No follow-up imaging data are reported, but despite the fact that the patients appeared to have advanced ischemia, there were no major amputations over a mean follow-up of 23 months. It is always difficult to be certain of the diagnosis of Buerger disease as the diagnosis can only be made with certainty pathologically. Nevertheless, in clinical practice, Buerger is a clinical diagnosis, and the authors did their best to confirm the diagnosis (Table 1). Given that most patients with Buerger can avoid major amputation with smoking cessation and that not all Buerger patients who continue to smoke will have major amputation, it is difficult to know how much of the longer-term clinical benefit in these patients was a result of the endovascular intervention or merely a reflection of the complexity of the natural history of

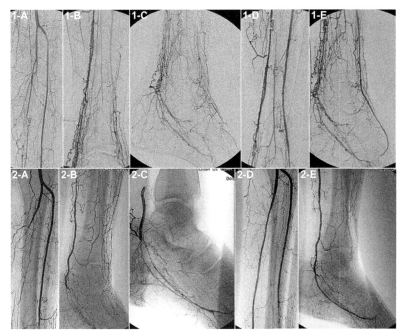

FIGURE 1.—Case 1 and 2: Typical angiographic findings in two patients with Buerger's disease before and after intervention. Case 1A—C: Diagnostic angiography showing distal vessel disease and corkscrew subcutaneous collaterals. 1D—E: Recanalization of both tibial vessels to obtain direct flow to the foot. Case 2A—C: Baseline angiography describing proximal occlusion of posterior tibial artery and distal tibial disease. 2D—E: Recanalization of posterior tibial artery directly to the lateral plantar artery, obtaining a straight flow to the foot. (Reprinted from the Annals of Vascular Surgery, Graziani L, Morelli L, Parini F, et al. Clinical outcome after extended endovascular recanalization in Buerger's disease in 20 consecutive cases. *Ann Vasc Surg.* 2012;26:387-395. Copyright 2012, with permission from Annals of Vascular Surgery, Inc.)

TABLE 1.—Diagnostic Criteria of Olin[1]

Age under 45 yr
Current or recent history of tobacco use
Presence of distal extremity ischemia indicated by claudication, pain at rest, ischemic ulcers, or gangrenes
   and documented by noninvasive vascular testing
Exclusion of autoimmune diseases, hypercoagulable states, and diabetes mellitus
Exclusion of a proximal source of emboli by echocardiography or arteriography

   Editor's Note: Please refer to original journal article for full reference.

this disease. What the article does show is that it is possible for skilled operators to achieve remarkable technical success with very distal catheter-based interventions in a population of likely Buerger patients (Fig 1). Studies correlating imaging outcomes with clinical outcomes are required to determine just how durable these procedures are and whether long-term durability is even necessary to sustain clinical benefit in Burger patients.

G. L. Moneta, MD

Functional Popliteal Entrapment Syndrome in the Sportsperson

Lane R, Nguyen T, Cuzzilla M, et al (Dalcross Adventist Hosp, Sydney, New South Wales, Australia; Royal North Shore Hosp, Sydney, New South Wales, Australia; et al)
Eur J Vasc Endovasc Surg 43:81-87, 2012

Objective.—To define the clinical syndrome of functional popliteal entrapment comparing pre and post surgical clinical outcomes with pre and post-operative provocative ultrasonic investigations. Further, to suggest a management pathway to differentiate chronic exertional compartment syndromes and concomitant venous popliteal compression.

Methods.—In 32 claudicant sportspersons, 55 limbs were characterised pre-surgery clinically, with provocative testing including hopping, and following a series of non-invasive tests. The clinical findings, ankle brachial indices (ABI) and duplex outcomes were compared pre-operatively, at 3 months post-operatively ($n = 52$) and in the long term i.e. 16 months ($n = 17$).

Results.—At 3 months, all 55 limbs had clinical follow up. 52 of the 55 limbs had follow up with ultrasound with provocative manoeuvres. The ABIs normalised in 46 (88%). There were 40 of 52 (76%) that became asymptomatic post surgery with a normal scan. There were 4 of 52 (8%) who were clinically asymptomatic but with residual obstruction on duplex and who were able to resume their usual lifestyle. There were 4 (8%) that had abnormal findings both on post-operative scan and clinically. Re-operation on 2 limbs corrected the duplex findings and the symptoms. There were 4 (8%) limbs that had normal duplexes but continued with symptoms albeit varied from the presenting symptoms.

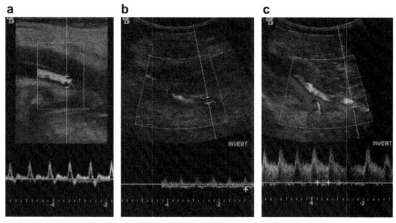

FIGURE 1.—Doppler findings with FPS a) Popliteal artery longitudinal duplex scan in neutral position. b) Same popliteal longitudinal scan with plantar flexion. c) Reactive hyperaemic response following resumption of normal position. (Reprinted from European Journal of Vascular and Endovascular Surgery, Lane R, Nguyen T, Cuzzilla M, et al. Functional popliteal entrapment syndrome in the sportsperson. *Eur J Vasc Endovasc Surg.* 2012;43:81-87. Copyright 2012, with permission from the European Society for Vascular Surgery.)

In the longer term, a further 2 became symptomatic at 2.8 years requiring a further successful intervention. (Concomitant popliteal venous obstruction was present in 5 limbs (10%) on standing.)

Conclusions.—In the claudicating sportsperson, where there are no well characterised specific anatomical abnormalities, the syndrome can be characterised by provocative clinical (particularly hopping) and non-invasive tests. A positive clinical outcome with surgery can be predicted by abnormal pre-surgical ultrasonic investigations and confirmed later by a similar normal post surgical study. Concomitant venous compression may occur while standing with both syndromes related to muscle hypertrophy (Figs 1 and 4).

▶ Functional popliteal entrapment (FPE) as described by Rignault and colleagues is commonly associated with classic claudication type symptoms in a young, active sportsperson in the absence of a definitive anatomic abnormality.[1] These authors present a helpful algorithm for both the diagnosis and management of these patients and present midterm follow-up for a large percentage of subjects (Fig 4). Unique to this series is the coupling of noninvasive duplex imaging, clinical findings, and exacerbation of symptoms with provocative "hopping" on the affected extremity (Fig 1).

Popliteal entrapment syndrome was described in the US military and later elucidated by Norm Rich and Jim Collins in 1979.[2] For those vascular surgeons who commonly diagnose and surgically treat patients with popliteal entrapment, this article may serve as a useful reference. One glaring weakness in the study is a lack of control subjects without symptoms of FPE who undergo the same provocative testing.

B. W. Starnes, MD

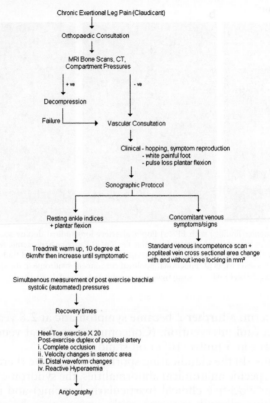

Chronic Exertional Leg Pain (Claudicant)

↓

Orthopaedic Consultation

↓

MRI Bone Scans, CT, Compartment Pressures

+ ve   - ve

Decompression

Failure → Vascular Consultation

↓

Clinical - hopping, symptom reproduction
- white painful foot
- pulse loss plantar flexion

↓

Sonographic Protocol

Resting ankle indices + plantar flexion   Concomitant venous symptoms/signs

↓   ↓

Treadmill: warm up, 10 degree at 6km/hr then increase until symptomatic   Standard venous incompetence scan + popliteal vein cross sectional area change with and without knee locking in mm²

↓

Simultaenous measurement of post exercise brachial systolic (automated) pressures

↓

Recovery times

↓

Heel-Toe exercise X 20
Post-exercise duplex of popliteal artery
i. Complete occlusion
ii. Velocity changes in stenotic area
iii. Distal waveform changes
iv. Reactive Hyperaemia

↓

Angiography

FIGURE 4.—Suggested clinical and investigative protocol for functional popliteal entrapment. (Reprinted from European Journal of Vascular and Endovascular Surgery, Lane R, Nguyen T, Cuzzilla M, et al. Functional popliteal entrapment syndrome in the sportsperson. *Eur J Vasc Endovasc Surg.* 2012;43:81-87. Copyright 2012, with permission from the European Society for Vascular Surgery.)

References

1. Rignault DP, Pailler JL, Lunel F. The "functional" popliteal entrapment syndrome. *Int Angiol.* 1985;4:341-343.
2. Rich NM, Collins GJ Jr, McDonald PT, Kozloff L, Clagett GP, Collins JT. Popliteal vascular entrapment. Its increasing interest. *Arch Surg.* 1979;114:1377-1384.

Endofibrosis and Kinking of the Iliac Arteries in Athletes: A Systematic Review

Peach G, Schep G, Palfreeman R, et al (St George's Vascular Inst, London, UK; Maxima Med Centre, Veldhoven, The Netherlands; Claremont Sports Medicine and Performance Centre, Sheffield, UK; et al)

Eur J Vasc Endovasc Surg 43:208-217, 2012

Introduction.—Kinking and endofibrosis of the iliac arteries are uncommon and poorly recognized conditions affecting young endurance athletes. Deformation or progressive stenosis of the iliac artery may reduce blood flow to the lower limb and adversely affect performance. The aim of this review was to examine the existing literature relating to these flow-limiting phenomena and identify a clear, unifying strategy for the assessment and management of affected patients.

Methods.—A systematic review of the literature was performed. A comprehensive search was carried out using Medline, Embase and The Cochrane Database to identify relevant articles published between 1950 and 2011 (last search date 05/08/2011). This search (and additional bibliography review) identified 413 articles, of which 367 were excluded. 46 articles were then studied in detail. Methodological quality of studies was assessed according to Scottish Intercollegiate Guideline Network criteria.

Results.—Focussed history and examination can successfully identify nearly 80% of patients with iliac flow limitation. However, both provocative exercise tests and detailed imaging are also necessary to identify those in need of intervention and establish most appropriate treatment. Provocative

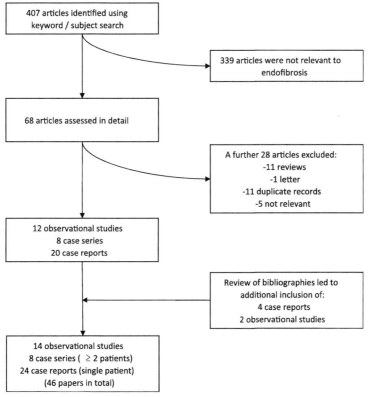

FIGURE 1.—PRISMA flow diagram representing the performed literature search. (Reprinted from European Journal of Vascular and Endovascular Surgery, Peach G, Schep G, Palfreeman R, et al. Endofibrosis and kinking of the iliac arteries in athletes: a systematic review. *Eur J Vasc Endovasc Surg.* 2012;43:208-217. Copyright 2012, with permission from the European Society for Vascular Surgery.)

exercise tests and duplex imaging can then be used to confirm flow limitation before detailed assessment of abnormal anatomy with MRA and DSA. These multiple imaging modalities are necessary to identify those most likely to benefit from surgery and clarify whether each patient should undergo arterial release, vessel shortening, endofibrosectomy or interposition grafting.

Conclusion.—We present a systematic review of the literature together with a proposed algorithm for diagnosis and management of these iliac flow limitations in endurance athletes (Figs 1 and 2).

▶ Endofibrosis has become an increasingly recognized entity among high-performance athletes in recent years. This systematic review is the best description to date of this rare phenomenon.

These authors conducted a literature review between 1950 and 2011 and identified 413 papers of which 46 met inclusion criteria based on PRISMA guidelines (Fig 1).[1] Because of the nature of the articles included, there were insufficient homogeneous data to allow for a meta-analysis. A systematic review was therefore undertaken. The resulting data are interesting.

Endofibrosis is estimated to have a prevalence of 10% to 20% in high-performance athletes. Competitive cyclists are most often affected, with intensity of training being at least as important as overall distance traveled. Males are affected more than females, and in more than 90% of patients, endofibrosis affects the external iliac artery, with the fibrotic segment measuring between 2

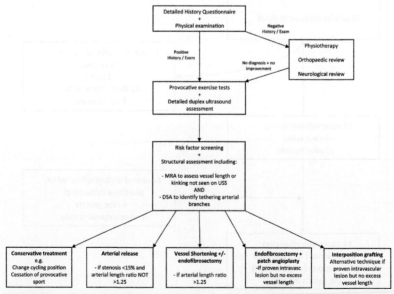

FIGURE 2.—Proposed strategy for the investigation and management of endofibrosis. (Reprinted from European Journal of Vascular and Endovascular Surgery, Peach G, Schep G, Palfreeman R, et al. Endofibrosis and kinking of the iliac arteries in athletes: a systematic review. *Eur J Vasc Endovasc Surg.* 2012;43:208-217. Copyright 2012, with permission from the European Society for Vascular Surgery.)

and 6 cm in length. Etiology is thought to include athletic position, psoas hypertrophy, arterial fixation, and excessive vessel length leading to kinking. Nicely presented is a proposed strategy for the investigation and management of endofibrosis (Fig 2).

B. W. Starnes, MD

Reference

1. Moher D, Liberati A, Tetzlaff J, Altman DG; The PRISMA Group. Preferred reporting items for systematic reviews and meta-analyses: the PRISMA statement. *Open Med.* 2009;3:e123-e130.

Importance of specimen length during temporal artery biopsy
Ypsilantis E, Courtney ED, Chopra N, et al (Queen Elizabeth Hosp, King's Lynn, UK, Conquest Hosp, Hastings, UK; et al)
Br J Surg 98:1556-1560, 2011

Background.—Variations in surgical technique of temporal artery biopsy (TAB) performed for diagnosis of giant cell arteritis (GCA) may contribute to high false-negative rates. This was a retrospective analysis of a large database that explored potential associations between specimen length and diagnostic sensitivity of TAB.

Methods.—Histopathological reports and medical records of patients who underwent TAB in six hospitals between 2004 and 2009 were reviewed.

Results.—A total of 966 biopsies were analysed. The median postfixation specimen length was 1 (range $0 \cdot 1 - 8 \cdot 5$) cm and 207 biopsies ($21 \cdot 4$ per cent) were positive for GCA. Significant variation in prebiopsy erythrocyte sedimentation rate (ESR), arterial specimen length and positive results was noted amongst hospitals. Multivariable analysis revealed that patient age, ESR value and specimen length were independent predictors of GCA. Positive biopsies had significantly longer median specimen length compared with negative biopsies: $1 \cdot 2$ (range $0 \cdot 3 - 8 \cdot 5$) *versus* $1 \cdot 0$ ($0 \cdot 2 - 8 \cdot 0$) cm respectively ($P = 0 \cdot 001$). Receiver operating characteristic (ROC) analysis identified postfixation specimen length of at least $0 \cdot 7$ cm as the cut-off length with highest positive predictive value for a positive biopsy (area under ROC curve $0 \cdot 574$). Biopsies with specimen length of $0 \cdot 7$ cm or more had a significantly higher rate of positive results than smaller specimens ($24 \cdot 8$ *versus* $12 \cdot 9$ per cent respectively; odds ratio $2 \cdot 17$, $P = 0 \cdot 001$).

Conclusion.—Specimen length and ESR were independent prognostic factors of a positive TAB result. A uniform referral practice and standard specimen length of approximately 1 cm could help eliminate discrepancies in the results of TAB.

▶ Giant cell arteritis (GCA) affects medium-sized and large arteries, most commonly the extracranial arteries of the head and neck. GCA has an incidence of 15 to 25×10^{-5} per year in individuals aged 50 years or older.[1] Incidence increases with age and, because of the potential for the complication of blindness, treatment with steroids is often relatively urgently indicated in such patients. Duplex ultrastenography is a reasonably accurate, noninvasive first-line investigation for GCA. However, treatment is generally based on a temporal artery biopsy (TAB) and is the recommended investigation for GCA.[2] The likelihood of a positive TAB may be related to whether an adequate length of temporal artery was obtained for analysis. The exact minimum length is debatable. The purpose of this retrospective study was to explore potential associations between TAB specimen length and diagnostic sensitivity. What the authors found was that, when it comes to TAB, longer is better! Length of temporal artery biopsy correlates positively in this study with diagnostic sensitivity. The study, in essence, provides a guideline for minimal length of a TAB. The data here would suggest that a length of at least 0.7 cm should be obtained. A uniform pattern of practice of obtaining a specimen of at least 1 cm in length should help eliminate discrepancies between hospitals and the results of TAB.

G. L. Moneta, MD

References

1. Bengtsson BA, Malmvall BE. The epidemiology of giant cell arteritis including temporal arteritis and polymyalgia rheumatica. Incidences of different clinical presentations and eye complications. *Arthritis Rheum.* 1981;24:899-904.
2. Dasgupta B, Borg FA, Hassan N, et al. BSR and BHPR guidelines for the management of giant cell arteritis. *Rheumatology (Oxford).* 2010;49:1594-1597.

Proposed Chronic Cerebrospinal Venous Insufficiency Criteria Do Not Predict Multiple Sclerosis Risk or Severity
Centonze D, Floris R, Stefanini M, et al (Univ Hosp Tor Vergata, Rome, Italy)
Ann Neurol 70:51-58, 2011

Objective.—It is still unclear whether chronic cerebrospinal venous insufficiency (CCSVI) is associated with multiple sclerosis (MS), because substantial methodological differences have been claimed by Zamboni to account for the lack of results of other groups. Furthermore, the potential role of venous malformations in influencing MS severity has not been fully explored. This information is particularly relevant, because uncontrolled surgical procedures are increasingly offered to MS patients to treat their venous stenoses.

Methods.—In the present study, CCSVI was studied in 84 MS patients and in 56 healthy subjects by applying the Zamboni method for CCSVI identification.

Results.—We found no significant differences ($p = 0.12$) in CCSVI frequency between MS and control subjects. Furthermore, no differences were found between CCSVI-positive and CCSVI-negative patients in terms of relevant clinical variables such as disease duration, time between onset and first relapse, relapsing or progressive disease course, and risk of secondary progression course. Statistically significant differences were not found between CCSVI-positive and CCSVI-negative MS subjects by analyzing direct measures of disability such as mean Expanded Disability Status Scale (EDSS) ($p = 0.07$), mean progression index ($p > 0.1$), and mean MS severity score ($p > 0.1$). The percentage of subjects who reached EDSS 4.0 and 6.0 milestones was not different among CCSVI-negative and CCSVI-positive subjects, and no significant correlation was found between severity of disability and number of positive CCSVI criteria.

Interpretation.—Our results indicate that CCSVI has no role in either MS risk or MS severity.

▶ Anatomic abnormalities of major neck and chest veins are proposed to cause impaired venous drainage of the central nervous system. Zamboni et al have proposed that chronic cerebrospinal venous insufficiency (CCSVI) has a strong association with multiple sclerosis,[1] finding CCSVI in basically all patients with MS and not in healthy subjects. Their results indicate that MS is caused by CCSVI and that CCSVI plays a substantial role in MS progression. Potentially, endovascular interventions directed to correct abnormalities of venous drainage instead that are reportedly characteristic of CCSVI can improve the clinical course of MS.[2] However, some question the very existence of CCSVI.[3]

There have been both confirmatory and nonconfirmatory associations between CCSVI and MS. It has been suggested that studies failing to demonstrate a significant association between CCSVI and MS use alternative approaches to define CCSVI than those used by Zamboni et al. The authors therefore used an experimental protocol they feel is identical to that developed by Zamboni and coworkers. This was applied to an independent population of MS patients and healthy control subjects studied by operators specifically trained by Zamboni in CCSVI identification who were unable to implicate CCSVI as having a role in MS. This is another in a series of articles disputing the Zamboni theory of CCSVI as the etiology of MS. By using ultrasound operators specifically trained by Zamboni and colleagues, the authors have sought to dissuade the arguments used to criticize previous negative studies of inappropriate operator training or skills. The results here, put simply, do not support a role of venous abnormalities as a source MS pathology. CCSVI was not found to be more prevalent in MS patients versus control subjects, and there was no association between CCSVI and disease severity in the MS subjects of this study. It is obviously premature, and in many respects perhaps irresponsible, to offer endovascular procedures to correct CCSVI in the MS patient population.

G. L. Moneta, MD

References

1. Zamboni P, Galeotti R, Menegatti E, et al. Chronic cerebrospinal venous insufficiency in patients with multiple sclerosis. *J Neurol Neurosurg Psychiatry.* 2009; 80:392-399.
2. Zamboni P, Galeotti R, Menegatti E, et al. A prospective open-label study of endovascular treatment of chronic cerebrospinal venous insufficiency. *J Vasc Surg.* 2009;50:1348-1358.
3. Doepp F, Paul F, Valdueza JM, Schmierer K, Schreiber SJ. No cerebrocervical venous congestion in patients with multiple sclerosis. *Ann Neurol.* 2010;68:173-183.

A Case of Pseudo-xanthoma Elasticum Presenting with Ischaemic Claudication

Lamb CM, Johns RA, Gallagher PJ, et al (Southampton Univ Hosps NHS Trust, UK)
Eur J Vasc Endovasc Surg 43:478-479, 2012

A 37-year-old man presented with symptoms of intermittent claudication. Investigations revealed atypical calf vessel disease but no obvious aetiology. Ten years later he re-presented with worsening symptoms. CT angiography confirmed the atypical pattern of lower limb arterial disease but also noted calcification of the renal parenchyma, myocardium and scrotum. A diagnosis of pseudo-xanthoma elasticum was confirmed by skin biopsy. Pseudo-xanthoma elasticum is a rare condition that presents

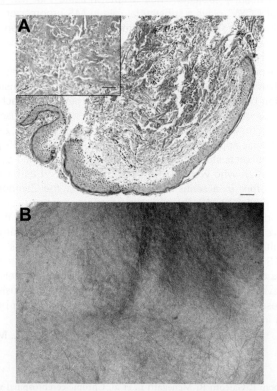

FIGURE 2.—(A) A low power view of a skin biopsy, stained with haematoxylin and eosin, taken from the neck lesion. Note that the epithelium is normal. The large mass of sub epithelial collagen shows degenerative change (Scale bar 1000 μm). A high power view of the abnormal collagen is shown in the upper left inset. The normal arrangement of the collagen bundles has been lost and many are clearly fragmented (Scale bar 250 μm). (B) Photograph showing typical PXE skin lesion superior to right clavicle. The patient, when questioned, had initially attributed this lesion to a childhood scald. (Reprinted from European Journal of Vascular and Endovascular Surgery, Lamb CM, Johns RA, Gallagher PJ, et al. A case of pseudo-xanthoma elasticum presenting with ischaemic claudication. *Eur J Vasc Endovasc Surg.* 2012;43:478-479. Copyright 2012, with permission from the European Society for Vascular Surgery.)

infrequently to vascular surgeons. Early recognition should prompt aggressive risk factor management to slow accelerated atherosclerosis. Clinicians should be aware of the clinical features of this condition to allow early diagnosis (Fig 2).

▶ Vascular surgeons seldom see a diagnosis of pseudoxanthoma elasticum. This article serves as a good review of several salient features of the treatment of these rare patients.

First, anytime a young patient presents with severe claudication, as in this case, several diagnoses should be considered: popliteal entrapment, cystic adventitial disease, or accelerated atherosclerosis due to either hyperhomocysteinemia or pseudoxanthoma elasticum.

Pseudoxanthoma elasticum is a rare, inherited disorder with an estimated incidence of 1:25 000 to 1:100 000. It is inherited in an autosomal recessive fashion and is caused by mutations in the ABCC6 gene on chromosome 16. The diagnosis is made by skin biopsy where, microscopically, lesions are characterized by the fragmentation and calcification of elastic fibers in the skin (Fig 2). Radiologically, ectopic microcalcifications are found throughout the body and, as in the presented case, commonly occur in the kidneys and testicles.

The three most important takeaway points for management of pseudoxanthoma elasticum are:

1. Current management is centered on risk-factor control: smoking cessation, control of diabetes and hypertension, and statin therapy.

2. Aspirin and other anticoagulants *should be avoided* due to the risk of mucosal and retinal hemorrhage.[1]

3. There is no specific contraindication to either bypass or angioplasty in this patient population.

B. W. Starnes, MD

Reference

1. Chassaing N, Martin L, Calvas P, Le Bert M, Hovnanian A. Pseudoxanthoma elasticum: a clinical, pathophysiological and genetic update including 11 novel ABCC6 mutations. *J Med Genet.* 2005;42:881-892.

15 Venous Thrombosis and Pulmonary Embolism

Dose-related Effect of Statins in Venous Thrombosis Risk Reduction
Khemasuwan D, Chae YK, Gupta S, et al (Albert Einstein Med Ctr, Philadelphia, PA; et al)
Am J Med 124:852-859, 2011

Background.—Atherosclerosis and venous thromboembolism share similar pathophysiology based on common inflammatory mediators. The dose-related effect of statin therapy in venous thromboembolism remains controversial. This study investigated whether the use of antiplatelet therapy and statins decrease the occurrence of venous thromboembolism in patients with atherosclerosis.

Methods.—We conducted a retrospective cohort study reviewing 1795 consecutive patients with atherosclerosis admitted to a teaching hospital between 2005 and 2010. Patients who had been treated with anticoagulation therapy were excluded. Patients who either used statins for <2 months or never used them were allocated to the nonuser group.

Results.—The final analysis included 1100 patients. The overall incidence of venous thromboembolism was 9.7%. Among statin users, 6.3% (54/861) developed venous thromboembolism, compared with 22.2% (53/239) in the nonuser group (hazard ratio [HR] 0.24; P <.001). After controlling for confounding factors, statin use was still associated with a lower risk of developing venous thromboembolism (HR 0.29; P <.001). High-dose statin use (average 50.9 mg/day) (HR 0.25; P <.001) lowered the risk of venous thromboembolism compared with standard-dose statins (average 22.2 mg/day) (HR 0.38; P <.001). Dual antiplatelet therapy with aspirin and clopidogrel decreased occurrence of venous thromboembolism (HR 0.19; P <.001). Interestingly, combined statins and antiplatelet therapy further reduced the occurrence of venous thromboembolism (HR 0.16; P <.001).

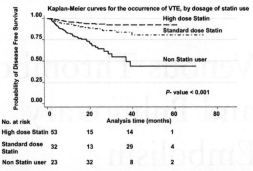

FIGURE 2.—Kaplan-Meier plot showing the occurrence of venous thromboembolism compared between nonstatin use, standard-dose statin use, and high-dose statin use. (Reprinted from The American Journal of Medicine, Khemasuwan D, Chae YK, Gupta S, et al. Dose-related effect of statins in venous thrombosis risk reduction. *Am J Med.* 2011;124:852-859. Copyright 2011, with permission from Elsevier.)

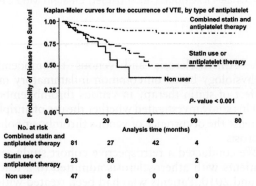

FIGURE 4.—Kaplan-Meier plot showing the occurrence of venous thromboembolism compared between combined statin and antiplatelet therapy, either use of statin and antiplatelet therapy, and non-user. (Reprinted from The American Journal of Medicine, Khemasuwan D, Chae YK, Gupta S, et al. Dose-related effect of statins in venous thrombosis risk reduction. *Am J Med.* 2011;124:852-859. Copyright 2011, with permission from Elsevier.)

Conclusions.—The use of statins and antiplatelet therapy is associated with a significant reduction in the occurrence of venous thromboembolism with a dose-related response of statins (Figs 2 and 4).

▶ Atherosclerotic plaques contain inflammatory cells that release cytokines such as interleukin-6 and interleukin-8 as well tumor necrosis factor alpha. These and other inflammatory mediators are thought to be involved in the basic mechanisms of atherosclerosis. It has also been determined, however, that the same inflammatory mediators are elevated in patients with venous thrombosis.[1,2] Indeed, there is now evidence that patients with a diagnosis of deep venous thrombosis and pulmonary embolism have higher risk of cardiovascular events over the next 20 years. In addition patients with myocardial infarction or stroke have an increased risk of venous thromboembolism (VTE) within 3 months of diagnosis.[3]

It now also appears that patients with the metabolic syndrome and those with elevated levels of low-density lipoprotein are also at increased risk of VTE.[4] Based on a possible emerging relationship between atherosclerosis and VTE with respect to underlying biochemical etiologic factors, the authors hypothesized that statins and antiplatelet therapy may have a role in preventing VTE in patients at high risk for atherosclerosis. The author's findings have potentially huge ramifications. The article indicates there are shared biochemical risk factors for VTE and atherosclerosis that are more than just coincidental. In addition, the data contradict the popular perception that aspirin is ineffective in the prevention of VTE (Fig 4). Finally, it is the first article to suggest a possible dose-response relationship of statins in prevention of VTE (Fig 2).

G. L. Moneta, MD

References

1. van Aken BE, den Heijer M, Bos GM, van Deventer SJ, Reitsma PH. Recurrent venous thrombosis and markers of inflammation. *Thromb Haemost.* 2000;83: 536-539.
2. Sørensen HT, Horvath-Puho E, Pedersen L, Baron JA, Prandoni P. Venous thromboembolism and subsequent hospitalisation due to acute arterial cardiovascular events: a 20-year cohort study. *Lancet.* 2007;370:1773-1779.
3. Sørensen HT, Horvath-Puho E, Søgaard KK, et al. Arterial cardiovascular events, statins, low-dose aspirin and subsequent risk of venous thromboembolism: a population-based case-control study. *J Thromb Haemost.* 2009;7:521-528.
4. Ageno W, Becattini C, Brighton T, Selby R, Kamphuisen PW. Cardiovascular risk factors and venous thromboembolism: a meta-analysis. *Circulation.* 2008;117: 93-102.

The utility of screening for deep venous thrombosis in asymptomatic, non-ambulatory neurosurgical patients

Dermody M, Alessi-Chinetti J, Iafrati MD, et al (Tufts Med Ctr, Boston, MA)
J Vasc Surg 53:1309-1315, 2011

Objectives.—Decisions regarding deep venous thrombosis (DVT) prophylaxis are complicated in neurosurgical patients because of the potential for catastrophic bleeding complications. Screening with venous duplex ultrasound (VDUS) may improve outcomes, but can strain hospital resources. Since there is little data to guide VDUS surveillance, we investigated the utility of a comprehensive VDUS screening program in neurosurgical patients.

Methods.—Medical records of patients admitted to the neurosurgical service at a university-affiliated hospital from October 2007 through January 2010 who underwent weekly VDUS of the lower extremities until ambulatory or discharged were retrospectively reviewed. Demographics, comorbidities, interventions, and use of DVT prophylaxis were recorded. All patients in this study were asymptomatic for clinical evidence of DVT. When DVT was identified, VDUS reported its location and progression.

Results.—One hundred seventy-four consecutive patients were screened according to the established protocol. They had 312 VDUS studies, 68

(21.8%) of which were positive in 40 (23%) unique patients; 10 were bilateral and two catheter-related. There were no documented pulmonary emboli in this series. Seventeen patients (37.7%) had isolated calf DVT, four of which were bilateral (totaling 21 thrombi), and 9 (20%) had coexistent thrombi in calf and proximal veins. Of the 21 isolated calf DVTs, 15 had follow-up studies and two progressed to the popliteal or ileofemoral vein on follow-up (13.3%). Mechanical prophylaxis was uniformly utilized, but chemical prophylaxis varied based on surgeons' assessment of bleeding risk. DVT developed in 19.3% (28/145) of patients receiving prophylactic medication (unfractionated heparin or low-molecular weight heparin) and 41.4% (12/29) receiving no chemoprophylaxis ($P < .001$). The only patient characteristic that correlated with DVT risk was a body mass index <30 (9.1% vs 29.4%, $P = .01$).

Conclusions.—Despite the uniform application of mechanical DVT prophylaxis and the use of chemoprophylaxis in a majority of patients, we found a 23% incidence of DVT in these hospitalized, nonambulatory, neurosurgical patients. No patients with isolated calf DVT had an embolic complication but 13.3% progressed proximally in short-term follow-up. While chemical prophylaxis significantly reduced DVT risk, no factor was sufficiently predictive to exclude patients from screening. These data substantiate the importance of full leg VDUS screening and maximizing DVT prophylaxis in this high risk population.

▶ Balancing the risk of deep venous thrombosis (DVT) and secondary bleeding from anticoagulation prophylaxis in neurosurgical patients continues to be problematic. Although all patients in this study received mechanical prophylactic measures, and 83% received pharmacologic thromboprophylaxis (most received heparin 5000 units subcutaneously twice a day, while 2 received enoxaparin subcutaneously once a day), overall DVT rate was still high at 23%, with 43% isolated to calf veins. Those receiving pharmacologic thromboprophylaxis compared with mechanical options only did have lower risk of DVT (19% vs 41%). And, most importantly, there were no pulmonary embolisms in the entire series, and secondary intracranial bleeding complications occurred in only 3 patients (1.7%). Given the high reported rate of DVT even with prophylactic measures in place, screening is supported in this study as a decision point for conversion to therapeutic anticoagulation or placement of vena cava filter if DVT is documented. Although an approach that utilizes routine ultrasound screening is not cost effective, with the special concern for balancing effective DVT prevention and treatment with potential secondary intracranial hemorrhage risk from anticoagulation, clinical usefulness may outweigh cost issues. Until more effective DVT prophylactic measures in neurosurgical patients are defined that can lower the rate of DVT to more acceptable levels, routine ultrasound screening at weekly intervals may be justified.

M. A. Passman, MD

Venous Lower-Limb Evaluation in Patients With Acute Pulmonary Embolism

Pomero F, Brignone C, Serraino C, et al (Santa Croce and Carle General Hosp, Cuneo, Italy; Univ of Turin, Italy)
South Med J 104:405-411, 2011

Objectives.—Compressive ultrasonography (CUS) of the lower limbs is the first choice for identifying deep venous thrombosis (DVT) in patients with symptomatic pulmonary embolism (PE). The aim of this study was to uncover clinical characteristics and CUS findings in patients with proven PE and their correlations with PE extent.

Methods.—A total of 524 consecutive cases of proven symptomatic PE diagnosed between January 1996 and December 2006 were reviewed.

Results.—Mean age was 71.06 ± 14.43 SD years; 244 patients (46.6%) were men. DVT signs or symptoms were present in 30.9% of patients and were associated with the femoral site ($P = 0.029$). CUS was performed in 383 patients (73.1%) and DVT was found in 75.5%. In 94.1% of patients DVT was proximal (popliteal and/or femoral), which would have been then identified by simplified CUS. CUS was performed significantly more often in presence of signs or symptoms of DVT ($P < 0.001$), less often in presence of medical illnesses ($P = 0.040$), age ≥75 years ($P = 0.001$) and death in hospital ($P < 0.001$). Signs or symptoms of DVT were predictors of positive CUS ($P < 0.001$), presence of medical illnesses ($P = 0.020$), central venous catheter ($P = 0.035$), death in hospital ($P = 0.032$) were predictors of negative CUS findings. Neither clinical findings nor CUS were associated with PE extent.

Conclusions.—In patients with proven symptomatic PE, signs or symptoms of DVT are present only in 1/3 of cases and are significantly more frequent when DVT is extended to the femoral vein. Simplified CUS of the lower limbs has a high sensitivity in finding proximal DVT. CUS is not able to predict PE extent.

▶ Both deep venous thrombosis (DVT) and pulmonary embolism (PE) are clinical manifestations of venous thromboembolism (VTE). The large majority of cases of symptomatic PE (90%) are felt to be caused by lower limb DVT.[1] Duplex ultrasonography is frequently used as the first method to search for venous thrombosis in patients with suspected PE or DVT. In addition, presence of DVT as diagnosed by duplex ultrasound is independently associated with adverse outcome of PE.[2] The authors sought to determine in patients with a diagnosis of PE whether clinical characteristics and thrombosis site in lower extremity veins are able to predict PE extent. It is noteworthy that 69% of the patients with proven PE had no DVT signs or symptoms on clinical examination. A positive duplex ultrasound finding did not correlate with a major PE ($P = .98$). Conversely DVT was found in only 75.6% of patients with proven PE. Ultrasound examination of the lower extremities in patients with suspected PE therefore cannot by itself rule out PE. However, it may still be useful to perform such a study in that the concordance of lower-extremity DVT with proven PE is still high. There is also evidence to suggest that early compressive therapy and mobilization of patients with acute

DVT may decrease long-term postphlebitic syndrome. Thus the reason to perform a duplex examination of the lower extremities in patients with suspected PE is not to try and diagnosis PE but to diagnosis DVT and potentially institute treatment directed to the DVT that may reduce long-term morbidity of DVT.

G. L. Moneta, MD

References

1. Kearon C. Natural history of venous thromboembolism. *Circulation.* 2003;107: 122-130.
2. Wicki J, Perrier A, Perneger TV, Bounameaux H, Junod AF. Predicting adverse outcome in patients with acute pulmonary embolism: a risk score. *Thromb Haemost.* 2000;84:548-552.

Heart Disease May Be a Risk Factor for Pulmonary Embolism Without Peripheral Deep Venous Thrombosis

Sørensen HT, Horvath-Puho E, Lash TL, et al (Aarhus Univ Hosp, Denmark; et al)
Circulation 124:1435-1441, 2011

Background.—Heart diseases increase the risk of arterial embolism; whether they increase the risk of pulmonary embolism without peripheral venous thrombosis is less certain.

Methods and Results.—We conducted a nationwide, population-based case-control study in Denmark using patients diagnosed with pulmonary embolism and/or deep venous thrombosis between 1980 and 2007. We computed odds ratios to estimate relative risks associating preceding heart disease with pulmonary embolism, pulmonary embolism and deep venous thrombosis, or deep venous thrombosis alone. In this study, 45 282 patients had pulmonary embolism alone, 4680 had pulmonary embolism and deep venous thrombosis, and 59 790 had deep venous thrombosis alone; 541 561 were population controls. Myocardial infarction and heart failure in the preceding 3 months conferred high risks of apparently isolated pulmonary embolism (odds ratio, 43.5 [95% confidence interval (CI), 39.6−47.8] and 32.4 [95% CI, 29.8−35.2], respectively), whereas the risks of combined pulmonary embolism and deep venous thrombosis (19.7 [95% CI, 16.0−24.2] and 22.1 [95% CI, 18.7−26.0], respectively) and deep venous thrombosis alone (9.6 [95% CI, 8.6−10.7] and 12.7 [95% CI, 11.6−13.9], respectively) were lower. Left-sided valvular disease was associated with an odds ratio of 13.5 (95% CI, 11.3−16.1), whereas the odds ratio was 74.6 (95% CI, 28.4−195.8) for right-sided valvular disease. Restricting the analysis to cases diagnosed after 2000 led to lower risk estimates but the same overall pattern.

Conclusion.—Heart diseases increase the near-term risk for pulmonary embolism not associated with diagnosed peripheral vein thrombosis.

▶ It is well known that up to 40% of patients with pulmonary embolism (PE), despite careful venous examination, will not have evidence of peripheral venous thrombosis.[1] One explanation for this observation is that the emboli have been dislodged from the lower extremity and are no longer visible by routine diagnostic methods. However, an additional explanation may be that there are other sources of emboli, including the heart itself, that may serve as an embolic source to the lung. This may be especially true in the setting of cardiac disease. It is well known that left-sided cardiac thrombi predispose to arterial embolization. Autopsy series have shown, however, that right-sided intercardiac thrombosis may be as common as thrombosis on the left side.[2] Echocardiographic studies have reported significant incidences of right-sided cardiac thrombi in patients with acute PE.[3] Recently, it has also been suggested that there is a higher prevalence of heart disease in patients with PE and no detected peripheral deep vein thrombosis (DVT) compared with patients who have PE and peripheral DVT.[4] It immediately stands out that the proportion of apparently isolated PE is much higher than one would normally expect. The authors did not have data on how often the presence of DVT was assessed in patients with a diagnosis of PE. However, multiple previous studies have also indicated that not everyone with confirmed PE has a diagnosable DVT. The authors' observations as to the timing of pulmonary embolism in relationship to cardiac disease, previous studies indicating a significant prevalence of right-sided cardiac thrombi, and the strong odd ratios in this study implicating right-sided cardiac sources for PE all combine to suggest their conclusion is correct that the right side of the heart can serve as a source of PE. A similar analysis performed in patients with PE simultaneously assessed for preexisting cardiac disease and DVT is needed to precisely determine what proportion of PE originates from the right side of the heart.

G. L. Moneta, MD

References

1. Hull RD, Hirsh J, Carter CJ, et al. Pulmonary angiography, ventilation lung scanning, and venography for clinically suspected pulmonary embolism with abnormal perfusion lung scan. *Ann Intern Med.* 1983;98:891-899.
2. Ogren M, Bergqvist D, Eriksson H, Lindblad B, Sternby NH. Prevalence and risk of pulmonary embolism in patients with intracardiac thrombosis: a population-based study of 23 796 consecutive autopsies. *Eur Heart J.* 2005;26:1108-1114.
3. Goldhaber SZ. Optimal strategy for diagnosis and treatment of pulmonary embolism due to right atrial thrombus. *Mayo Clin Proc.* 1988;63:1261-1264.
4. Prandoni P, Pesavento R, Sørensen HT, et al. Prevalence of heart diseases in patients with pulmonary embolism with and without peripheral venous thrombosis: findings from a cross-sectional survey. *Eur J Intern Med.* 2009;20:470-473.

Long-term outcome after additional catheter-directed thrombolysis versus standard treatment for acute iliofemoral deep vein thrombosis (the CaVenT study): a randomised controlled trial
Enden T, on behalf of the CaVenT Study Group (Oslo Univ Hosp, Norway; et al)
Lancet 379:31-38, 2012

Background.—Conventional anticoagulant treatment for acute deep vein thrombosis (DVT) effectively prevents thrombus extension and recurrence, but does not dissolve the clot, and many patients develop post-thrombotic syndrome (PTS). We aimed to examine whether additional treatment with catheter-directed thrombolysis (CDT) using alteplase reduced development of PTS.

Methods.—Participants in this open-label, randomised controlled trial were recruited from 20 hospitals in the Norwegian southeastern health region. Patients aged 18—75 years with a first-time iliofemoral DVT were included within 21 days from symptom onset. Patients were randomly assigned (1:1) by picking lowest number of sealed envelopes to conventional treatment alone or additional CDT. Randomisation was stratified for involvement of the pelvic veins with blocks of six. We assessed two co-primary outcomes: frequency of PTS as assessed by Villalta score at 24 months, and iliofemoral patency after 6 months. Analyses were by intention to treat. This trial is registered at ClinicalTrials.gov, NCT00251771.

Findings.—209 patients were randomly assigned to treatment groups (108 control, 101 CDT). At completion of 24 months' follow-up, data for clinical status were available for 189 patients (90%; 99 control, 90 CDT). At 24 months, 37 (41·1%, 95% CI 31·5—51·4) patients allocated additional CDT presented with PTS compared with 55 (55·6%, 95% CI 45·7—65·0) in the control group (p=0·047). The difference in PTS corresponds to an absolute risk reduction of 14·4% (95% CI 0·2—27·9), and the number needed to treat was 7 (95% CI 4—502). Iliofemoral patency after 6 months was reported in 58 patients (65·9%, 95% CI 55·5—75·0) on CDT versus 45 (47·4%, 37·6—57·3) on control (p=0·012). 20 bleeding complications related to CDT included three major and five clinically relevant bleeds.

Interpretation.—Additional CDT should be considered in patients with a high proximal DVT and low risk of bleeding.

▶ In patients with deep vein thrombosis (DVT), antithrombotic therapy prevents thrombus extension, pulmonary embolism, death, and DVT recurrence. Many patients, however, develop venous dysfunction, so called postthrombotic syndrome (PTS). PTS is associated with decreased quality of life and adverse economic situation. Patients with symptomatic DVT of the popliteal and more proximal veins have a nearly 50% incidence of some degree of PTS.[1] PTS may develop from either venous obstruction, venous reflux, or a combination of both. A recent systematic review suggests accelerated removal of thrombus material can prevent vein dysfunction and PTS.[2] Systemic thrombolysis is associated with an unacceptable incidence of hemorrhagic complications, while case series of catheter-based thrombolysis have suggested effective lysis with decreased bleeding. The catheter-directed venous thrombolysis study evaluated whether the addition of catheter-directed thrombolysis (CDT) to standard anticoagulation for acute iliofemoral venous thrombosis improved long-term outcome through a reduction of PTS. For the first time there is now a randomized trial to show clinically significant reductions in PTS after the use of CDT compared to conventional treatment alone. The effect was modest, with an absolute risk reduction of 14.4% and a treatment rate of 7 to prevent 1 PTS. There was a small additional risk of bleeding in patients treated with CDT. Overall, however, the results seem clinically significant and support recent guidelines that CDT can be considered in patients with proximal DVT and a low risk of bleeding. The ATTRACT (Acute Venous Thrombosis: Thrombus Removal with Adjunctive Catheter-Directed Thrombolysis) trial is currently underway in the United States to evaluate catheter-directed thrombolysis for iliofemoral DVT.

G. L. Moneta, MD

References

1. Prandoni P, Lensing AW, Prins MH, et al. Below-knee elastic compression stockings to prevent the post-thrombotic syndrome: a randomized, controlled trial. *Ann Intern Med.* 2004;141:249-256.
2. Watson LI, Armon MP. Thrombolysis for acute deep vein thrombosis. *Cochrane Database Syst Rev.* 2004;(4). CD002783.

Placement and Removal of Inferior Vena Cava Filters: National Trends in the Medicare Population

Duszak R Jr, Parker L, Levin DC, et al (Mid-South Imaging and Therapeutics, Memphis, TN; Thomas Jefferson Univ Hosp and Jefferson Med College, Philadelphia, PA)

J Am Coll Radiol 8:483-489, 2011

Purpose.—The aim of this study was to evaluate trends in the placement and removal of inferior vena cava (IVC) filters in the Medicare population.

Methods.—Summary Medicare claims data from 1999 through 2008 were used to identify the frequency of IVC filter placement procedures by specialty (radiology, surgery, cardiology, and all others) and site of service. Claims from 2003 (the first year the FDA cleared retrievable labeling for filters) through 2008 were used to identify intravascular foreign body retrieval procedures, and modeling was used estimate a frequency range of removal procedures. Trends over time were evaluated.

Results.—Between 1999 and 2008, total Medicare fee-for-service beneficiary frequency of IVC filter placement procedures increased by 111.5% (30,756 to 65,041). Volumes increased for radiologists (16,531 to 36,829 [+122.8%]), surgeons (11,295 to 22,606 [+100.1%]), and cardiologists (1,025 to 4,236 [+313.3%]). Relative specialty market shares changed little over time. Volumes increased by 114.2% (26,511 to 56,774) and 229.1% (2,286 to 7,524) for hospital inpatients and outpatients, respectively, and decreased by 62.1% (1,959 to 743) for those in all other locations combined. In 2008, with 65,041 filters placed, only an estimated 801 to 3,339 (1.2 to 5.1%) were removed.

Conclusion.—The frequency of IVC filter placement has doubled over the past decade, and radiologists continue to perform more than half of all procedures. Although volume has more than tripled in hospital outpatients,

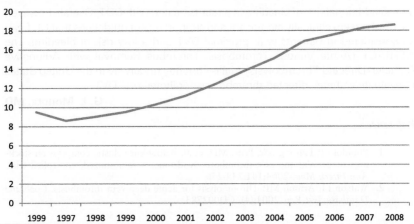

FIGURE 1.—Annual rate of IVC filter placement procedures by all providers per 10,000 Medicare. (Reprinted from the Journal of the American College of Cardiology, Duszak R Jr, Parker L, Levin DC, et al. Placement and removal of inferior vena cava filters: National trends in the medicare population. *J Am Coll Radiol.* 2011;8:483-489. Copyright 2011, with permission from American College of Radiology.)

the inpatient setting remains by far the most common site of service. In the Medicare population, IVC filters are not commonly removed (Fig 1).

▶ There seems little doubt that the recent availability of retrievable inferior vena cava (IVC) filters has, in many physicians' practices, lowered the threshold for filter placement. Recent studies of frequency of IVC filter placement have focused largely on patients with trauma.[1,2] The Medicare population, however, represents a much larger group than trauma patients, and thus patterns of filter placement in these patients should be of interest in the discussion of utilization of health care resources. Therefore, the authors sought to evaluate placement and removal of IVC filters in the Medicare population. They found that the number of IVC filters placed in the Medicare population has increased dramatically (Fig 1). Few were removed, suggesting, hopefully, that the indications for placement mirror traditional indications for placement of permanent IVC filters. In addition, the presence of a higher prevalence of comorbidities may also contribute to a lower retrieval rate for IVC filters in the Medicare population. It is rumored that reimbursement for placement of IVC filters will soon be dramatically reduced. However, because a large percentage of filters are still placed by radiologists, who generally do not make the decision to place the filter, decreased reimbursement for filters may lower the overall cost to Medicare but may not influence many referring physicians' choice to have the filter placed. It is therefore likely that with the aging population, the trend of more filters being placed will continue.

G. L. Moneta, MD

References

1. Antevil JL, Sise MJ, Sack DI, et al. Retrievable vena cava filters for preventing pulmonary embolism in trauma patients: a cautionary tale. *J Trauma.* 2006;60: 35-40.

2. Karmy-Jones R, Jurkovich GJ, Velmahos GC, et al. Practice patterns and outcomes of retrievable vena cava filters in trauma patients: an AAST multicenter study. *J Trauma*. 2007;62:17-25.

A Method for Following Patients with Retrievable Inferior Vena Cava Filters: Results and Lessons Learned from the First 1,100 Patients
Lynch FC (Penn State Univ College of Medicine, Hershey, PA)
J Vasc Interv Radiol 22:1507-1512, 2011

Purpose.—Patients who have undergone implantation of a retrievable inferior vena cava (IVC) filter require continued follow-up to have the device removed when clinically appropriate and in a timely fashion to avoid potential long-term filter-related complications. The efficacy of a method for patient follow-up was evaluated based on a retrospective review of a single-institutional retrievable IVC filter experience.

Materials and Methods.—Patients with retrievable IVC filters were tracked via a prospectively collected database designed specifically for patient follow-up. Follow-up consisted of periodic review of the electronic medical record. Patients were contacted by mail (at regular intervals one or more times) when removal of the filter was deemed appropriate. A retrospective review of the ultimate fate of the first 1,127 retrievable IVC filters placed at a single institution was performed. Retrieval rates were compared with those seen in the initial experience, during which no structured follow-up was performed.

Results.—Of 1,127 filters placed, 658 (58.4%) were removed. Filter removal or declaration of the device as permanent was achieved in 860 patients (76.3%). Filter removal, declaration of the device as permanent, or establishment of the need for continued follow-up was achieved in 941 patients (83.5%). Only 186 patients (16.5%) were lost to follow-up.

Conclusions.—The follow-up method described in the present study resulted in a statistically significant difference ($P < .001$) in the likelihood of a patient returning for IVC filter removal compared with a lack of follow-up (59% vs 24%) (Fig 1).

▶ In August of 2010 the US Food and Drug Administration (FDA) issued an alert regarding complications and adverse events associated with inferior vena cava (IVC) filters. Vascular surgeons have been aware for years that IVC filters are not without long-term complications but apparently complications reached the FDA's "radar" as a result of the sheer numbers of filters implanted once the so-called retrievable devices were approved for implantation. The epidemic of IVC filters likely resulted from the allure of a retrievable device and possibly also from relative favorable reimbursement for the procedure and fear of missing an opportunity to prevent a fatal pulmonary embolism. Many IVC filters were thus implanted for what could be considered very marginal indications. Unfortunately, once implanted, many of these temporary filters became unintentionally permanent devices leading to longer-term complications that could be avoided if the

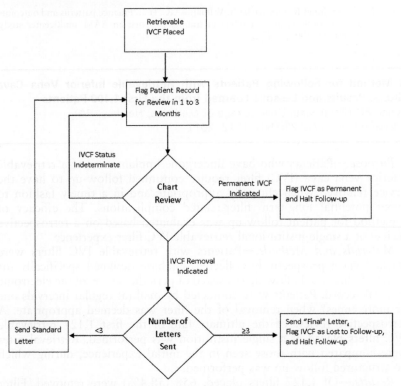

FIGURE 1.—Algorithm for retrievable IVC filter follow-up. IVCF = inferior vena cava filter. (Reprinted from Journal of Vascular and Interventional Radiology, Lynch FC. A method for following patients with retrievable inferior vena cava filters: results and lessons learned from the first 1,100 patients. *J Vasc Interv Radiol.* 2011;22:1507-1512. Copyright 2011, with permission from Elsevier.)

filter had never been implanted or had been removed once it was no longer necessary. This article shows it is possible to improve the dismal retrieval rates of IVC filters documented in previous reports. However, the program implemented in rural Pennsylvania (Fig 1) is not likely to achieve the same results in an inner city trauma population. The best way to avoid the problem of the unretrieved IVC filter and subsequent filter-related complications is not to place the filter in the first place unless it is truly needed, and that need is supported by data.

G. L. Moneta, MD

Stenting of chronically obstructed inferior vena cava filters

Neglén P, Oglesbee M, Olivier J, et al (River Oaks Hosp, Flowood, MS; Univ of New South Wales, Sydney, Australia)
J Vasc Surg 54:153-161, 2011

Objectives.—A protective inferior vena cava (IVC) filter may later be incorporated into a chronic postthrombotic ilio-caval obstruction (occlusive, requiring recanalization, or nonocclusive). This study aims to assess the safety and stent-related outcome following stenting across an obstructed filter.

Methods.—From 1997 to 2009, 708 limbs had stenting for postthrombotic ilio-caval outflow obstruction (occlusion in 121 limbs). In 25 patients, an IVC filter was obstructed (Group X). The site was crossed by a guidewire and balloon dilated. The filter was markedly displaced sidewise or remodeled. A stent was placed across the IVC filter and redilated. In 28 other patients, the cephalad stenting terminated below a patent IVC filter (Group B). The remaining 655 patients had no previous IVC filter placement (Group no IVC filter present [NF]). The patients were followed to assess patency. The types of reintervention were noted.

Results.—The stenting maneuver through a variety of previously inserted IVC filters was safely performed without an apparent tear of the IVC, no clinical bleeding or abdominal symptoms, or pulmonary embolism. Mortality was nil; morbidity minimal. The primary and secondary cumulative patency rates at 54 months for limbs with postthrombotic obstruction were with and without IVC filter (38% and 40%; $P = .1701$ and 79% and 86%; $P = .1947$, respectively), and for limbs with stenting across the filter (Group X) and stent termination below the filter (Group B; 32% and 42%; $P = .3064$ and 75% and 84%; $P = .2788$, respectively), not statistically different. When Group X alone was compared with Group NF, the secondary patency rate was, however, significantly lower (75% vs 86%; $P = .0453$), suggesting that crossing of the stent was associated with reduced patency. Occlusive postthrombotic disease requiring recanalization was more frequent in Group X than in Group B and Group NF (68%, 25%, and 15%, respectively; $P = .004$). A comparison was therefore performed only between limbs stented for recanalized occlusions with (n = 23) and without IVC filters (n = 92) showing no difference (cumulative primary and secondary patency rates 30% and 35%; $P = .9678$ and 71% and 73%; $P = .9319$, respectively). Multiple logistic regression analysis also supported a significant association between patency rate and occlusive disease (odds ratio, 6.9; 95% confidence interval, 3.4-13.9; $P < .0001$), but not between patency rate and presence of an IVC filter ($P = .5552$).

Conclusions.—Stenting across an obstructed IVC filter is safe. It appears that patency is not influenced by the fact that an IVC filter is crossed by a stent, but is related to the severity of postthrombotic disease (occlusive or nonocclusive obstruction) and the associated recanalization procedure.

▶ This is an insightful analysis by Drs Nelgen and Raju of a cohort of their patients with severe thrombotic disease of the iliocaval system secondary to the adverse effects of inferior vena cava filters. From 1997 to 2009, this group treated 121 patients who had symptomatic inferior vena cava (IVC) occlusion secondary to IVC filter thrombosis. This group accounts for 17% of their 708 limbs associated with venous thromboembolic disease treated over this timeframe. The reported incidence of caval thrombosis varies from filter to filter but is roughly 2% to 5%. Despite this low figure, the prevalence of this entity is becoming more frequent because of the exponential increase in the insertion of IVC filters. As such, vascular surgeons should become more familiar with the techniques used to treat this entity and become involved in its process improvement. In this study, thrombosed Greenfield filters accounted for 44% of the caval thromboses encountered. The authors don't mention if these were titanium or stainless steel Greenfield filters. The authors used standard techniques of venous stenting to reestablish venous outflow in these patients, typically, Wallstent sizes 14-24 as guided by intravascular ultrasonography. The authors don't comment on the incidence of thrombophilia in these patients or whether these patients were maintained on chronic anticoagulation with warfarin or low-molecular-weight heparin. They do report an early stent occlusion rate of 12% at 30 days and a late stent occlusion rate at 12%. With this they report a primary and secondary cumulative patency rate at 54 months for limbs with postthrombotic obstruction of 38% and 79%, respectively. Further analysis was performed using logistic regression analysis showing that when compared with stenting patients with nonocclusive thrombus, the presence or absence of an IVC filter had no influence on long-term patency as long as the stent remained widely patent. This analysis did show, however, that patients with occlusion versus stenosis had significantly worse outcomes.

As stated previously, it is important for clinicians to continue to collect and analyze data regarding this patient population, as treatment options for them are severely limited. More than half of the patients in this series had active or healed venous ulceration. In my clinician's experience, these patients also suffer from severely debilitating lower extremity pain and venous claudication, which is severely lifestyle limiting. Future studies on the role of anticoagulation, bifurcation stenting, and long-term follow-up are needed to help this severely underserved patient population.

D. L. Gillespie, MD, FACS

16 Chronic Venous and Lymphatic Disease

The care of patients with varicose veins and associated chronic venous diseases: Clinical practice guidelines of the Society for Vascular Surgery and the American Venous Forum
Gloviczki P, Comerota AJ, Dalsing MC, et al (Mayo Clinic, Rochester, MN; Jobst Vascular Ctr, Toledo, OH; Indiana Univ School of Medicine, Indianapolis; et al)
J Vasc Surg 53:2S-48S, 2011

The Society for Vascular Surgery (SVS) and the American Venous Forum (AVF) have developed clinical practice guidelines for the care of patients with varicose veins of the lower limbs and pelvis. The document also includes recommendations on the management of superficial and perforating vein incompetence in patients with associated, more advanced chronic venous diseases (CVDs), including edema, skin changes, or venous ulcers. Recommendations of the Venous Guideline Committee are based on the Grading of Recommendations Assessment, Development, and Evaluation (GRADE) system as strong (GRADE 1) if the benefits clearly outweigh the risks, burden, and costs. The suggestions are weak (GRADE 2) if the benefits are closely balanced with risks and burden. The level of available evidence to support the evaluation or treatment can be of high (A), medium (B), or low or very low (C) quality. The key recommendations of these guidelines are: We recommend that in patients with varicose veins or more severe CVD, a complete history and detailed physical examination are complemented by duplex ultrasound scanning of the deep and superficial veins (GRADE 1A). We recommend that the CEAP classification is used for patients with CVD (GRADE 1A) and that the revised Venous Clinical Severity Score is used to assess treatment outcome (GRADE 1B). We suggest compression therapy for patients with symptomatic varicose veins (GRADE 2C) but recommend against compression therapy as the primary treatment if the patient is a candidate for saphenous vein ablation (GRADE 1B). We recommend compression therapy as the primary treatment to aid healing of venous ulceration (GRADE 1B). To decrease the recurrence of venous ulcers, we recommend ablation of the incompetent superficial veins in addition to compression therapy (GRADE 1A). For treatment of the incompetent great saphenous vein (GSV), we recommend endovenous thermal ablation (radiofrequency or laser) rather than high ligation and inversion stripping of the saphenous vein to the level of the knee (GRADE 1B). We recommend phlebectomy or sclerotherapy to treat varicose tributaries (GRADE 1B) and suggest foam sclerotherapy as an option for the treatment of the incompetent saphenous vein (GRADE 2C). We recommend against selective treatment of perforating vein incompetence in patients with simple varicose veins (CEAP class C_2; GRADE 1B), but we suggest treatment of pathologic perforating veins (outward flow duration ≥ 500 ms, vein diameter ≥ 3.5 mm) located underneath healed or active ulcers (CEAP class C_5-C_6; GRADE 2B). We suggest treatment of pelvic congestion syndrome and pelvic varices with coil embolization, plugs, or transcatheter sclerotherapy, used alone or together (GRADE 2B).

▶ These clinical practice guidelines developed by the Society for Vascular Surgery and the American Venous Forum are a must read for any practitioner providing care to patients with varicose veins of the lower legs and pelvis. Essential current information is provided on clinical classification, comprehensive evaluation, testing, and treatment recommendations as supported by evidence-based grading and consensus assessment of important literature. The extent of review is well beyond the scope of this commentary. Readers are encouraged to review the source document and apply these guidelines to current clinical practice standards.

M. A. Passman, MD

The Influence of Abdominal Pressure on Lower Extremity Venous Pressure and Hemodynamics: A Human In-vivo Model Simulating the Effect of Abdominal Obesity

Willenberg T, Clemens R, Haegeli LM, et al (Univ Hosp, Berne, Switzerland; Univ Hosp Zurich, Switzerland)
Eur J Vasc Endovasc Surg 41:849-855, 2011

Objective.—To demonstrate that abdominal pressure impacts venous flow and pressure characteristics.

Methods.—Venous pressure at the femoral vein was measured in 6 non-obese subjects (mean BMI 22 ± 2 kg/m^2) that were exposed to a circumferential cuff placed around the abdominal trunk and inflated to 20 and 40 mmHg. In a second step non-obese subjects ($n = 10$, BMI 21.8 ± 1.8 kg/m^2) exposed to this cuff compression were studied for duplexsonographic parameters at the femoral vein. Duplexsonographic results were compared to subjects with abdominal obesity ($n = 22$, BMI 36.2 ± 5.9 kg/m^2) in whom duplexsonographic parameters at the femoral vein were studied without cuff compression.

Results.—Intravenous pressure increased with pressure application in all participants ($p = 0.0025$). Duplex examination of 10 non-obese subjects revealed increasing venous diameter ($p < 0.0001$) and decreasing venous peak and mean velocity (all $p < 0.0001$) when cuff pressure was applied. Duplex parameters with cuff pressure application of 20 and 40 mmHg respectively, were similar to those in obese subjects that were studied without pressure application.

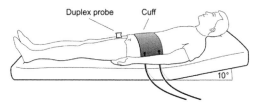

FIGURE 1.—Test arrangement for duplexsonographic assessment of venous flow characteristics of the lower extremities in non-obese participants (BMI 20—25 kg/m²). All subjects were examined in a supine position with 10° degree trunk elevation. The pressure cuff was placed at the mid abdomen. Assessment was performed with the cuff deflated and with the cuff inflated at 20 mmHg and 40 mmHg. (Reprinted from European Journal of Vascular and Endovascular Surgery, Willenberg T, Clemens R, Haegeli LM, et al. The influence of abdominal pressure on lower extremity venous pressure and hemodynamics: a human in-vivo model simulating the effect of abdominal obesity. *Eur J Vasc Endovasc Surg.* 2011;41:849-855. Copyright 2011, with permission from the European Society for Vascular Surgery.)

Conclusions.—External abdominal pressure application creates venous stasis in lower limbs. Results of this study indicate that abdominal obesity might induce resistance to venous backflow from the lower limbs (Fig 1).

▶ Central obesity appears to result in increased intra-abdominal pressure.[1] Pressure in the iliofemoral veins in morbidly obese patients is higher compared with that in the iliofemoral veins of nonobese subjects (19.1 cm H_2O vs 8.5 cm H_2O). In addition, it appears there is a significant difference in venous hemodynamics between obese and nonobese subjects when studied with duplex ultrasound.[2] Finally, epidemiologic studies suggest abdominal obesity is associated with an increased prevalence of chronic venous insufficiency (CVI) and an increased risk of venous thromboembolism.[3,4] This article presents a model in the nonobese patient to mimic intra-abdominal pressures found in the obese patient (Fig 1). The model described in this article appears to simulate the effects of abdominal obesity on venous physiology and lends strong evidence to the concept that abdominal obesity impairs lower extremity venous outflow. It is, however, unclear whether impairment in lower extremity venous outflow alone is sufficient to increase the risk of venous thromboembolism or CVI. Whereas, as noted above, obesity is associated with increased risk of venous thromboembolism and CVI, there are also many confounding factors such as ambulatory activity, ankle and joint function, gait pattern, and levels of vascular inflammation, as well as various genetic predispositions that may, to a greater or lesser extent, influence the risk of venous thromboembolism or CVI in the obese patient. Nevertheless, the model described here provides a means of measuring the effects of varying levels of abdominal pressure on lower extremity venous flow patterns.

G. L. Moneta, MD

References

1. Arfvidsson B, Eklof B, Balfour J. Iliofemoral venous pressure correlates with intra-abdominal pressure in morbidly obese patients. *Vasc Endovascular Surg.* 2005;39: 505-509.
2. Willenberg T, Schumacher A, Amann-Vesti B, et al. Impact of obesity on venous hemodynamics of the lower limbs. *J Vasc Surg.* 2010;52:664-668.

3. Hansson PO, Eriksson H, Welin L, Svärdsudd K, Wilhelmsen L. Smoking and abdominal obesity: risk factors for venous thromboembolism among middle-aged men: "the study of men born in 1913". *Arch Intern Med.* 1999;159:1886-1890.
4. Darvall KA, Sam RC, Silverman SH, Bradbury AW, Adam DJ. Obesity and thrombosis. *Eur J Vasc Endovasc Surg.* 2007;33:223-233.

Trends in Patient Reported Outcomes of Conservative and Surgical Treatment of Primary Chronic Venous Disease Contradict Current Practices

Lurie F, Kistner RL (Univ of Hawaii, Honolulu)
Ann Surg 254:363-367, 2011

Objective.—To analyze patient-reported quality of life (QOL) and symptoms in a prospective cohort of CVD patients who was managed within the framework of existing policies.

Design Study.—Prospective cohort study of 150 patients with C2–C4 clinical class of primary chronic venous disease (CVD). Management consisted of initial conservative measures, following which, the patients were given a choice of continuing conservative therapy, or surgical treatment. Patients completed Specific Quality of Life and Outcome Response–Venous (SQOR-V) tool before initial visit, after completion of conservative treatment, and at 1 and 12 month follow up visits after surgical treatment. Management consisted of initial conservative measures. QOL score and symptom score (SS) part of this instrument was analyzed separately.

Results.—Conservative treatment resulted in improvement of symptom score in 85(57%) patients, and the QOL in 111(74%) patients. Despite this improvement, the majority of patients (121) chose surgical option. At the 1-month follow up after surgical treatment 97 (80%) patients reported significant improvement of their symptoms and 114 (94%) in the QOL compare to their status after conservative therapy. The QOL improvement was due mainly to improvement in symptom score. Patients who improved after conservative therapy were more than 15 times more likely to have symptoms relief at 1 month (RR = 15.6, 95% CI 4.3–56.5), and 21 times higher at 1 year after surgery (RR = 21.3, 95% CI 4.7–96.9) compared with those who did not change the SS.

Conclusions.—Surgical treatment resulted in a better relief of symptoms compare to conservative therapy. The relief of symptoms after conservative therapy predicts better outcomes of surgical treatment. These findings suggest that success of conservative therapy should be considered as an indication, and the failure of conservative therapy should not be an indication to surgical treatment.

▶ Most insurance policies will approve treatment for varicose veins only when medically necessary. Medical necessity is usually defined as failure to obtain symptom relief after a period of conservative management. Conservative management is generally the use of a graduated compression stockings for 1 to 6 months. There is, however, no significant evidence that conservative therapy obviates the need for invasive treatment. The percentage of patients who actually receive adequate relief with conservative therapy and who have primary chronic venous disease is not well documented. The potential of further improvement in symptoms with surgical therapy for patients who have improved with conservative therapy is also not known. In assessment of the effects of conservative therapy for chronic venous disease, there have also been relatively few studies using patient-reported outcome instruments. Patient-centered medicine however, in essence, requires examination of practice guidelines and polices from the patient perspective of disease severity and treatment outcomes. The data suggest that conservative therapy for patients with primary chronic venous disease improves symptoms and quality of life. This finding would be consistent with conventional wisdom. The provocative piece of this article is to suggest that improvement with conservative therapy should not be used to withhold surgical therapy but actually serves as a marker for those patients who will improve further with surgical therapy. The findings thus contradict the current practice of insurance companies that interpret success of conservative measures as a contraindication to surgical treatment. In essence, success of conservative therapy is an indication for surgical therapy.

G. L. Moneta, MD

Compression Stockings with a Negative Pressure Gradient Have a More Pronounced Effect on Venous Pumping Function than Graduated Elastic Compression Stockings

Mosti G, Partsch H (Clinica MD Barbantini, Lucca, Italy; Private Practice, Wien, Austria)
Eur J Vasc Endovasc Surg 42:261-266, 2011

Objectives.—To measure the effect on the venous pumping function of a stocking providing a negative pressure gradient with higher pressures over the calf in comparison to a conventional graduated elastic compression stocking (GECS) in patients with advanced venous insufficiency.

Design.—Experimental study.

Material.—30 patients with severe superficial chronic venous insufficiency were enrolled. Two elastic stocking designs exerting a pressure at ankle between 15 and 25 mm Hg were compared; a conventional GECS and a stocking exerting a higher pressure over the calf than over the ankle producing a "progressive" increase in compression (PECS).

Method.—The venous calf pumping function was assessed by measuring the ejection fraction (EF) from the lower leg by a plethysmographic method during a standardised exercise. Interface pressure of the 2 compression devices was simultaneously recorded both at B1 = 12 cm above ankle, C = just above widest part of calf.

Results.—The mean increase of EF produced by PECS was +75% (95 CI 48,7-101,3) compared with +32% (95%CI 16,8-48,6) with GECS ($P < 0.001$). There was a significant correlation between EF and the stocking pressure measured at calf level during standing and walking.

Conclusion.—Stockings exerting a higher pressure on the calf than on the ankle show a greater efficacy in increasing the venous ejection fraction from the leg.

▶ Compression therapy has been the standard of care in patients with chronic venous insufficiency (CEAP classes C3-C6), but this concept has been debated in the case of varicose veins (C2) for which studies have demonstrated that surgery is more cost effective.[1] Compression therapy is often instituted in the United States because third-party payers require a period of compression prior to reimbursement for surgical procedure. One of the biggest issues with compression therapy has been patient compliance with using the stockings. Many elderly patients have a difficult time applying the stocking without assistance, which is a common complaint we have noted from this group of patients. The graduated compression stockings (GECS) with a decreasing pressure gradient distally to proximally are the standard stockings that are used with the concept, which mimics the normal venous circulation. The amount of exertional pressure required to overcome the hydrostatic pressure diminishes from the distal leg proximally. The authors of this study describe their experience with standard GECS and new stockings that provide a higher compression over the calf than the ankle (progressive elastic compression stockings [PECS]).

The concept is opposite to that of the graduated (degressive) compression therapy and based on studies evaluating the local blood volume in the leg and demonstrating that the highest amount of blood is in the midcalf, with the content of blood in the distal portion of the leg much lower. Objective data were obtained using an interface pressure measurement monitor and strain gauge plethysmography. The mean ejection fraction of the calf increased with both compression stockings, but with the PECS, it was significantly higher (52.5% with PECS vs 44.5% with GECS). Pressure measurements in the supine position were, as expected, the opposite between the 2 stockings, with the GECS exerting a higher pressure at the ankle and a lower pressure at the calf; however, when standing and exercising, the PECS exerted a pressure higher than the GECS at the calf. The authors describe that an ankle pressure of 44 to 60 mm Hg would be required to achieve this same pressure profile with GECS and that this would again likely lead to compliance issues in patients attempting to use it. Although the study had a group of patients who likely did not need compression (11 C2 patients), this study reveals a potential method to increase compliance with compression therapy.

N. Singh, MD

Reference

1. Gloviczki P, Comerota AJ, Dalsing MC, et al. The care of patients with varicose veins and associated chronic venous diseases: clinical practice guidelines of the Society for Vascular Surgery and the American Venous Forum. *J Vasc Surg.* 2011; 53:2S-48S.

Clinical and technical outcomes from a randomized clinical trial of endovenous laser ablation compared with conventional surgery for great saphenous varicose veins

Carradice D, Mekako AI, Mazari FAK, et al (Univ of Hull, UK)
Br J Surg 98:1117-1123, 2011

Background.—This report describes the clinical effectiveness and recurrence rates from a randomized trial of endovenous laser ablation (EVLA) and surgery for varicose veins.

Methods.—Some 280 patients were randomized equally using sealed opaque envelopes to two parallel groups: surgery and EVLA. Inclusion criteria included symptomatic disease secondary to primary, unilateral, isolated saphenofemoral junction incompetence, leading to reflux into the great saphenous vein (GSV). Outcomes were: technical success, recurrent varicose veins on clinical examination, patterns of reflux on duplex ultrasound examination, and the effect of recurrence on quality of life, assessed by the Aberdeen Varicose Vein Questionnaire (AVVQ). Assessments were at 1, 6, 12 and 52 weeks after the procedure.

Results.—Initial technical success was greater following EVLA: 99·3 *versus* 92·4 per cent ($P = 0·005$). Surgical failures related mainly to an inability to strip the above-knee GSV. The clinical recurrence rate at 1 year was lower after EVLA: 4·0 *versus* 20·4 per cent ($P < 0·001$). The number of patients needed to treat with EVLA rather than surgery to avoid one recurrence at 1 year was 6·3 (95 per cent confidence interval 4·0 to 12·5). Twelve of 23 surgical recurrences were related to an incompetent below-knee GSV and ten to neovascularization. Of five recurrences after EVLA, two were related to neoreflux in the groin tributaries and one to recanalization. Clinical recurrence was associated with worse AVVQ scores ($P < 0·001$).

Conclusion.—EVLA treatment had lower rates of clinical recurrence than conventional surgery in the short term. Registration number: NCT00759434 (http://www.clinicaltrials.gov).

▶ Conventional surgical treatment of superficial venous incompetence has recurrence rates as high as 30% at 1 year, 40% at 2 years, and up to 66% beyond 10 years.[1,2] Requests for intervention following recurrence are not as common as recurrence itself, with about 15% to 20% of varicose vein procedures performed for recurrence.[3] This article reports relative rates of clinical recurrence and patterns of treatment failure of patients enrolled in a nonblinded, randomized trial of endovenous laser ablation (EVLA) versus conventional surgery in treatment of great saphenous vein (GSV) varicose veins. Results were better with EVLA. There are several other interesting points. One can question the widely practiced principal of only stripping the GSV to the knee, as the largest number of recurrences in the surgical group were associated with incompetence of the below knee GSV. Perhaps length of GSV stripping should more reflect the length of the refluxing vein and not concerns about injuring the saphenous nerve? Another interesting point is that neovascularization, thought to be the leading cause of recurrence of varicosities in patients with traditional open surgical treatment of GSV varicosities, appears rare after EVLA. The reason for this is unclear, but may be due to decreased extravenous inflammation following EVLA versus conventional surgery. Finally, all patients with recanalization after EVLA in this trial were treated with an 810-nm laser with energy density of 60 J/cm. No recanalization was seen when energy densities were above 115 J/cm.

G. L. Moneta, MD

References

1. Campbell WB, Vijay Kumar A, Collin TW, Allington KL, Michaels JA. The outcome of varicose vein surgery at 10 years: clinical findings, symptoms and patient satisfaction. *Ann R Coll Surg Engl.* 2003;85:52-57.
2. van Rij AM, Jiang P, Solomon C, Christie RA, Hill GB. Recurrence after varicose vein surgery: a prospective long-term clinical study with duplex ultrasound scanning and air plethysmography. *J Vasc Surg.* 2003;38:935-943.
3. Gibbs PJ, Foy DM, Darke SG. Reoperation for recurrent saphenofemoral incompetence: a prospective randomised trial using a reflected flap of pectineus fascia. *Eur J Vasc Endovasc Surg.* 1999;18:494-498.

Three-year European follow-up of endovenous radiofrequency-powered segmental thermal ablation of the great saphenous vein with or without treatment of calf varicosities
Proebstle TM, for the European Closure Fast Clinical Study Group (Univ of Mainz, Germany; et al)
J Vasc Surg 54:146-152, 2011

Background.—Radiofrequency segmental thermal ablation (RSTA) has become a commonly used technology for occlusion of incompetent great saphenous veins (GSVs). Midterm results and data on clinical parameters are still lacking.

Methods.—A prospective multicenteral trial monitored 295 RSTA-treated GSVs for 36 months. Clinical control visits included flow and reflux analysis by duplex ultrasound imaging and assessment of clinical parameters according to the CEAP classification and Venous Clinical Severity Score (VCSS).

Results.—A total of 256 of 295 treated GSVs (86.4%) were available for 36 months of follow-up. At 36 months, Kaplan-Meier survival analysis showed the probability of occlusion was 92.6% and the probability of no reflux was 95.7%, and 96.9% of legs remained free of clinically relevant axial reflux. If complete occlusion was present at the 12-month follow-up, the risk of developing new flow by 24 and 36 months of follow-up was 3.7% and 4.1%, respectively. Diameters of the GSV measured 3 cm distal to the saphenofemoral junction reduced from 5.8 ± 2.1 mm at screening to 2.2 ± 1.1 mm at 36 months. The average VCSS score improved from 3.9 ± 2.1 before treatment to 0.9 ± 1.5 at 3 months ($P < .0001$) and stayed at an average <1.0 during the complete 36 months of follow-up. Only 41.1% of patients were free of pain before treatment;

at 36 months, 251 (98.0%) reported no pain and 245 (95.7%) did not experience pain during the 24 months before. At 36 months, 189 of 255 legs (74.1%) showed an improvement in CEAP class compared with the clinical assessment before treatment ($P < .001$). Stages C_3 and C_4 combined to 46% before treatment and dropped constantly to a combined level of 8% at 36 months. However, the proportion of C_2 legs that dropped from 52.3% before treatment to <10% at 12 months showed a constant increase thereafter, reaching 33.3% at 36 months.

Conclusion.—RSTA showed a high and durable success rate in vein ablation in conjunction with sustained clinical efficacy.

▶ As a 3-year follow-up study from the European Closure Fast Study Group, radiofrequency segmental thermal ablation (RSTA) showed durable sustained occlusion (92.6%), absence from reflux (95.7%), and freedom from clinically relevant reflux (96.9%), which are much improved over the results previously published for radiofrequency ablation using prior catheter technology and techniques. Side effects reported at 1 week, such as ecchymosis (5.8%), paresthesias (3.4%), pigmentation (2.4%), erythema (2.0%), hematoma (1.4%), phlebitis (1.0%), and DVT (0%), also improved to negligible levels, although this would have been expected at the longer follow-up interval. While initial decrease was seen in clinical class CEAP in the first year, this increased slightly at 3 years, but a drop in mean venous clinical severity scoring (VCSS) was sustained. Part of this finding likely represents the more static nature of CEAP compared with VCSS, although it is important to note that a large portion of patients (41%) had no pain at time of operation, which improved to 98% at 3 years. But because only mean VCSS is reported, change in individual VCSS attributes, such as pain and its effect on mean VCSS, is lacking. While concomitant treatment of varicose veins (57% phlebectomy; 12% foam sclerotherapy) was additionally performed, it is difficult to determine impact on clinical outcomes of these additional procedures. Overall, as a single-arm, nonrandomized study with extended follow-up from a prior study, these findings support that with refinement of radiofrequency ablation catheter technology and technique allowing segmental ablation along with judicious use of combined treatments for varicosities when indicated, excellent outcomes can be achieved.

M. A. Passman, MD

Late follow-up of a randomized trial of routine duplex imaging before varicose vein surgery
Blomgren L, Johansson G, Emanuelsson L, et al (Karolinska Univ Hosp, Stockholm, Sweden; Capio St Göran's Hosp, Stockholm; et al)
Br J Surg 98:1112-1116, 2011

Background.—Routine preoperative duplex examination led to an improvement in results 2 years after surgery for primary varicose veins. The aim of the present study was to evaluate the impact of preoperative duplex imaging after 7 years, in relation to other risk factors for varicose vein recurrence.

Methods.—Patients with primary varicose veins were randomized to operation with (group 1), or without (group 2) preoperative duplex imaging. The same patients were invited to attend follow-up with interview, clinical examination and duplex imaging. Quality of life (QoL) was measured with the Short Form 36 questionnaire.

Results.—Some 293 patients (343 legs) were included initially; after 7 years 227 were interviewed, or their records reviewed: 114 in group 1 and 113 in group 2. One hundred and ninety-four legs (95 in group 1 and 99 in group 2) were examined clinically and with duplex imaging. Incompetence was seen at the saphenofemoral junction and/or saphenopopliteal junction in 14 per cent of legs in group 1 and 46 per cent in group 2 ($P < 0.001$). QoL was similar in both groups. After a mean follow-up of 7 years (and including patients who underwent surgery after the review), 15 legs in group 1 needed reoperation and 38 in group 2 ($P = 0.001$).

Conclusion.—Routine preoperative duplex imaging improved the results of surgery for primary varicose veins for at least 7 years. Registration number: NCT01195623 (http://www.clinicaltrials.gov).

▶ Inadequate surgery secondary to inadequate preoperative investigation contributes to high recurrence rates following surgery for primary varicose veins.[1] One study found no clear benefit of duplex imaging before uncomplicated varicose vein surgery.[2] The authors here, however, previously reported the rate of recurrence and reoperation 2 years after varicose vein surgery was lower with preoperative duplex examination than without. It has also been suggested recently that groin surgery induces recurrence through neovascularization. If neovascularization is an important contributor to recurrence following primary varicose vein surgery, 2 years of follow-up may be inadequate to judge true effectiveness or lack of effectiveness of duplex scanning to reduce long-term recurrence following primary varicose vein surgery. The aim of this study was to evaluate the impact of preoperative duplex imaging after 7 years with respect to other risk factors for varicose vein recurrence. The study shows preoperative duplex imaging before primary varicose vein surgery results, even after 7 years, in lower recurrence and reoperation rates. Indirectly, the study also addresses a controversial topic in varicose vein treatment, that of neovascularization. In this study, at 7 years, neovascularization did not appear to cause recurrence with symptoms that required reoperation. The current thought that catheter-based techniques provide better long-term results than open surgery because of decreased neovascularization associated with nonoperative obliteration of the greater saphenous vein may not be true.

G. L. Moneta, MD

References

1. Blomgren L, Johansson G, Bergqvist D. Randomized clinical trial of routine preoperative duplex imaging before varicose vein surgery. *Br J Surg.* 2005;92:688-694.

2. Smith JJ, Brown L, Greenhalgh RM, Davies AH. Randomised trial of pre-operative colour duplex marking in primary varicose vein surgery: outcome is not improved. *Eur J Vasc Endovasc Surg.* 2002;23:336-343.

Air versus Physiological Gas for Ultrasound Guided Foam Sclerotherapy Treatment of Varicose Veins

Beckitt T, Elstone A, Ashley S (Derriford Hosp, Plymouth, UK)
Eur J Vasc Endovasc Surg 42:115-119, 2011

Objectives.—We have used Ultrasound Guided Foam Sclerotherapy (UGFS) to treat varicose veins in 2029 limbs since 2006. In 2009 we introduced physiological gas (30% O_2 and 70% CO_2) for making foam with sodium tetradecyl sulphate (Fibrovein, STD Pharmaceutical Products Ltd, Hereford UK) instead of air. The aim of this study was to compare our early experience of UFGS using CO_2/O_2 with our prior experience using air.

Methods.—Data were collected in a prospectively maintained database. In this series 470 limbs were treated with UGFS and followed up at 6 weeks with clinical and duplex ultrasound assessment. The 235 consecutive limbs undergoing UGFS immediately before and the 235 after the introduction of CO_2/O_2 were selected for comparison.

Results.—The age, gender and CEAP classifications for the two groups were not significantly different. 73% were primary veins and 70% great saphenous, with no differences between the groups. Transient neurological events are rare in our experience (0.7%) with only one visual disturbance occurring in this series. There was a significant reduction in the incidence of skin staining in the CO_2/O_2 (7.2% vs 3.3%, $p = 0.02$, χ^2 test) as compared to the air treated group, but no difference in the incidence of thrombophlebitis. The total volume of foam injected was similar in both groups but use of CO_2/O_2 foam was associated with a significant improvement in the truncal occlusion rate, from 86% to 91% ($p < 0.05$, χ^2 test).

Conclusion.—UGFS with CO_2/O_2 instead of air was associated with a slightly increased saphenous truncal occlusion rate and reduced the incidence of skin staining without increasing thrombophlebitis in this clinical series. We observed only one transient neurological event in this series so could not evaluate the effect of CO_2/O_2 foam in reducing these events (Fig 1).

▶ Foam sclerotherapy has a potential advantage over radiofrequency ablation or endoluminal thermal techniques for treatment of varicose veins in that a single technique can address truncal incompetence and varicose vein tributaries. Potential side effects of foam sclerotherapy include thrombophlebitis and skin pigmentation. Systemic side effects are also possible, especially in patients with patent foramen ovale. Stroke is a theoretic possibility in patients undergoing foam sclerotherapy because bubbles have been tracked experimentally to the middle cerebral artery using transcranial Doppler during foam sclerotherapy. Frequency of side effects may be related to the volume of foam injected as well

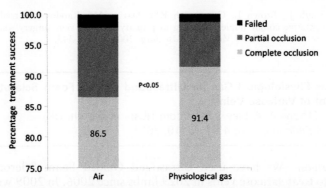

FIGURE 1.—The Proportion of duplex documented occlusions following UGFS at 8 weeks of follow-up. Complete occlusion was observed in 91.4% of subjects treated with physiological gas as compared to 86.5% treated with air, $p < 0.05$. Please note axis range is from 75% to 100%. (Reprinted from European Journal of Vascular and Endovascular Surgery, Beckitt T, Elstone A, Ashley S. Air versus physiological gas for ultrasound guided foam sclerotherapy treatment of varicose veins. *Eur J Vasc Endovasc Surg.* 2011;42:115-119. Copyright 2011, with permission from the European Society for Vascular Surgery.)

as the composition of the foam. A European Consensus document recommends limiting foam to less than 10 mL per treatment.[1] There is also some evidence that using CO_2 in place of air may reduce the incidence of side effects.[2] In this study, the authors compared their use of foam sclerotherapy when foam was prepared with physiologic gas and when foam was prepared using a mixture of 70% CO_2 and 30% O_2. They wished to determine whether the introduction of physiologic gas for foam sclerotherapy reduces the incidence of side effects. The data showed that foam sclerotherapy with CO_2/O_2 instead of air was associated with a slightly increased saphenous trunk occlusion rate but reduced the incidence of skin staining without increasing thrombophlebitis. The data confirmed that foam sclerotherapy is effective (Fig 1) and safe in that there was only 1 incident of a significant systemic side effect (0.2% of patients). In addition, there was only a 0.2% incidence of deep venous thrombosis associated with foam sclerotherapy. The incidence of systemic side effects in this study is clearly far less than that reported by Morrison and colleagues.[2] In the Morrison study, larger volumes of foam were used with a median volume of 25 mL (range 6–57). In addition, foam was injected following thermal ablation of the greater saphenous vein. Overall, it appears that low volumes of foam sclerotherapy using physiologic gas for preparation of the foam increases treatment efficacy and may reduce the incidence of skin staining. Based on cost, safety, and efficacy parameters, foam sclerotherapy using physiologic gas for preparation of the foam appears to be an effective technique for control of lower extremity varicosities.

G. L. Moneta, MD

References

1. Breu FX, Guggenbichler S, Wollmann JC. 2nd European consensus meeting on foam sclerotherapy 2006, Tegernsee, Germany. *Vasa.* 2008;37:1-29.
2. Morrison N, Neuhardt DL, Rogers CR, et al. Comparisons of side effects using air and carbon dioxide foam for endovenous chemical ablation. *J Vasc Surg.* 2008;47: 830-836.

Longevity and Outcomes of Axillary Valve Transplantation for Severe Lower Extremity Chronic Venous Insufficiency

Kabbani L, Escobar GA, Mansour F, et al (Univ of Michigan, Ann Arbor; St Joseph Mercy, Ypsilanti, MI)
Ann Vasc Surg 25:496-501, 2011

Background.—To assess the efficacy of axillary vein transplantation in the treatment of severe chronic venous insufficiency (CVI).

Methods.—Among 139 complex venous reconstructions performed between 1991 and 2007 for CVI, 18 patients underwent upper extremity to lower extremity venous valve transplantation. An upper extremity valve was transplanted to the popliteal vein in 13 cases, to the common femoral vein in six cases, and to the saphenofemoral junction in two cases for a total of 21 procedures. All patients had follow-up with duplex scanning to assess valve competency and clinical visits to assess clinical improvement. Mean follow-up period was 37 months.

Results.—Mean patient age was 44 years, and 57% were men. Clinically, 57% of the limbs were Clincal (C) class C5-C6. The mean preoperative venous disability score was 2.95. Most of the patients (66%) had post-thrombotic valvular dysfunction. At the time of valve transplantation, there was no proximal venous obstruction documented. A successful operation was defined as a competent valve at the end of the procedure and was achieved in 20 of 21 (95%) patients. Eight patients had at least one postoperative complication, primarily bleeding. The mean postoperative venous disability score was 2.65 and this increased to 2.75 (p = not significant as compared with baseline) at the last postoperative visit. Median time to return of symptoms was 12 months, and median reflux-free survival period was 15 months.

Conclusion.—Despite initial technical and symptomatic success with venous valve transplantation, there is a poor long-term valve competency rate and symptomatic control. These data suggest that a better understanding and therapy for severe CVI associated with valvular incompetence needs to be found.

▶ Venous valve reconstruction, either by internal or external valvuloplasty, and venous valve transplantation are surgical techniques to treat a small subset of patients with chronic venous insufficiency (CVI) who fail exercise treatment, elevation, compression therapy, or more standard techniques of superficial venous surgery or perforator ligation. Axillary valve transplant has been advocated as a potential technically less-demanding form of venous valve reconstruction than direct valvuloplasty. However, it appears axillary valve transplantation to lower extremity veins is another example of a theoretically sound but poorly performing procedure to treat deep venous insufficiency in patients with CVI who have failed conservative management. The operation is not as easy to perform as it would seem. Some axillary valves are incompetent, and in 6 of the authors' patients, the valves needed to be repaired in the primary operation to achieve competency. As in any surgical procedure, patient selection is likely important in achieving long-term success. Nearly three-quarters of the patients in this series were postthrombotic patients, arguably the most difficult subset of patients with refractory CVI. Whereas it appears axillary valve transplantation does not work well for postthrombotic CVI, there may be some subsets of patients (ie, those with primary deep venous insufficiency) who potentially could benefit from the procedure.

G. L. Moneta, MD

17 Technical Notes

Advanced Catheter Technology: Is This the Answer to Overcoming the Long Learning Curve in Complex Endovascular Procedures
Riga CV, Bicknell CD, Sidhu R, et al (Imperial College London, UK)
Eur J Vasc Endovasc Surg 42:531-538, 2011

Introduction.—Advanced endovascular procedures require a high degree of skill with a long learning curve. We aimed to identify differential increases in endovascular skill acquisition in novices using conventional (CC), manually steerable (MSC) and robotic endovascular catheters (RC).

Materials/Methods.—10 novices cannulated all vessels within a CT-reconstructed pulsatile-flow arch phantom in the Simulated Endovascular Suite. Subjects were randomly assigned to conventional/manually-steerable/robotic techniques as the first procedure undertaken. The operators repeated the task weekly for 5 weeks. Quantitative (cannulation times, wire/catheter-tip movements, vessel wall hits) and qualitative metrics (validated rating scale (IC3ST)) were compared.

Results.—Subjects exhibited statistically significant differences when comparing initial to final performance for total procedure times and catheter-tip movements with all catheter types. Sequential non-parametric comparisons identified learning curve plateau levels at weeks 2 or 3 (RCs, MSCs), and at week 4 (CCs) for the majority of metrics. There were significantly fewer catheter-tip movements using advanced catheter technology after training (Week 5: CC 74 IQR (59−89) versus MSC 62 (44−81); $p = 0.028$, and RC 33 (28−44); $p = 0.012$). RCs virtually eliminated wall hits at the arch (CC 29 (28−76) versus RC 8 (6−9); $p = 0.005$) and produced significantly higher overall performance scores ($p < 0.02$).

Conclusion.—Advanced endovascular catheters, although more intricate, do not seem to take longer to master and in some areas offer clear advantages with regards to positional control, at a faster rate. RCs seem to be the most intuitive and advanced skill acquisition occurs with minimal training. Robotic endovascular technology may have a significantly shorter path to proficiency allowing an increased number of trainees to attempt more complex endovascular procedures earlier and with a greater degree of safety.

▶ As endovascular surgery continues to evolve, procedures are becoming increasingly advanced. Often, the rate-limiting step is selective cannulation of a diseased or occluded branch vessel; navigating complex vascular anatomy in a 2-dimensional angiographic image can take several years to master. Steerable catheters and robotic catheters may improve technical outcomes.

The current study evaluates performance measures of 3 catheter systems in a phantom aortic arch model: conventional catheters, mechanical steerable catheters, and robotic catheters. Intuitively, robotic catheters resulted in less catheter movement in the arch and minimized interaction of the catheter with the aortic wall. Conventional catheters and mechanical steerable catheters were clinically comparable. In addition, the authors evaluated individual improvement, and surgeons' learning curves plateaued first with robotic catheters, followed by mechanical steerable catheters and then conventional catheters. All metrics suggest that advanced catheters improve individual performance measures.

Z. M. Arthurs, MD

Endurance Athletes with Intermittent Claudication Caused by Iliac Artery Stenosis Treated by Endarterectomy with Vein Patch — Short- and Mid-term Results
Bender MHM, Schep G, Bouts SW, et al (Máxima Med Centre, Veldhoven, The Netherlands; et al)
Eur J Vasc Endovasc Surg 43:472-477, 2012

Introduction.—Endurance athletes may suffer from intermittent claudication. A subgroup of 16% has severe iliac artery stenosis due to endofibrosis. In this study we report the short- and mid-term results of endarterectomy with venous patching.

Patients/Methods.—Athletes with claudication-like complaints were analysed using a protocol including cycling test and provocative echo-Doppler. Thirty-six athletes were diagnosed with serious iliac flow limitation (one bilateral), confirmed by additional magnetic resonance (MR) angiography. Endarterectomy with venous patching was performed for 32 iliac artery stenosis and five occlusions. Postoperative (mean 15.6 months) 33 legs

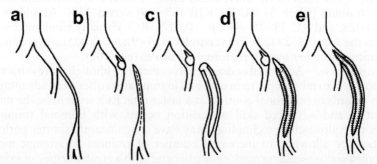

FIGURE 1.—External iliac artery stenosis (EIA) corrected by endarterectomy and vein patch (a) EIA stenosis, (b) dissection and trans-section of the EIA at the iliac bifurcation, (c) longitudinal incision after exteriorisation with endarterectomy, (d) reconstruction of the EIA by vein patch, (e) re-anastomosis of the EIA to the iliac bifurcation. (Reprinted from European Journal of Vascular and Endovascular Surgery, Bender MHM, Schep G, Bouts SW, et al. Endurance athletes with intermittent claudication caused by iliac artery stenosis treated by endarterectomy with vein patch — short- and mid-term results. *Eur J Vasc Endovasc Surg.* 2012;43:472-477. Copyright 2012, with permission from the European Society for Vascular Surgery.)

were evaluated using the same diagnostic protocol. A complete follow-up after mean 29 months was obtained by questionnaire.

Results.—Twenty-eight athletes were symptom free or could perform on a desired level with minor remaining complaints. Two athletes were satisfied though minor complaints prohibited high competition performance. Two athletes developed a re-stenosis and became symptom free after an additional operation. Three athletes had objective improvement but limited decrease in symptoms. One was unsatisfied but refused postoperative tests. The only major surgical complication was a postoperative bleeding necessitating re-operation. Postoperative tests showed significant increase in maximal workload and post-exercise ankle—brachial index. No aneurysm formation was detected.

Conclusions.—Precise diagnosis and meticulously performed endarterectomy with vein patching have satisfactory results in mid-term follow-up

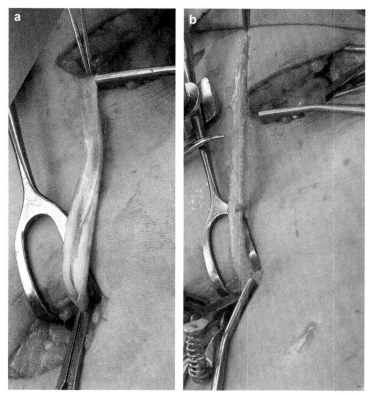

FIGURE 2.—(a) External iliac artery exteriorised though groin incision with ventral arteriotomy revealing severe stenosis by endofibrosis, (b) Closure of the endarterectomised external iliac by long vein patch. (Reprinted from European Journal of Vascular and Endovascular Surgery, Bender MHM, Schep G, Bouts SW, et al. Endurance athletes with intermittent claudication caused by iliac artery stenosis treated by endarterectomy with vein patch — short- and mid-term results. *Eur J Vasc Endovasc Surg.* 2012;43:472-477. Copyright 2012 with permission from the European Society for Vascular Surgery.)

with acceptable risk in endurance athletes complaining of intermittent claudication due to iliac artery stenosis (Figs 1 and 2).

▶ Endofibrosis of the external iliac artery develops in endurance athletes—most commonly cyclists and speed skaters in whom strong hip flexion is combined with strenuous leg exercise. There are a number of small case series in the literature describing treatments for this condition. This is among the largest series and is somewhat unique in that a single technique of external iliac artery endarterectomy combined with saphenous vein patch angioplasty was used as operative treatment. There were reasonably good functional results in what is undoubtedly a difficult-to-please patient population given that basically only a perfect result will allow these athletes to return to their same level of competition. The technique described is basically used for performance of an eversion endarterectomy of the external iliac artery. The procedure is adapted to this particular patient group by opening the artery in a longitudinal fashion and enlarging it with a saphenous vein patch (Figs 1 and 2). There were only 2 restenotic lesions, and aneurysm dilatation of the repair was not observed. Long-term data are still needed, but endarterectomy combined with long vein patch angioplasty of the external iliac artery seems to be gaining favor as the operative procedure of choice for sufficiently symptomatic external iliac artery endofibrosis.

G. L. Moneta, MD

How to Avoid a Difficult Groin in Redo Arterial Surgery: Eversion Endarterectomy of the Proximal Superficial Femoral Artery Versus Profunda Femoris Artery as Inflow for Distal Bypass

Cavallaro A, Sterpetti AV, Sapienza P, et al (Università di Roma la Sapienza, Italia)

Ann Vasc Surg 26:383-386, 2012

Background.—The aim of the study was to describe and analyze the results of a technique in which the inflow for distal bypasses is provided by the proximal superficial femoral artery, reopened through an eversion endarterectomy, to avoid a "difficult groin."

Material and Methods.—Twenty-one patients who underwent distal bypass for severe lower-limb ischemia and in whom the proximal superficial femoral artery was reopened with an eversion endarterectomy to provide inflow for the bypass itself were included in the study. As a comparison group, 20 patients in whom the inflow for a distal bypass was obtained by the distal deep femoral artery were randomly selected. In all 41 patients, the groin was considered "difficult" because of multiple previous operations.

Results.—Five-year cumulative patency rates were 53% for femoropopliteal bypasses and 40% for femorotibial bypasses. Similar patency rates were obtained when the distal deep femoral artery was used as inflow.

Conclusions.—Eversion endarterectomy of the proximal superficial femoral artery provides a valid source of inflow for distal bypasses, and it should be kept in the armamentarium of the vascular surgeon, to be used in selected cases.

▶ The article addresses potential methods of avoiding redissection of the vascular structures in the groin in a patient who requires a lower extremity bypass that must originate from the ipsilateral groin arteries. Redo vascular surgery is certainly more difficult than primary vascular surgery, but it is not much more difficult. Redo groin dissections are frequently necessary in almost everyone's vascular practice. In our practice, we frequently originate an infrainguinal bypass from the profunda femoris artery not so much to stay out of the groin per se but rather because this is often the best artery from which to originate the bypass. The common femoral may be thicker walled and is frequently diseased, whereas the profunda, especially beyond the circumflex profunda vein, is generally soft and easy to work with. The principle in our practice is to use the best conduit possible and best proximal and distal anastomotic sites possible. The principle is not to avoid difficulty of dissection as suggested in this article. The techniques described in this article should be used as adjuncts to achieve the best anastomotic site for the proximal anastomosis of an infrainguinal bypass given the availability of conduit. Using the techniques described can allow the use of shorter autogenous conduits when there is limited vein available. These are good techniques to keep in mind to maximize the use of autogenous infrainguinal reconstruction. Avoiding work of dissection is a far secondary consideration in my opinion. In my experience, the profunda is a more reliable proximal anastomotic site than endarterectomized proximal superficial femoral artery.

G. L. Moneta, MD

A percutaneous aortic device for cerebral embolic protection during cardiovascular intervention

Carpenter JP, Carpenter JT, Tellez A, et al (Robert Wood Johnson Med School, Camden, NJ; Jack H. Skirball Ctr for Cardiovascular Res of the Cardiovascular Res Foundation, Orangeburg, NY; et al)
J Vasc Surg 54:174-181, 2011

Background.—Embolic stroke is a major cause of morbidity in aortic and cardiac interventional procedures. Although cerebral embolic protection devices have been developed for carotid interventions and for open heart surgery, a percutaneous device for cerebral embolic protection during aortic and cardiac interventions would be desirable.

Methods.—The Embrella Embolic Deflector (Embrella Cardiovascular Inc, Wayne, Pa) is a percutaneously placed embolic protection device, inserted by a 6F access in the pig's right forelimb, and deployed in the aorta, covering the brachiocephalic vessel origins. The device functions by deflecting embolic debris downstream in the aortic circulation. A swine model (n = 3) was developed for testing the deployment, retrieval, and efficacy of the device using a carotid filtration circuit for collection of emboli.

Human atheromatous material was prepared as embolization particles with diameters between 150 and 600 μm. Deflection efficiency of the device was calculated by comparing numbers of embolic particles in the carotid circulation during protected and unprotected injections.

Results.—The device was reliably deployed, positioned, and retrieved (n = 24). There was no significant drop in blood pressure across the membrane of the device to suggest reduction of cerebral blood flow. The device did not become occluded by embolic debris despite an embolic load many times that encountered in the clinical situation. Particles entering the carotid circulation after aortic injection of emboli were reduced from 19% of total (unprotected) to 1.3% (protected, $P < .0001$), with 98.7% of all injected particles being deflected downstream. There was no evidence of arterial injury related to the device found at necropsy.

Conclusion.—The Embrella Embolic Deflector performs safely and reliably in the swine model of human atheroembolism. It effectively deflects almost all emboli downstream, away from the carotid circulation. The deflector shows promise as an aortic embolic protection device and merits further investigation.

▶ The authors present a commendable study of a novel embolic protection device based on a current clinical need related to percutaneous aortic and cardiac procedures and periprocedural cerebral infarcts. While they clearly prove efficacy of the device in a swine model, there are 2 key elements that make human translation more difficult: (1) swine arch anatomy relative to human arch anatomy and (2) testing the device in an undiseased arch versus a diseased arch. The approximately 10 cm^2 surface area of the Embrella, adequate for coverage of a common origin of brachiocephalic and left circumflex coronary artery, may not be large enough to cover separate origins. Resizing of the device will change delivery mechanics and sheath size. Deployment and gentle retraction to seal the great curvature in an arch with large atherosclerotic burden could generate emboli distal to the filter, resulting in stroke from the device itself. This device will be important to follow as human trials are considered.

A. Chandra, MD

Early use conversion of the HeRO dialysis graft
Schuman E, Ronfeld A (Legacy Oregon Surgical, Portland)
J Vasc Surg 53:1742-1744, 2011

Although more challenging to place, the HeRO device (Hemosphere Inc, Eden Prairie, Minn) provides the dialysis access-challenged patient the opportunity to have an upper extremity graft rather than being dependent on a catheter or requiring a lower extremity access. A major difficulty with the HeRO is the need for a concomitant dialysis catheter until the graft matures. This has been associated with a large number of bacteremia episodes. Currently available early-access grafts have patency rates similar to standard polytetrafluoroethylene. We have modified the HeRO insertion technique to combine its attributes with those of an early-use graft. In the five patients presented in this report, we confirm that this new technique can give the patient a graft that is functional ≤72 hours and obviate the need for a concomitant catheter. This results in an infection-free access over the follow-up period.

▶ Maintaining a functional and infection-free access site is paramount in patients on hemodialysis. A major challenge is not having adequate vein and having to resort to tunneled lines for immediate dialysis. A major complication of tunneled lines is malfunction and infection. In addition, in patients with axillary-subclavian vein stenosis, the challenges for dialysis can become significant. The Hemodialysis Reliable Outflow (HeRO) device consists of a 6-mm expanded polytetrafluoroethylene graft attached to a 5-mm nitinol-reinforced silicone outflow component designed to bypass venous stenoses and enter the central venous system directly, providing continuous arterial blood flow into the right atrium. The device is designed such that the expanded polytetrafluoroethylene is placed in the upper arm over the biceps muscle. The silicone outflow component is placed similarly to a tunneled line, and by way of a counter-incision at the deltopectoral groove, the 2 components are brought together entirely subcutaneously with a titanium connector. The device provides continuous arterial blood flow into the central venous system, forming a subcutaneous arterial-venous access that bypasses central venous stenosis and the need for a graft-to-vein anastomosis.

One drawback of the HeRO catheter is that it requires concomitant tunneled line placement while the polytetrafluoroethylene graft incorporates. In the pivotal trial by Katzman HE et al,[1] bacteremia rates went from 2.3 per 1000 days with tunneled lines, to 0.70 per 1000 days with the HeRO catheters. All HeRO-related bacteremias occurred during the bridging period when a tunneled line was still implanted.

The HeRO device patency at a mean follow-up of 8.6 months was 38.9% primary, 86.1% assisted primary, and 72.2% secondary, which is similar to conventional arterial-venous grafts. In this study, the authors propose a modification in the insertion technique, obviating the need for placement of a concomitant tunneled line catheter and offering the ability to use the HeRO catheter within 72 hours. The authors followed all the steps in placing the HeRO graft, including connecting the titanium component joining the silicone to the polytetrafluoroethylene graft. Here, the graft was transected at the lateral end of the ringed segment of this connecting section, and an early-access graft (Flixene Grafts Atrium Medical, Hudson, NH) was then sutured to this part of the HeRO graft, tunneled to the selected artery, and anastomosed. The study consisted of 5 patients undergoing this modification (except 1 patient had the transected HeRO graft sutured to a previously placed arm polytetrafluoroethylene graft). Although access for dialysis was obtained either immediately or at 1, 2, and 3 days, 3 of the 5 grafts occluded within days to several months, 2 of which were thrombectomized and functioning at short-term follow-up and one which was completely removed. There were no graft-related infections at 6-month follow-up. Although conceptually the HeRO graft should provide a direct arterial flow in the right atrium and modification of the graft allows for early access without the need for temporary tunneled catheters, graft occlusions and infections still occur. In addition, these are only short-term data, and the consequences of direct and chronic arterial flow into the right atrium are unknown. Having said this, there are patients with central venous stenosis who have exhausted all possible options for dialysis access; for these individuals, one of the few options remaining may be insertion of a HeRO catheter graft or peritoneal dialysis.

J. D. Raffetto, MD

Reference

1. Katzman HE, McLafferty RB, Ross JR, Glickman MH, Peden EK, Lawson JH. Initial experience and outcome of a new hemodialysis access device for catheter-dependent patients. *J Vasc Surg.* 2009;50:600-607.

18 Miscellaneous

Validity of Selected Patient Safety Indicators: Opportunities and Concerns
Kaafarani HMA, Borzecki AM, Itani KMF, et al (Tufts Univ School of Medicine, Boston, MA; Boston Univ School of Medicine, MA; et al)
J Am Coll Surg 212:924-934, 2011

Background.—The Agency for Healthcare Research and Quality (AHRQ) recently designed the Patient Safety Indicators (PSIs) to detect potential safety-related adverse events. The National Quality Forum has endorsed several of these ICD-9-CM-based indicators as quality-of-care measures. We examined the positive predictive value (PPV) of 3 surgical PSIs: postoperative pulmonary embolus and deep vein thrombosis (pPE/DVT), iatrogenic pneumothorax (iPTX), and accidental puncture and laceration (APL).

Study Design.—We applied the AHRQ PSI software (v.3.1a) to fiscal year 2003 to 2007 Veterans Health Administration (VA) administrative data to identify (flag) patients suspected of having a pPE/DVT, iPTX, or APL. Two trained nurse abstractors reviewed a sample of 336 flagged medical records (112 records per PSI) using a standardized instrument. Inter-rater reliability was assessed.

Results.—Of 2,343,088 admissions, 6,080 were flagged for pPE/DVT (0.26%), 1,402 for iPTX (0.06%), and 7,203 for APL (0.31%). For pPE/DVT, the PPV was 43% (95% CI, 34% to 53%); 21% of cases had inaccurate coding (eg, arterial not venous thrombosis); and 36% featured thromboembolism present on admission or preoperatively. For iPTX, the PPV was 73% (95% CI, 64% to 81%); 18% had inaccurate coding (eg, spontaneous pneumothorax), and 9% were pneumothoraces present on admission. For APL, the PPV was 85% (95% CI, 77% to 91%); 10% of cases had coding inaccuracies and 5% indicated injuries present on admission. However, 27% of true APLs were minor injuries requiring no surgical repair (eg, small serosal bowel tear). Inter-rater reliability was >90% for all 3 PSIs.

Conclusions.—Until coding revisions are implemented, these PSIs, especially pPE/DVT, should be used primarily for screening and case-finding. Their utility for public reporting and pay-for-performance needs to be reassessed (Figs 2-4).

▶ In 2000, the Institute of Medicine published 2 landmark reports: "To Err Is Human" and "Crossing the Quality Chasm." These reports served as a stimulus to numerous studies aimed at measuring adverse events, safety-related events, and medical errors. The Agency for Healthcare Research and Quality (AHRQ) has designed a set of evidence based ICD-9 based algorithms termed Patient

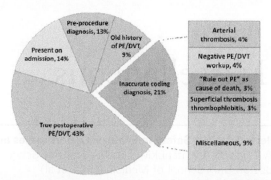

FIGURE 2.—Positive predictive value and analysis of false positives of postoperative pulmonary embolus or deep vein thrombosis (pPE/DVT). Numbers might not add to totals due to rounding. The percentages reported in the figure refer to the percentage of the total number of cases; those reported in the text of the manuscript refer to the percentage of the false positive cases only. (Reprinted from Journal of American College of Surgeons, Kaafarani HMA, Borzecki AM, Itani KMF, et al. Validity of selected patient safety indicators: opportunities and concerns. *J Am Coll Surg*. 2011;212:924-934. Copyright 2011, with permission from the American College of Surgeons.)

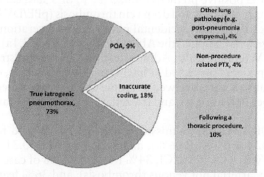

FIGURE 3.—Positive predictive value and analysis of false positives of iatrogenic pneumothorax (iPTX). Numbers might not add to totals due to rounding. The percentages reported in the figure refer to the percentage of the total number of cases; those reported in the text of the manuscript refer to the percentage of the false positive cases only. POA, present on admission. (Reprinted from Journal of American College of Surgeons, Kaafarani HMA, Borzecki AM, Itani KMF, et al. Validity of selected patient safety indicators: opportunities and concerns. *J Am Coll Surg*. 2011;212:924-934. Copyright 2011, with permission from the American College of Surgeons.)

Safety Indicators (PSIs). PSIs are potentially readily obtainable from hospital discharge data and can be used to screen for patient safety events among inpatients. Whereas the intent of PSIs is to use them as screening tools to identify safety-related events, they have been adopted by several organizations for hospital profiling and pay- for- performance purposes. Eight PSIs have been endorsed by the National Quality Forum as hospital performance measures. Four have been adopted by CMS for hospital comparisons with quality and safety potentially tied to financial reimbursement. However, many question the validity of data derived from large administrative databases. If one uses chart abstractions as gold standards, rather than reporting data, the calculated

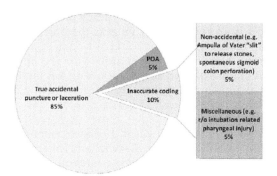

FIGURE 4.—Analysis of false positive cases of accidental punctures or lacerations (APLs). The percentages reported in the figure refer to the percentage of the total number of cases; those reported in the text of the manuscript refer to the percentage of the false positive cases only. POA, present on admission; r/o, rule out. (Reprinted from Journal of American College of Surgeons, Kaafarani HMA, Borzecki AM, Itani KMF, et al. Validity of selected patient safety indicators: opportunities and concerns. *J Am Coll Surg.* 2011;212: 924-934. Copyright 2011, with permission from the American College of Surgeons.)

positive predicted values of PSIs can range between 44% and 91%.[1-3] In essence the data here also indicate that it may be premature to use PSIs for public reporting or pay- for- performance measures. (Figs 2-4) While the concept of PSIs as means to identify potential ways to improve patient safety is reasonable, one can certainly argue that the accuracy of the data, especially for venous thromboembolic events, must be improved before at least some PSIs can be appropriately used for public reporting or tied to reimbursement.

G. L. Moneta, MD

References

1. White RH, Sadeghi B, Tancredi DJ, et al. How valid is the ICD-9-CM based AHRQ Patient Safety Indicator for postoperative venous thromboembolism? *Med Care.* 2009;47:1237-1243.
2. Utter GH, Zrelak PA, Baron R, et al. Positive predictive value of the AHRQ accidental puncture or laceration patient safety indicator. *Ann Surg.* 2009;250: 1041-1045.
3. Zhan C, Battles J, Chiang YP, Hunt D. The validity of ICD-9-CM codes in identifying postoperative deep vein thrombosis and pulmonary embolism. *Jt Comm J Qual Patient Saf.* 2007;33:326-331.

The von Willebrand Inhibitor ARC1779 Reduces Cerebral Embolization After Carotid Endarterectomy: A Randomized Trial
Markus HS, McCollum C, Imray C, et al (St Georges Univ of London, UK; Univ Hosp of South Manchester, Manchester, UK; Univ Hosps Coventry and Warwickshire NHS Trust & Warwick Med School, UK; et al)
Stroke 42:2149-2153, 2011

Background and Purpose.—Inhibition of von Willebrand factor offers a novel approach to prevention of stroke and myocardial ischemia but has not yet been demonstrated to show efficacy on clinically relevant end points. ARC1779 is an aptamer that inhibits the prothrombotic function of von Willebrand factor by binding to the A1 domain of von Willebrand factor and thereby blocking its interaction with glycoprotein. Phase 1 studies suggest it inhibits platelet aggregation with less increase in bleeding than conventional antiplatelet agents. The effect of ARC 1779 on cerebral emboli immediately after carotid endarterectomy was investigated in a randomized clinical trial.

Methods.—Patients undergoing carotid endarterectomy were randomized double-blind to ARC1779 or placebo administered intravenously. Transcranial Doppler recording, to detect cerebral embolic signals, was performed in the first 3 hours postoperatively. The primary end point was time to first embolic signals.

Results.—Thirty-six patients were recruited, 18 in each arm. The Kaplan-Meier median time to first embolic signals was 83.6 minutes for ARC1779 compared with 5.5 minutes for placebo. Using Cox proportional hazards embolic signals occurred statistically significantly later on ARC1779 ($P=0.007$). Reduced embolic signals counts were correlated with inhibition of von Willebrand factor activity ($P=0.03$). Increased perioperative bleeding and anemia were seen with ARC1779.

Conclusions.—von Willebrand factor inhibition reduces thromboembolism in humans. It may play a role in treatment of stroke and myocardial ischemia. The extent to which bleeding complications occur in nonoperated patients needs to be assessed in further studies.

Clinical Trial Registration.—URL: http://clinicaltrials.gov. Unique identifier: NCT00742612 (Fig).

▶ Minor stroke and transient ischemic attacks are followed by a high early risk of recurrent stroke. Risk is highest in patients with larger artery disease. Aspirin can reduce recurrent stroke but actually fails to prevent 80% of stroke recurrences.[1] Therapy with clopidogrel or combination therapy of aspirin and dipyridamole also fails to prevent many recurrences.[2] Other combined therapies such as aspirin with clopidogrel or triple therapy with aspirin, dipyridamole, and clopidogrel are being considered and explored. Alternatively there are also novel antiplatelet therapies that may be considered. It appears inhibition of platelet receptor glycoprotein or absence of von Willebrand factor (vWF) may, in an animal model, protect against brain infarction without increasing intercerebral hemorrhage despite prolongation of bleeding time.[3] ARC1779 is an aptamer-inhibiting prothrombotic function of vWF. It blocks to the A-1 domain of vWF, blocking interaction with glycoprotein. The authors investigated the effect of ARC1779 on cerebral emboli following carotid endarterectomy (CEA) in a randomized clinical trial. This study introduces a new class of antithromboitic (aptamer) in a new therapeutic mechanism (vWF antagonism). Aptamers are oligonucleotides that share some attributes of monoclonal antibodies as well as some of those of low-molecular, chemically synthesized drugs. ARC1779 is aptamer that blocks the A1 domain of vWF and therefore inhibits vWF factor—dependent platelet function. The model of efficacy here was to reduce cerebral embolism after

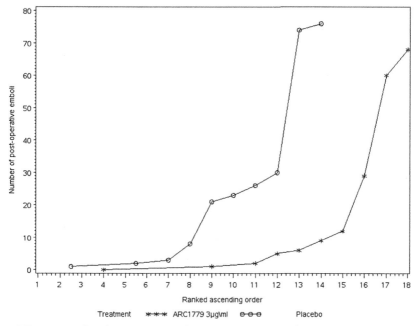

FIGURE.—Number of postoperative embolic signals (ES) during the 3 hours monitoring after carotid endarterectomy (CEA) in the 2 treatment groups ranked in ascending order. (Reprinted from Markus HS, McCollum C, Imray C, et al. The von willebrand inhibitor ARC1779 reduces cerebral embolization after carotid endarterectomy: a randomized trial. *Stroke*. 2011;42:2149-2153.)

CEA. However, whereas embolic signals appear to be reduced with ARC1799 (Fig), there was one stroke in both the ARC1779 group and the placebo group. There was 1 serious case of bleeding in the ARC1779 patients. The data suggest a possibility of a new therapeutic class of drugs for patients with carotid artery occlusive disease. Additional work with truly meaningful reductions of clinically significant endpoints without increased bleeding will be needed before one can consider the use of an ARC1779 type drug in clinical practice. Some platelet-inhibiting drugs may be just too good at what they do!

G. L. Moneta, MD

References

1. Antithrombotic Trialists' Collaboration. Collaborative meta-analysis of randomised trials of antiplatelet therapy for prevention of death, myocardial infarction, and stroke in high risk patients. *BMJ*. 2002;324:71-86.
2. ESPRIT Study Group, Halkes PH, van Gijn J, Kappelle LJ, Koudstaal PJ, Algra A. Aspirin plus dipyridamole versus aspirin alone after cerebral ischaemia of arterial origin (ESPRIT): randomised controlled trial. *Lancet*. 2006;367:1665-1673.
3. Kleinschnitz C, De Meyer SF, Schwarz T. Deficiency of von Willebrand factor protects mice from ischemic stroke. *Blood*. 2009;113:3600-3603.

Reinterventions for stent restenosis in patients treated for atherosclerotic mesenteric artery disease

Tallarita T, Oderich GS, Macedo TA, et al (Mayo Clinic, Rochester, MN)
J Vasc Surg 54:1422-1429.e1, 2011

Objective.—Mesenteric artery angioplasty and stenting (MAS) has been plagued by high restenosis and reintervention rates. The purpose of this study was to review the outcomes of patients treated for mesenteric artery in-stent restenosis (MAISR).

Methods.—The clinical data of 157 patients treated for chronic mesenteric ischemia with MAS of 170 vessels was entered into a prospective database (1998-2010). Fifty-seven patients (36%) developed MAISR after a mean follow-up of 29 months, defined by duplex ultrasound peak systolic velocity >330 cm/s and angiographic stenosis >60%. We reviewed the clinical data, radiologic studies, and outcomes of patients who underwent reintervention for restenosis. End points were mortality and morbidity, patient survival, symptom recurrence, reintervention, and patency rates.

Results.—There were 30 patients (25 female and five male; mean age, 69 ± 14 years) treated with reintervention for MAISR. Twenty-four patients presented with recurrent symptoms (21 chronic, three acute), and six had asymptomatic preocclusive lesions. Twenty-six patients (87%) underwent redo endovascular revascularization (rER) with stent placement in 17 (13 bare metal and four covered) or percutaneous transluminal angioplasty (PTA) in nine. The other four patients (13%) had open bypass, one for acute ischemia. There was one death (3%) in a patient treated with redo stenting for acute mesenteric ischemia. Seven patients (27%) treated by rER developed complications, including access site problems in four patients, and distal embolization with bowel ischemia, congestive heart failure and stent thrombosis in one each. Symptom improvement was noted in 22 of the 24 symptomatic patients (92%). After a mean follow-up of 29 ± 12 months, 15 patients (50%) developed a second restenosis, and seven (23%) required other reintervention. Rates of symptom recurrence, restenosis, and reinterventions were 0/4, 0/4, and 0/4 for covered stents, 2/9, 3/9, and 2/9 for PTA, 5/13, 8/13, and 5/13 for bare metal stents, and 1/4, 4/4, and 0/4 for open bypass. For all patients, freedom from recurrent symptoms, restenosis, and reinterventions were 70% ± 10%, 60% ± 10% and 50% ± 10% at 2 years. For patients treated by rER, secondary patency rates were 72 ± 12 at the same interval.

Conclusions.—Nearly 40% of patients developed mesenteric artery in-stent restenosis, of which half required reintervention because of symptom recurrence or progression to an asymptomatic preocclusive lesion. Mesenteric reinterventions were associated with low mortality (3%), high complication rate (27%), and excellent symptom improvement (92%).

▶ The use of endovascular options has expanded for treatment of chronic mesenteric occlusive disease, but there has been some concern regarding durability. This study raises caution regarding potential of restenosis in 36% of patients undergoing primary mesenteric artery stenting, most of which presented with symptomatic recurrence or asymptomatic preocclusive lesion. Although 87% of these were retreated with endovascular techniques, this high recurrence rate highlights potential limitations of current bare metal stent technology for mesenteric position. The authors note in the discussion that the covered stents used to treat some of the recurrences may offer promise as a primary option, but this is purely conjecture. Clearly, current stent designs may perform differently when used in other vascular territories, and until there is a specific stent designed for mesenteric artery use, adaptation of the current technology will be limited. With the high recurrence rate noted here, the need for ongoing surveillance follow-up is important, although optimal surveillance criteria, intervals, and protocols are still variable.

M. A. Passman, MD

M. A. Passman, MD

Article Index

Chapter 1: Basic Considerations

Chapter 2: Epidemiology

Chapter 3: Vascular Laboratory and Imaging

Chapter 4: Perioperative Considerations

Chapter 5: Grafts and Graft Complications

Chapter 6: Aortic Aneurysm

Chapter 7: Abdominal Aortic Endografting

Chapter 8: Visceral and Renal Artery Disease

Chapter 9: Thoracic Aorta

Chapter 10: Leg Ischemia and Aortoiliac Disease

Chapter 11: Upper Extremity Ischemia/Dialysis Access

Chapter 12: Carotid and Cerebrovascular Disease

Chapter 13: Vascular Trauma

Chapter 14: Nonatherosclerotic Conditions

Chapter 17: Technical Notes

Chapter 18: Miscellaneous

Author Index

Printed and bound by CPI Group (UK) Ltd, Croydon, CR0 4YY

08/05/2025

01864679-0002